A Lover's Pinch

A Lover's Pinch

A Cultural History of Sadomasochism

Peter Tupper

ROWMAN & LITTLEFIELD
Lanham • Boulder • New York • London

Published by Rowman & Littlefield
A wholly owned subsidiary of The Rowman & Littlefield Publishing Group, Inc.
4501 Forbes Boulevard, Suite 200, Lanham, Maryland 20706
www.rowman.com

Unit A, Whitacre Mews, 26-34 Stannary Street, London SE11 4AB

Copyright © 2018 by Peter Tupper

All rights reserved. No part of this book may be reproduced in any form or by any electronic or mechanical means, including information storage and retrieval systems, without written permission from the publisher, except by a reviewer who may quote passages in a review.

British Library Cataloguing in Publication Information Available

Library of Congress Cataloging-in-Publication Data

Names: Tupper, Peter, author.
Title: A lover's pinch : a cultural history of sadomasochism / Peter Tupper.
Description: Lanham : Rowman & Littlefield, [2018] | Includes bibliographical references and index.
Identifiers: LCCN 2017055887 (print) | LCCN 2017058499 (ebook) | ISBN 9781538111185 (Electronic) | ISBN 9781538111178 (cloth : alk. paper)
Subjects: LCSH: Sadomasochism—History. | Sex—History.
Classification: LCC HQ79 (ebook) | LCC HQ79 .T87 2018 (print) | DDC 306.77/509—dc23
LC record available at https://lccn.loc.gov/2017055887

∞™ The paper used in this publication meets the minimum requirements of American National Standard for Information Sciences—Permanence of Paper for Printed Library Materials, ANSI/NISO Z39.48-1992.

Printed in the United States of America

"The stroke of death is as a lover's pinch,
Which hurts and is desir'd."

   —Shakespeare, *Antony and Cleopatra*, Act V, Scene 2, Ln. 292–93

"You never know what is enough unless you know what is more than enough."

> —William Blake, "Proverbs of Hell," *The Marriage of Heaven and Hell*

Contents

List of Illustrations		ix
Introduction: The Marriage of Heaven and Hell		1
1	Saints and Shamans	13
2	The Pornography of the Puritan	33
3	Virtue in Distress	49
4	Orientalism	71
5	The Peculiar Institution	89
6	Romance of the Rod	115
7	Class and Classification	131
8	Every Woman Adores a Fascist	149
9	The Velvet Underground	173
10	Unknown Pleasures	195
11	alt.sex	217
12	Sex and Power	229
Conclusion		251
Notes		263

Bibliography	299
Index	311
About the Author	329

Illustrations

Figure 1.1.	Detail of the mural in Villa of the Mysteries, Pompeii.	15
Figure 1.2.	Detail of the mural in Villa of the Mysteries, Pompeii.	16
Figure 1.3.	Broadsheet, c. 1470, "Jesus Courting the Christian Soul."	28
Figure 1.4.	"Of the Innermost Soul, How God Chastises Her and Makes Her Suited to Him," c. 1500.	31
Figure 3.1.	Plate 3 of William Hogarth's *A Harlot's Progress*, 1732.	55
Figure 4.1.	*The Bitter Draught of Slavery*, by Ernest Normand, 1885.	81
Figure 4.2.	Photograph of Hiram Powers's *The Greek Slave*.	85
Figure 4.3.	*The Greek Slave*, publicly displayed and viewed by men, women, and children.	86
Figure 5.1.	*The Voyage of the Sable Venus, from Angola to the West Indies*.	91
Figure 5.2.	Arthur Munby and Ellen Grounds, aged 22, a broo wench at Pearson and Knowles's Pits.	103
Figure 5.3.	Hannah Cullwick, 1867.	105
Figure 5.4.	Hannah Cullwick posing black and naked to the waist as a chimney sweep.	111
Figure 8.1.	Promotional poster, *Ilsa: She Wolf of the SS*, 1974.	158

Introduction
The Marriage of Heaven and Hell

It's a Saturday night in any major urban center in the Western world, in a darkened hall, in the early years of the twenty-first century. The people here are unmistakable in their hyper-skins of leather, rubber, and lace, their collars and cuffs, their boots, and of course, lots and lots of black.

As the music pulses, people hang suspended in webs of hemp rope from wood and metal frames. Leather straps smack against bare buttocks, evoking moans of pleasure. A man accepts dozens upon dozens of fine needles pierced through his skin. Cool blue alcohol flames ripple across a woman's naked body, only to be extinguished by the man standing over her. A woman carefully slips her entire, well-lubricated fist into the vagina of another, and they never break eye contact. A man leans against a wall, shuddering in pleasure each time another man snaps a single-tailed whip at his bare back, with a sound like a rifle shot. A French maid in black-and-white rubber minces across the room on six-inch heels. A man rains his fists down on the soft, meaty parts of his lover's body, and stops the instant she says "Yellow."

Their actions are paradoxical. They speak of "punishment" and "torture," and their bodies are beaten, cut, pierced, burned, and bound, but the mutual goal is pleasure. They precisely measure sensation, exploring to find the outer limits. There is endless variation, innovation, experimentation, transformation. The weak become strong, the old become young, men become women, women become men, pain becomes pleasure, confinement becomes freedom. This is a laboratory for developing new pleasures and intimacies that cannot be had any other way. Yet there is an order to this, a precise etiquette that regulates but does not confine.

Beyond these night rituals, sadomasochism has spread into the greater culture. Surf through channels, page through magazines, click through the web. Heroes and villains wear black leather and rubber. Whip-wielding dominatrices sell everything from cars to breath mints. Pop singers rhapsodize over pain mixed with pleasure, captivity, submission, and dominance. Every fashion designer has their momentary dalliance with high-heeled boots; dark, shiny coats; wasp-waisted corsets. The aesthetic is so ubiquitous that it is scarcely noticeable, almost cliché.

The question I have to ask is: Where did all this come from? Where did the idea that pain and pleasure are intertwined begin? How did black leather acquire its potent erotic charge?

Today, there are many instructive works on BDSM, ranging from techniques to relationships. But to understand the history is difficult. In my readings and conversations, I usually found only myths and generalizations. Some people tell tall tales of slave-owning houses that date back to pre-Revolutionary France or even the Roman Empire. Others allude to physical ordeal rituals in indigenous cultures but are vague about any connection to modern practices. Some recite a list of the usual suspects—Sade, Sacher-Masoch, motorcycle gang culture, medieval flagellants, *Story of O*—but there is no coherent history, no genealogy linking these people, groups, texts, and artifacts together and showing how they grew together into the modern BDSM culture. The name itself is a slightly awkward portmanteau of Bondage and Discipline, Dominance and Submission, Sadism and Masochism, and Slave and Master. It is apt for a subculture and a style that conglomerated together haphazardly instead of being designed.

Michel Foucault, the French philosopher and practicing sadomasochist, wrote,

> Sadism [and masochism] is not a name finally given to a practice as old as Eros; it is a massive cultural fact which appeared precisely at the end of the eighteenth century, and which constitutes one of the greatest conversions of Western imagination: unreason transformed into delirium of the heart, madness of desire, the insane dialogue of love and death in the limitless presumption of appetite. Sadism appears at the very moment that unreason, confined for over a century and reduced to silence, reappears, no longer as an image of the world, no longer as a *figura*, but as language and desire.[1]

However, nothing is created spontaneously. There are always antecedents and contributing circumstances. Before "the end of the eighteenth century" there must have been, and were, people and things who contributed. This book will examine customs and relationships that may resemble BDSM, and may be the source material for the fantasy that drives BDSM, but are not. This is a story of transformation.

Somewhere, hidden beneath secrecy and mythology and ignorance, is the network that connects all those different things together and leads to other, unexplored worlds. These are not the main thoroughfares of history, but the "cunning passages, [and] contrived corridors."[2]

The hidden history of consensual sadomasochism needs to be told.

CRIMINALITY

Modern advocates of the BDSM community are quick to state that consensual sadomasochism is not rape or abuse, and that terms like "master and slave" or "punishment" should not be taken literally. However, to explore this particular branch of history requires confronting humanity's legacy of violence and oppression. The grotesque crimes of the Marquis de Sade, the tyranny of American slavery, the corporal punishment of Victorian children, and the atrocities of fascism are just a few of the disturbing subjects that must be examined to discover the links between them and consensual sadomasochism.

Acknowledging the relationships between modern BDSM and this history is not to condone or excuse these events. The link between the horrors of slavery and the consensual, pleasurable Master-slave relationships of the early twenty-first century is long and winding. It is comparable to the connection between the athleticism and discipline of modern Olympic fencing and the brutal business of thrusting a piece of sharpened steel through the vital organs of a fellow human being on the battlefield. They are related, but one is violence and the other is an art or game, an indirect reflection of reality, bounded by rules.

There are few, if any, straight lines in the history of BDSM. The most apt metaphor for this particular field of human endeavor is not a branching tree, or a labyrinth, or even Foucault's "archeology," but a house of mirrors. Instead of direct imitation, there is endless reflection, distortion and mimicry, collage and parody, copies of copies. The sadomasochistic imagination is both *mobile* and *transformative*.

In Sigmund Freud's essay "A Child Is Being Beaten" (1919), he explored his patients' masochistic fantasies, asking:

> Who was the child that was being beaten? The one who was himself producing the phantasy or another? Was it always the same child or as often as not a different one? Who was it that was beating the child? A grown-up person? And if so, who? Or did the child imagine that he himself was beating another one? Nothing could be ascertained that threw any light upon all these questions—only the hesitant reply: "I know nothing more about it: a child is being beaten." . . .
>
> In these circumstances it was impossible at first even to decide whether the pleasure attaching to the beating-phantasy was to be described as sadistic or masochistic.

Freud later established that the fantasizer is constantly shifting their point of view, and the meaning they attach to the fantasy. Even if the fantasizer explicitly identifies with one position, the subjective experience of the other does matter. In a sadomasochistic relationship, the masochist/submissive's subjective experience matters very much to the sadist/dominant's involvement. There's no point in playing with an automaton that merely goes through the motions. The submissive also has his or her expectations about the dominant's subjectivity.

Freud's daughter, Anna Freud, wrote another essay that explored the sadomasochistic imagination, "Beating Fantasies and Daydreams" (1922),[3] which showed how the fantasizer repeatedly revises the fantasy scenario.

She described a girl (herself), who buried her childhood beating fantasies under a layer of "nice stories," full of affectionate, orderly families. In her adolescence, she happened across a boy's book about the Middle Ages and read a story, which she only remembered in vague detail, that she then turned into the master narrative for a new set of fantasies. These bore only slight resemblance to the original story.

> The original story had been so cut up into separate pieces, drained of their content, and overlaid by new fantasy material that it was impossible to distinguish between the borrowed and the spontaneously produced elements. All we can do therefore—and that was also what the analyst had to do—is to drop this distinction, which in any event has no practical significance,

and deal with the entire content of the fantasied episodes regardless of their sources.

The material she used in this story was as follows: A medieval knight has been engaged in a long feud with a number of nobles who are in league against him. In the course of a battle a fifteen-year-old noble youth (i.e., the age of the daydreamer) is captured by the knight's henchmen. He is taken to the knight's castle where he is held prisoner for a long time. Finally, he is released.

Instead of spinning out and continuing the tale (as in a novel published in installments), the girl made use of the plot as a sort of outer frame for her daydream. Into this frame she inserted a variety of minor and major episodes, each a completed tale that was entirely independent of the others, and formed exactly like a real novel, containing an introduction, the development of a plot which leads to heightened tension and ultimately to a climax.[4]

There are only two essential characters in this variable scenario: the innocent youth and the brutish knight. The fantasizer plays the narrative out in many different ways. For example:

The prisoner has strayed beyond the limits of his confine and meets the knight, but the latter does not as expected punish the youth with renewed imprisonment. Another time the knight surprises the youth in the very act of transgressing a specific prohibition, but he himself spares the youth the public humiliation which was to be the punishment for this crime. The knight imposes all sorts of deprivations and the prisoner then doubly savors the delights of what is granted again.

All this takes place in vividly animated and dramatically moving scenes. In each the daydreamer experiences the full excitement of the threatened youth's anxiety and fortitude. At the moment when the wrath and rage of the torturer are transformed into pity and benevolence—that is to say, at the climax of each scene—the excitement resolves itself into a feeling of happiness.[5]

The narrative was rewritten to suit the momentary desires of the fantasizer. Rape became ravishment became seduction became love. The stereotypical rape fantasy does not mean the fantasizer wants to be raped, but that the imagination takes a real-world experience (directly experienced or not) and revises it until it becomes a scenario for personal satisfaction that allows pleasures that are not available in other ways. The fantasizer re-channels anxiety into a source of pleasure by heightening dramatic tension and delaying the release.

Thus, early twenty-first-century consensual Master-slave relationships are not a direct imitation of antebellum American slavery (or any other form of violence throughout history), but a scenario that has been told and retold, with certain elements subtracted and others added, until it bears only the slightest resemblance to the original. The relationship between reality and BDSM cannot be reduced to simple imitation. It is a process of interpretation, becoming a performance or ritual.

Over the centuries, people have drawn upon different cultural anxieties to derive fantasy pleasures, such as the fears of the Roman Catholic Church, the Islamic societies of North Africa and the Middle East, antebellum American slavery, the Nazis, alien invaders, and others. All of these fantasies have little to do with the historical realities, and are instead more like myths, archetypal stories with different set dressing and costumes.

DEFINITION

A fundamental problem is the question of what is and isn't sadomasochism? American Justice Potter Stewart famously said, "I know it when I see it," with regards to pornography, but that won't suffice. Were Chinese foot binders or medieval Christian flagellants practicing sadomasochism? Or were they doing something else that resembled sadomasochism but wasn't? "Just erotic. Nothing kinky. It's the difference between using a feather and using a chicken," as the saying goes.[6] For some people, kinky is sex with the lights on.

Like "pornography," "sadomasochism" is strongly defined by the legal and medical attempts to regulate it. "Sadism" and "masochism" were originally like "homosexuality," medical terms that designated aberrant sexual behaviors exhibited by individuals. However, this book is less interested in sadistic or masochistic individuals than in sadomasochistic interactions between individuals, which are the root of sadomasochistic culture.

Kinky can be defined as the opposite of vanilla—that is, "normal," but that definition is tautological. Scientists don't even like to use the term "normal" anymore. They prefer words like "normative." Alfred Kinsey and his followers showed that what "normal" people do is quite varied, and shifts throughout lives and over time. Kink as a distinct entity becomes even fuzzier when it starts to influence the mainstream. Some fetishes are so common they have effectively become normative: high-heeled shoes, for instance. Other fetishes, such as corsets or smoking, were once nearly universal in common life and are now rare. For nineteenth-century European women, corsets were everyday wear, but now are worn almost solely as costume. Only a few generations ago, smoking was a ubiquitous habit, but it has become increasingly rare in North America. We may one day see smoking become primarily or solely a fetishized practice, done as an erotic performance.

To create a working definition as a starting point: "BDSM is a form of consensual erotic play."

While "erotic" may seem self-evident, it is actually more complex. Sadomasochism and fetishism, along with homosexuality, became visible in the late nineteenth century because certain people were being aroused by things that did not fit the standard definition of "normal" sex: heterosexual coitus leading to conception. However, many people practice BDSM or similar activities for reasons other than sexual arousal or release, and prefer to keep their sexuality separate from their play.

In a broader definition, BDSM is playing with the body: testing, modifying, experimenting. The goal of this may be physical pleasure, which may or may not include sexual arousal, or it may produce other sensations that the person desires. Implicit in the definition of BDSM is the idea that people have a right to do with their bodies as they wish, and to pursue pleasure by whatever means. That can be expanded to mean that people have a right to use their bodies to pursue things other than pleasure.

Many people who practice BDSM also participate in the modern primitive and body modification subcultures. For them, sadomasochism is a spiritual practice, not sexual. I once witnessed a suspension piercing event, which involved people being suspended by metal hooks embedded in their bodies. This was not considered a sexual event; teenage minors were allowed into the space to observe, though not participate. I likened the practice to BDSM to the organizer. "It's not SM," she told me indignantly. "It's just people playing around with their pain thresholds."

"That sounds like SM to me," I told her.

She disagreed.

Throughout human history, there are many examples of people voluntarily undergoing physical ordeals. However, for the most part these are religious or military practices. They must be performed at certain times and in certain ways by people who are properly authorized. While they are technically consensual, they are culturally prescribed, and to refuse them is to face social disapproval.

BDSM is a form of human play, however, and therefore is optional, not obligatory. There is no social cost to not doing BDSM. Play also allows for experimentation and variation. Participants can try new things, invent new roles, props, and techniques. People enter a BDSM interaction with the tacit understanding that they choose their role, one that has nothing to do with the role society assigns to them. To be dominant or submissive, top or bottom, is recognized as a personal choice, not determined by a person's gender, race, or other characteristics.

Roger Callois, in his book *Man, Play and Games* (1961),[7] defined four different modes of play which can be combined in various ways. The modes are *agon*, or competition; *alea*, or randomness; *mimesis*, or mimicry and playing roles; and *ilinx*, meaning the alteration of perception. Sadomasochism is a form of play that includes one or both of *ilinx*, as perception is altered by bondage, flagellation, sexual stimulation, or other methods; and *mimesis*, as the participants perform the roles of master/slave, cop/criminal, interrogator/prisoner, et cetera.

Callois also defined a continuum between *ludus*, structured activities with rules, and *paidia*, unstructured and spontaneous activities. BDSM falls towards the *ludus* end of that continuum, and the most important rule is consent.

Unlike the other elements mentioned above, this one is not optional. In both "Safe, Sane and Consensual" and "Risk-Aware Consensual Kink" philosophies, consent is essential. Without consent in the interaction, it isn't BDSM. It is brutality and victimization. Consent can turn what would be a traumatizing experience into a life-affirming one. Consent, as we define it, couldn't really exist until the creation of modern liberal ideas of personhood, self-determination, and rights.

Though this definition doesn't cover the full range of topics this book will discuss, it is enough to identify a core group of symbols and practices.

PROBLEMS TO SURMOUNT

There are many difficulties in uncovering the history of a subculture buried beneath layers of shame, secrecy, and censorship.

The history of alternative sexuality is full of holes left by records lost or destroyed by their owners out of shame, or by others trying to suppress the ideas and images. For every person in the past who left evidence of their sexual interests and activities, there are untold numbers who didn't. We can only guess how many other Victorians led secret lives like Arthur Munby and Hannah Cullwick, or whoever really wrote *The Lustful Turk* or *Memoirs of Dolly Morton*.

During the excavation of Pompeii, unearthed erotic art and phallic icons were destroyed on the spot, locked up in secret collections in museums, or hidden away from tourists.[8] The complete, unpublished manuscript of Richard Francis Burton's *The Perfumed Garden* was burnt after his death by his wife Isabel. The bulk of Henry Spencer Ashbee's collection of erotica was destroyed by the trustees of the British Museum. In 1913, the American censor Anthony Comstock bragged he had disposed of 160 tons of "obscene literature" over his career.[9] The Nazis immolated a hundred thousand books and manuscripts from the library of Dr. Magnus Hirschfeld's Institute of Sexology, while a brass band played.[10] Even in recent times, a corset aficionado's collection was destroyed after his death by his family.[11] It's more by luck than anything else that the evidence of the secret lives of Hannah Cullwick and Arthur Munby has survived.

Simple neglect has caused the loss of even more records. Most people consider pornographic broadsheets, magazines, newspapers, films, and other media unworthy of archiving. Only a few institutions, such as the Kinsey Institute, the Leather Archives and Museum, or the Carter-Johnson Memorial Library, work to preserve such material.

Even the records that do survive may not be truthful. *My Secret Life*, a massive sexual autobiography of a Victorian gentleman, is frequently cited by scholars of sexual history, but its authorship is a mystery. Stephen Marcus, in *The Other Victorians* (1964), says that the author was a real person, while Ian Gibson's *The Erotomaniac* (2001) says it is a composite of anecdotes and fantasies from upper-middle-class gentlemen, compiled by Henry Spencer Ashbee. The true identity of the author, "Walter," will probably never be known.

Some sources may exaggerate out of bravado. Was Richard Burton sincere in his offer to bring back the skin of an African maiden (preferably taken while she was alive) so that his friend Frederick Hankey would have something to bind his copy of the Marquis de Sade's *Justine*?[12] Or was it just a bit of colonialist black humor?

Other sources may misrepresent out of wishful thinking. Henry Spencer Ashbee, perhaps the first person to study pornography academically, was an exhaustive bibliographer, but he wasn't a critical reviewer. He described a novel called *The Mysteries of Verbena House; or, Miss Bellasis Birched for Thieving* as "a most minute and truthful description of a fashionable Brighton seminary for young ladies, of the present day, and the tale turns upon the corporal punishments administered to the fair inmates."[13] Whether he actually believed this, or just played along with the fantasy, is impossible to say.

This investigation requires a balance between sticking to the historical record and erring on the side of caution, and drawing connections between the different sources to tell the story.

In the absence of hard facts about the history of sadomasochism, people have filled in the gaps with mythology. In her keynote speech at the 2005 South Plains Leatherfest, erotica writer Laura Antoniou asked the question, "And how can we even begin to address [BDSM] history seriously when so much of who and what we are is partial—if not purely—fiction?" Antoniou wrote the *Marketplace* books, which draw upon the widespread and long-running fantasy of a secret network of modern-day slave markets and aristocratic estates.[14] This put Antoniou in the awkward position of the debunker of a myth she helped spread.

Thus, we have a culture of people with self-chosen titles, rules, and roles, often based on fictitious sources, such as the *Marketplace* books or John Norman's *Gor* novels. The BDSM scene has persistent legends of "training houses," secret establishments where masters, mistresses, and slaves are trained in "*real*" BDSM. If such institutions ever existed, they conceal themselves better than the CIA and the Mafia.

The so-called Old Guard, the first generation of leathermen that grew out of the post–World War II biker culture, is frequently invoked to proclaim some way of doing BDSM as more authentic or "real" than others. The early leather culture was far from monolithic, with a wide variation in customs, symbols, and practices, and also far less diverse in membership and interests than the modern BDSM scene.

Myths can make for entertaining and arousing fantasies, but they can also obscure understanding. Twisted Monk, one of the leading bondage rope suppliers in North America, wrote on his blog in 2006:

> Honorable samurai and secret European houses did not write our history; rather it was born in back alleys and leather bars by pornographers, queers and sexual outlaws. We should celebrate this rather than attempt to re-imagine it.[15]

The true history of consensual sadomasochism is a story of misfits, hustlers, and visionaries, dreams and nightmares, and the strange vicissitudes of human nature, transforming pain and hatred into pleasure and love. To understand it requires the human ability to accept and embrace irony and paradox. The connection between the self-flagellating Christians of the first century and the twenty-first-century bondage burlesque performers is long and winding, but it is there.

Gay writers speak of "your first lover's first lover," a lineage of chosen bonds instead of familial ties, which in principle can go back for centuries. I would like to find a similar lineage of shared desire and imagination for kinky people, "your first play partner's first play partner." This is that untold story.

Chapter One

Saints and Shamans

Where to begin? A researcher can't just start with the BDSM subculture of the early twenty-first century and proceed backwards. The historical record soon dissolves into clouds of myth and speculation, if not ignorance. The problem can be approached from another angle: Take what we know of early societies and look for examples of sadomasochistic activity. That has its own problems, as other cultures have very different views of pain and pleasure, or sex and religion.

That humans fear and avoid pain would seem to be obvious, hence the use of pain in punishment throughout history. But a moment's thought shows that humans have willingly accepted pain in many times and in many places. Not only do they engage in activities to which pain and suffering is incidental, such as surgical treatment, warfare, or athletic competition, but they also do things in which pain is essential. Depending on the context, experiencing pain can be seen as having positive value.

TRANSCENDENCE THROUGH PAIN

The most common example of this is religious customs. Many faiths have some form of physical ordeal ritual, performed in both ancient times and the present day, both individually and collectively, privately and publicly.

The Sioux and other Plains peoples of North America perform the Sun Dance, a complex four-day ritual of spiritual renewal in which some participants pierce the skin of their chests with sticks or eagle claws and then lean away from a sacred tree until the piercings rip free. Other participants drag buffalo skulls or even hang suspended off the ground from their piercings.[1]

In India, the Tamil people celebrate Thaipusam in honor of the war god Murugan, and perform the Kavadi Attam dance of carrying burdens. Devotees ritually fast, abstain from alcohol, and perform other austerities in preparation. While most of the worshipers carry small pots of milk on their heads or other offerings, a few practice more radical devotions involving piercing their cheeks or tongues with *vel* skewers, hanging weights from hooks embedded in their back or chest, or carrying the *vel kavadi*, a portable altar supported by 108 *vels* embedded into the bearer's chest and back. Their symbolic labor is made sacred by doing it in as difficult and painful a way as possible.[2]

On the Day of Ashura in the Islamic calendar, some Shiite Muslims mourn the death of the prophet Mohammed's grandson by practicing *Tatbir*, striking themselves on the head with a blade or hitting their back and chest with blades attached to chains.[3]

The Yoruba people of West Africa engage in mutual flagellation with whips, switches, or staves as part of their festivals.[4]

In these examples, people voluntarily receive pain as part of a religious experience, and not as a sexual act. It's important to note that these are not "primitive" forms of religious expression that certain human cultures have evolved beyond. These acts of flagellation and other forms of asceticism occur in specific religious contexts as well-established customs, in order to minimize lasting injury.

Western Classical societies had their own uses for the physical in the sacred. For example, the Etruscan "Tomb of the Whipping," built circa 490 BCE, includes frescoes of people in sexual acts. One of the frescoes shows two men in intercourse with one woman. One man appears to be slapping the woman's back with an open hand, while the other man has raised a small stick or cane over the woman's buttocks. Etruscans added erotic art to their tombs to repulse demons, suggesting that flagellation and spanking had both sexual and spiritual aspects.

Plutarch described the Roman festival of Lupercalia: "At this time many of the noble youths and of the magistrates run up and down through the city naked, for sport and laughter striking those they meet with shaggy thongs. And many women of rank also purposely get in their way, and like children at school present their hands to be struck, believing that the pregnant will thus be helped in delivery, and the barren to pregnancy."[5]

The ancient Roman city of Pompeii, buried by a volcanic eruption in CE 79 and rediscovered in 1749, is rife with sexual art. The ubiquity of sexual imagery led early archaeologists to theorize that Pompeii was full of brothels and that ancient Rome was a sex-obsessed culture. Later archaeologists stated that these phalli were symbols of protection, health, and fertility, something the Romans just felt comfortable having around.

Flagellation appears in a semi-erotic context in a fresco in one of the city's buried houses. The Villa of the Mysteries is a large house that scholars initially thought to be a brothel or temple because of the nude frescoes on the walls. Later archaeologists decided it was actually a private home and the art depicted a sequential narrative about preparing a young bride for marriage in the mystery cult of Dionysius.

Reading the images around the room, the narrative starts with a woman in street clothes, then a mother with son, then a pregnant woman with a laurel crown carrying cakes, and so on. The images are tranquil until a

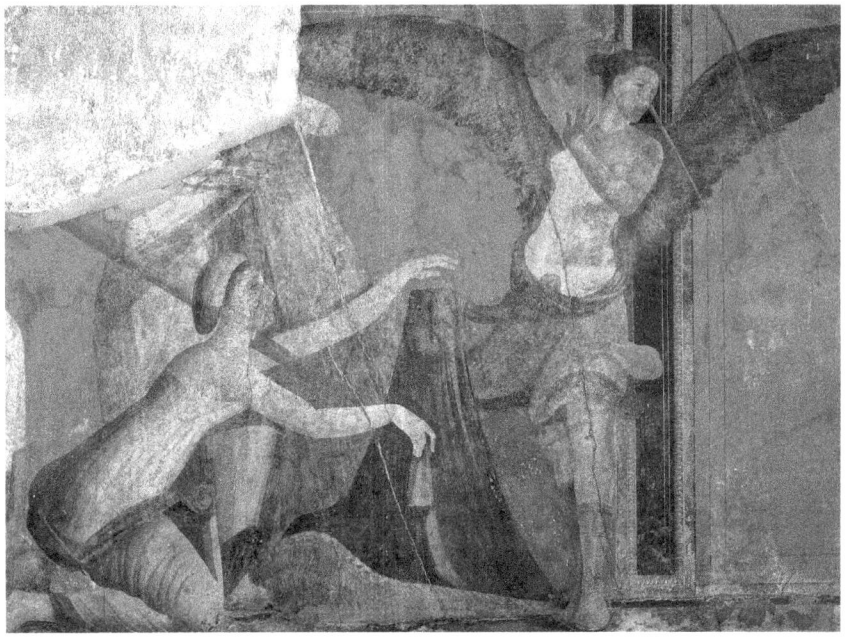

Figure 1.1. Detail of the mural in Villa of the Mysteries, Pompeii, showing woman in boots with black wings, whipping woman to right of frame. *Courtesy Wikimedia Commons*

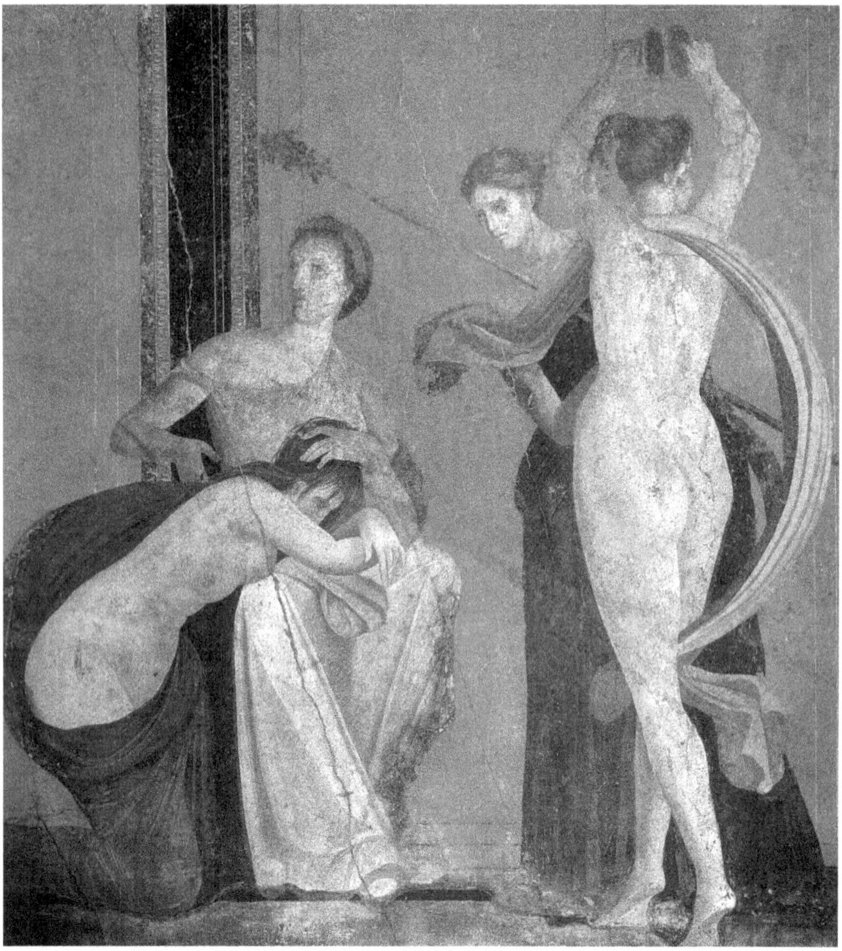

Figure 1.2. Detail of the mural in Villa of the Mysteries, Pompeii, showing woman in purple cloak, kneeling and being beaten by woman in panel to left. *Courtesy Wikimedia Commons*

woman is startled; she draws away from something in surprise, her cape in violent motion over her.

As one enters the room, the first image visible is Dionysius sitting with his head almost in the lap of his lover, Ariadne (see Figure 1.1). To the right of them is an undressed woman kneeling before a large phallus in a basket, covered with purple cloth. Immediately to the right of that is a standing female figure with dark wings, identified as a "female demon." Unlike the other female figures in the fresco, who are nude or in dresses, she wears boots or sandals, a knee-length skirt, and a belt suitable for fighting or another athletic activity. Her right hand wields a cane or switch, in full backswing, apparently beating the kneeling woman on the other side of the room's corner (see Figure 1.2). Here, a woman kneels, back and buttocks exposed, resting her face in the lap of another, clothed woman. After that, a nude woman dances with cymbals. The final image is a maidservant arranging a young woman's hair in the style reserved for brides.

Although there are other interpretations to this work, the connection between sexual pleasure, physical pain, and fertility is clear. The narrative shows flagellation as part of the marriage/fertility rite.[6]

RITUAL

These voluntary physical ordeals, found across the world and throughout history, are aspects of rituals. Ritual is a powerful force in human affairs, used to resolve conflicts, regulate social change, and guide individuals and societies through their lives. In some rituals, individuals transition from one social role to another, such as weddings, initiations into military, religious or fraternal orders, or graduations from school. Other rituals are periodic events in which social roles change for prescribed periods of time, such as holidays or sporting events. Rituals may be widespread social practices of a given culture, or small groups or individuals may develop their own rituals for their purposes. By viewing sadomasochistic practice as ritual, we can understand how sadomasochism works in the context of culture, instead of viewing it as a pathology of individuals.

Anthropologist Victor Turner, in his book *The Ritual Process* (1969), defined ritual as a three-step process of separation, liminality (derived from *limen* or threshold), and aggregation. Fittingly, a modern sadomasochistic interaction is often called a "scene," suggesting the theatricality and performance that is a key aspect of ritual. The archetypal BDSM scene repeats the three stages of the ritual.

In separation, ritual participants break from their usual routine and their social role in it by fasting, changing clothing, or traveling away from regular places. In the BDSM scene, participants abandon their regular attire and dress in a particular fashion (leather or latex fetishwear, lingerie, costume, or nudity), travel to a particular place of seclusion (a dungeon or playspace), adopt different names or titles (scene names, "Master," "Mistress"), and otherwise separate from their everyday lives.

In the liminal phase of the ritual, participants inhabit a social space with new social rules that can be inversions of normal society (e.g., women dominate men, blacks dominate whites) or exaggerations (e.g., wives become slaves). People experience a heightened awareness, a sense of expressing their true selves. Sexual arousal may be a part of this, but the release from the usual social roles is the bigger appeal. Mundane objects acquire great symbolic value; for example, bread and wine becomes the body and blood of Christ, to be consumed as a symbolic act of cannibalism. States that are avoided and discouraged in the regular world are embraced and encouraged: dirtiness, sexual aggression, captivity, dependency, and so on. Turner writes:

> Liminal entities, such as neophytes in initiation or puberty rites, may be represented as possessing nothing. They may be disguised as monsters, wear only a strip of clothing, or even go naked, to demonstrate that as liminal beings they have no status, property, insignia, secular clothing indicating rank or role, position in a kinship system—in short, nothing that may distinguish them from their fellow neophytes or initiands. Their behavior is normally passive or humble; they must obey their instructors implicitly, and accept arbitrary punishment without complaint. It is as though they are being reduced or ground down to a uniform condition to be fashioned anew and endowed with additional powers to enable them to cope with their new station in life.[7]

Turner contrasts social structure, the rules and roles of society, with what he calls communitas, the sense of being emotionally, intuitively integrated into humanity, soul to soul contact. The purpose of a rite of passage is to take a person out of structure, make them experience communitas so they understand that society is more than just rules and roles, and put them back into society.

People can experience liminality without necessarily reaching communitas, and may not want to. Liminality may be its own reward, as in liminoid rituals, in which the participants don't experience lasting changes in social status. As Turner wrote, "For the hippies—as indeed for many millenarian and 'enthusiastic' movements—the ecstasy of spontaneous communitas is seen as the end of human endeavor."[8]

Liminality is not always achieved through gentle means, and may employ literal or symbolic ordeals of discomfort, deprivation, or outright pain.

> We very often do find that the concept of threat or danger to the group—and, indeed, there is usually real danger in the form of a circumciser's or cicatrizer's knife, many ordeals, and severe discipline—is importantly present. And this danger is one of the chief ingredients in the production of existential communitas, like the possibility of a "bad trip" for the narcotic communitas.[9]

Radically changing a person's sensory experience is a common method of altering his or her consciousness to experience liminality. There are many techniques toward this end, including dancing, chanting, drumming, flagellation, burning, cutting, fasting, dehydration, immersion in cold water, ingesting psychoactive drugs, sweat lodges, or piercing; paradoxically, the same effect may be achieved by under-loading the sensorium by blindfolding, psychoactive drugs, or isolation.

Ariel Glucklich's book *Sacred Pain* (2001) explains how pain, or other disruptions in a person's sensorium, is used in ritual.

> To sum up three chapters in three sentences, the more irritation one applies to the body in the form of pain, the less output the central nervous system generates from the areas that regulate the signals on which a sense of self relies. Modulated pain weakens the individual's feeling of being a discrete agent; it makes the "body-self" transparent and facilitates the emergence of a new identity. Metaphorically, pain creates an embodied "absence" and makes way for a new and greater "presence."[10]

Pain is both a sign that psychological transformation is happening and an agent of that change. The anticipation of pain, such as from the sight of weapons, even if they are not used, can have the same effect.

> Hurting initiates in rites of passage and initiations is a form of applying force on them. Force, or power, is brought to bear by those who already belong to the adult world, or to the society of the initiated. But initiates are not simply brutalized, and highly ritualized force becomes sacrificial pain. Rites of passage are rites of supercession. In order to become adults, the initiates sacrifice or give up their lesser identity as boys or girls. Instead of being

victims—however symbolic—the children must hurt in a voluntary manner. Only then can the psychological mechanism of self-sacrifice become effective. . . . If adults were to hurt their children in a brutal manner and with no ritual, the pain would not be transformative.[11]

The ritual structure creates a social container for the violence, a time and place in which transgression from norms are prescribed and performed in a controlled manner, understood by the ritual's officiants.

In the BDSM scene, the participants inflict or experience deprivation, confinement, and threatened or actual violence, through bondage (such as rope, handcuffs, or restrictive clothing), sensory deprivation (such as blindfolds), impact play (such as spanking or flogging), sensation play (such as scratching or ice), or other methods. Particular objects are assigned great symbolic meanings, both of arousal and of power or submission: fetishized items like high-heeled shoes, leather or rubber clothing, or cigarettes. Social roles related to age, gender, race, and other categories may be radically different, exaggerated or even inverted, through ageplay, genderplay, or raceplay. Derogatory terms like "slut" or "whore" or "pig" become expressions of desire, worthiness, and even affection. Transgression is not just allowed, but encouraged.

In the final step, aggregation, the participants have achieved psychological renewal, and reintegrate into society, either in their new social status in liminal rituals or in original social status in liminoid rituals. The students graduate, the bride and groom become husband and wife, the sports or music fans take off their subcultural uniforms and return to everyday life until the next game or concert. After the BDSM scene, the arousal and endorphins fade, and the participants go through physical and emotional aftercare to ease the transition back into everyday life. The dominant may provide water, snacks, cuddling, or verbal reassurance to the submissive. At the end, they return to their original social roles. This transition is not always smooth, and sometimes, after intense scenes, participants experience "drop," feelings of depression, just as other people experience disappointment at having to shift from the heightened reality of a holiday or another major life event to mundane routine.

The sadomasochistic scene is a temporary ritual of transgression in which people take a vacation from everyday life and experience a radically different existence. It functions on the same ritual principles as other secular rituals, such as a fraternity initiation or a university graduation, or the religious rituals of many faiths, such as a wedding or a Catholic mass. Ritual is both a temporary rebellion against mundane life and a supporter of it.

> Cognitively, nothing underlines regularity so well as absurdity or paradox. Emotionally, nothing satisfies as much as extravagant or temporarily permitted illicit behavior. Rituals of status reversal accommodate both aspects. By making the low high, and the high low, they reaffirm the hierarchical principle. By making the low mimic (often to the point of caricature) the behavior of the high, and by restraining the initiatives of the proud, they underline the reasonableness of everyday culturally predictable behavior between the various estates of society.[12]

Sadomasochism is a ritual for the modern age.

VOLUNTARY SUFFERING IN CHRISTIANITY

The distant ancestors of modern consensual sadomasochism can be found in Christianity's own rituals of transgression and pain. Christianity has two conflicting ways of thinking about physical suffering: the penitential and the ascetic.

The first is the idea that physical punishment is a necessary means of disciplining a subordinate, be it a wife, slave, child, apprentice, or other underling. This is not just a self-serving means of ensuring that your orders are carried out. Physical discipline is supposed to be good for the subordinate, spiritually. This recurs all through Proverbs in the Bible: For example, "For whom the Lord loveth he correcteth; even as a father the son in whom you delighteth."[13] "He that spareth his rod hateth his son: but he that loveth him chasteneth him betimes."[14] "Thou shalt beat him with the rod, and shalt deliver his soul from hell."[15]

Early Christians thought God was an awe-inspiring, even terrifying being, and the fear and pain one would feel in the presence of God meant one was even closer to the divine. This was the driving idea behind penitential self-flagellation, that one would punish oneself for one's sins on behalf of the divine.

The second idea is attaining spiritual advancement by voluntarily accepting pain, in imitation of the Passion of Christ. This depends on the argument that Christ allowed himself to be beaten and crucified, and this must be spiritually significant. "Christ's suffering merged with the suffering of the believer and removed or mitigated it."[16] The image of Christ's suffering body was a means to healing and transcendence. The word "ascetic" comes from the Greek word *askein*, meaning "work," "to practice," or "to train." It is not merely suffering or the absence of comfort or pleasure, but an intentional undertaking. Thus Christianity adopted flagellation from other religions, just as it absorbed other pagan rituals and practices.

As explored earlier, intense physical sensations are a common method of achieving liminality. This opens the person experiencing them to altered states of consciousness, including sexual arousal. Niklaus Largier wrote in his history of flagellation:

> If we could state any specific thesis that emerges from this overview of flagellation, it would be that voluntary flagellation and the texts that cover it are concerned not so much with "sexuality" (as all the sexual pathologists hold), but with the arousal of emotion and imagination. . . . Erotica and religious flagellation emerge as rituals that aim to unfetter desire, imagination, and the passions.[17]

Early Christian mystics struggled with the content of those unfettered passions. Saint Jerome, who lived as an ascetic in the desert for years, wrote, "Yet that same I, who for fear of hell condemned myself to such a prison, I the comrade of scorpions and wild beasts was there, watching the maidens in their dance . . . and the Lord himself is witness, after many tears, and eyes that clung to heaven, I would sometimes seem to myself to be one with the angelic hosts."[18]

As Christianity became a more established religion, rituals became more regulated. In the great monastic orders that began in the eleventh century, life was a never-ending ritual, a permanent state of liminality, in which monks and nuns segregated themselves from profane, everyday life and lived according to rules that regulated every aspect of conduct. This included flagellation and self-mortification.

Saint Peter Damian, an eleventh-century reforming monk, was so known for his extreme self-mortification that he is traditionally depicted holding a knotted cord (*disciplina*). *Disciplina* originally meant living under monastic rule, but it gradually shifted to the knotted cord as a symbol of religious discipline.

Peter was part of a postmillennial movement in Christendom that believed divine judgment was imminent, and the body had to be renewed through suffering to make it acceptable to God.[19] To live the austere life of a monk or hermit was a good start, but to be truly purified, one had to go further. Members of Peter's monastic community wore iron bands next to their flesh, prayed with their arms extended in the form of a cross, and beat themselves with scourges.

Peter held up as example the hermit Dominic, known as Loricatus for the iron corselet and bands he wore. Peter described how Dominic completed nine psalters with flagellation in a day and a night, and "his whole appearance seemed to be so beaten with scourges and so covered with livid welts, as if he had been bruised like barley in a mortar."[20] Dominic's "whole life was for him a Good Friday crucifixion, but now with festive splendor he celebrates the eternal glory of the resurrection."[21] In other words, Dominic's life was a permanent state of ritual preparation for spiritual renewal.

Nuns could also practice mortification of the flesh, such as St. Rita of Cascia. In 1442, she prayed before an image of Christ, asking to participate in the pain caused by the Crown of Thorns. Reportedly, the image wounded her in the forehead, and the wound remained until her death.[22]

Lay worshipers also practiced flagellation and other mortifications. The Cistercian lay brother Arnulf was one such spiritual athlete. As an illiterate lay brother, Arnulf could not participate in most devotions, and compensated with elaborate discipline. He wore a hair shirt made of hedgehog pelts, with their quills inward. He self-flagellated, with a cane enhanced with quills or a scourge of thorny branches, while singing a vernacular song: "Got to be braver, got to be manly, manly I've got to be! Friends need it badly: this stroke for this one, that stroke for that one; take *that* in the name of God!"[23]

Arnulf also wrapped knotted ropes around his waist, supposedly so tight that his flesh began to rot. His biographer Goswin described this as purification from a feminine deity: "Oh, the happiness of this newborn child, for whom Mother Grace is so solicitous that she not only nourishes him with the sweetness of her milk but . . . there in his infant cradle, she swaddles him in the bands of these piercing cords, and with so sharp a flint-knife, she circumcises away any lewdness in his flesh."[24] Arnulf's "manly" self-inflicted violence paradoxically returned him to infancy, an echo of the moment in the Passion when Mary cradles her dead son, all part of a ritual of spiritual renewal.

The ascetics created a feedback loop: the disease of the flawed, pleasure-seeking body is cured by physical punishment and denial, which produces more pleasure, which requires more punishment. This cycle continues until the ecstatic climax, follow by relaxation, which is only temporary.[25]

The Catholic hierarchy remained highly ambivalent about flagellation and other physical ordeals, particularly when performed by lay worshipers outside of church control. Flagellation as a method of correction was acceptable, even sanctioned by the monastic Rule of Benedict and the laws of the Church, as was asceticism as spiritual exercise. But the voluntary self-mortification advocated by Peter Damian was seen as an overly radical innovation. The clerics of Florence argued that "if it is sanctioned and observed, all the sacred canons will surely be destroyed, the precepts of the ancient fathers will disappear, and, as the Jew said, the traditions of our fathers will be reduced to nothing." Peter Damian countered that flagellation was solidly grounded in Christian tradition, and the austerities of his followers were sanctioned by the lives of Christ, the apostles, and the early martyrs. He also critiqued the church's hypocrisy for sanctioning flagellation as punishment but not as devotion.[26]

In the thirteenth century, during the years of plagues and famines, radical lay Christians took flagellation as a sacrament. The leaders of the movement, lay "masters" and "fathers," claimed that God had written a heavenly letter threatening to destroy sinful humanity. The Virgin Mary interceded on man's behalf to save those who joined a flagellant procession for thirty-three and one-half days, representing the span of Jesus's life on Earth in years. Flagellants gathered into groups of fifty to five hundred members. The masters heard confession and granted absolution, and maintained strict discipline: no shaving, bathing, changing clothes, or interacting with women. People fed and lodged them as living saints. They gathered around churches to flog themselves with metal-tipped scourges, sing hymns, pray, and cry, while the master read aloud the alleged heavenly letter. Flagellants claimed that their suffering would absolve others, along with other supernatural powers such as exorcism and speaking with the Virgin Mary.

> Here it was not only a question of a penitential gesture, but of a system of actions in which the salvation of the world would be attained through flagellation and through a radical likeness to Christ. Thus, every flagellant would work on the spectator like "a new Christ" and thereby actually change the entire population into an image of Christ.[27]

The earliest organized flagellant processions emerged in Italian cities in 1260, and spread to Hungary, the Low Countries, and France by the mid-fourteenth century.[28]

By 1348, the flagellant movement had grown too large to be ignored. In response to the plague reaching southern France, Pope Clement VI approved and instituted public mass flagellations in the streets of Avignon in which men and women participated.

By October 1349, however, the movement had grown too large to be tolerated. Not only were the flagellants an organized populist movement that threatened both clergy and aristocracy, they committed grave doctrinal errors. Flagellation was an accepted monastic practice, common among Franciscan clergy. For the lay worshipers to use it as a sacramental penance, however, threatened the Church's monopoly on repentance. Clement VI issued a papal bull condemning the flagellants, ordering that their "masters of error" be arrested and burned if necessary. Clerical and secular authorities immediately forbade flagellant processions, punishable by excommunications and executions. Ironically, some members of the flagellant movements did penance by being beaten, by clerics instead of lay leaders, at St. Peter's in Rome.[29] However, the pope's ban explicitly excepted self-flagellation at home or elsewhere if not done in connection with heretic groups.[30]

Devotional manuals like Francis de Sales's *Introduction to the Devout Life* (1609) deemphasized religious empathy with the suffering body of Christ or saints in favor of viewing saints as moral exemplars.[31] Officially, the path to ecstasy through personal bodily experience had been closed.

In practice, it survived in many scattered forms. Despite persecution by church and state, secretive flagellant groups cropped up intermittently for centuries. The last covert group of flagellants were executed in the

1480s.[32] The lay confraternities of Renaissance Bologna included flagellation as part of their ritual devotions, though these were indoor, carefully regulated, collective activities by people who hardly considered themselves revolutionaries.[33] In early modern France, flagellant lay worshipers organized into confraternities, which accepted men from all social classes. Women were accepted into some confraternities, but they did not flagellate themselves in public. Supposedly, women already had their burden of pain, from menstruation and childbirth, so they didn't need additional self-inflicted pain.[34]

In the twenty-first century, lay members of the Catholic organization Opus Dei continue to practice mild forms of mortification of the flesh, such as fasting or wearing a cilice, a small version of the hair shirt, which has been reduced to a studded chain worn around the upper thigh.

RELIGIOUS ART AND LITERATURE

Christians who could not or would not practice flagellation or other mortification could vicariously experience spiritual renewal by contemplating art.

Beginning in the thirteenth century, the Franciscans developed a complex system of iconography detailing the *via crucis*, the fourteen stages of the Cross, depicted in a wide variety of formats, from wall-covering paintings inside churches to handheld devotional booklets. Later artists interpolated even more scenes of the familiar story. Images of the Passion were a key part of public and private devotional practice, creating a link from human suffering to Christ's suffering to the divine. The viewer suffered *with* Christ intimately, via imagining the same suffering, and experienced resurrection (spiritual renewal) in the same way.[35] Instead of being a mortal coil, the suffering body was the medium by which the believer knew God. The narrative of the Passion and Resurrection of Christ forms a ritual cycle of separation, liminality, and integration, and to read or see it is to vicariously experience the ritual. The image of the Passion was ubiquitous throughout Christian Europe and spread to the Americas in the colonial era centuries later.

While some artists depicted Christ with supernatural endurance, smiling and serene through his torments, other artists emphasized his human vulnerability, his mental and physical anguish, depicting him as the Man of Sorrows. Mathias Grünewald's *The Crucifixion* (1500–1508) depicted Christ as dead, or as good as, his skin gray, his face anguished, his body contorted in agony, his five wounds visible in great detail.[36] Other artists literalized the connection between suffering Christ and viewer. Francisco Ribalta's *Saint Francis Embracing the Crucified Christ* (c. 1620) showed Francis literally drinking blood from the wound in Christ's side, while Christ placed the crown of thorns on his follower's head.[37] Diego Velazquez's *Christ after the Flagellation Contemplated by the Christian Soul* (c. 1630) showed Christ tied to the pillar with chords, just after his beating, with a winged angel guiding a child (representing the soul) to look at him; a ray of light reached from Christ's head to the child's heart.[38]

The *Legenda aurea*, or *Golden Legend*, is a collection of biographies of Christian saints, created in the late thirteenth century. It is full of stories of the martyrdom of saints: Laurence is roasted alive, Sebastian is pierced with arrows, Agatha's breasts are severed, and others are stabbed, stoned, boiled, and decapitated. Such a book was used by preachers as a reference for sermons and readings on feast days. It became one of the most widely read and reproduced works of the period.

The manuscript of the *Golden Legend* kept in the Huntington Library is notable for its lavish illuminations, which contain many graphic images of violence. In fact, the imagery is far more violent than the text, which may only describe the saint's torture briefly after telling of his or her acts of faith, good works, and miracles. For example, the text only says that St. Felicula was "tortured on the rack" after rejecting the sexual advances of a nobleman, but the illustration shows the martyr suspended from a rack, nude from the waist up with sharp combs being raked across her body and orange-red blood evident.

These images of violence and death had mnemonic functions, fixing each saint's method of torture and/or death in the reader's mind as a memory device. Thomas Aquinas wrote that "we are less able to remember things that have subtle and spiritual aspect, while those that are gross and sensible are able to be remembered." A book like the Huntington Library's *Golden Legend* would likely have been used for meditative personal devotion, not public display, with the graphic images intensifying the experience of contemplating these moral exemplars.[39]

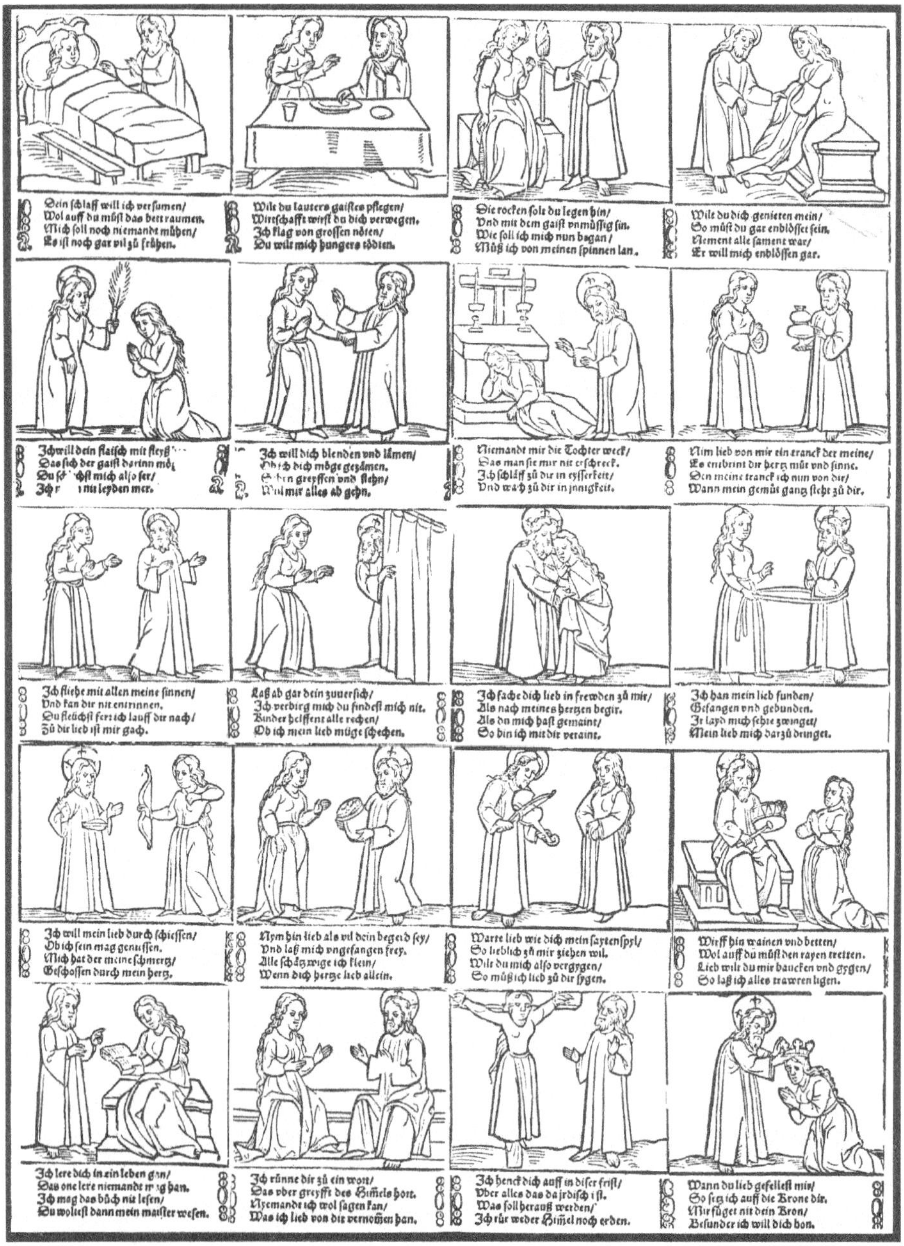

Figure 1.3. Broadsheet, c. 1470 *Die Minnende Seele* ("Jesus Courting the Christian Soul"). *Courtesy David Kunzle Collection*

The concepts of religious ordeal appeared in religious art for the masses as well, in scenes that have no basis in the Gospels or other scripture.

"Jesus Courting the Christian Soul," a broadsheet printed in German sometime between 1460 and 1480, shows the relationship between Jesus (a bearded man with a halo) and the Christian soul (a young woman) in terms that are not only sensual, but sadomasochistic (see Figure 1.3). Each of the twenty panels in this narrative contains a simple woodcut illustration and accompanying text, like an early comic strip.

Jesus wakes the Soul out of bed (panel 1), says she must forgo food (2) and other pursuits, symbolized by the distaff (3), and has her strip bare (4). The Soul complains: "I do not wish to be disturbed, it is too early yet." "I suffer in dire necessity, you will starve me to death." "Look at the way he wants to strip me bare."

Jesus ramps things up in panels 5 and 6:

Jesus: "I shall castigate your flesh severely, to let the spirit thrive."

Soul: "You are beating me so sorely, I cannot bear it anymore."

Jesus: "I will blind and cripple you, so as to tame you."

Soul: "I am unable to walk, stand or grasp."

However, in panel 7, Jesus proves he's a good dominant by looking after the Soul while she sleeps before an altar:

Jesus: "Let no-one waken the girl, lest she be frightened."

Soul: "I go to sleep before you in outwardness, and awaken to you in inwardness."

The relationship takes an unexpected turn when the Soul chases after Jesus (9) and finds where he is hiding (10). At first they are reconciled harmoniously (11), then the positions reverse. In 12, the Soul ties a cord around Jesus's waist.

Soul: "I have found my love, caught him and bound him."

Jesus: "Her pain overpowers me, my love forces me (to submit)."

In panel 13, she shoots arrows into Jesus.

Soul: "I shoot arrows at my love, so that I may enjoy him."

Jesus: "The pains of love have pierced my heart."

Jesus turns seductive again. He offers her gold, which she refuses out of love (14), then plies her with music (15, 16).

Jesus: "Stop your weeping and praying, come and join the dance."

Soul: "Love, if you thus entice me with drum and fiddle, all my sorrow is gone."

In panels 17 and 18, their bond is close again, with Jesus as teacher/dominant.

Jesus: "I'll teach you to lead a life that no-one can have without my teaching."

Soul: "I cannot read a book unless you are my master."

Jesus: "I shall whisper a word to you that surpasses the treasure of heaven."

Soul: "I will tell no-one, love, what I have heard from you."

Finally, Jesus puts the Soul up on a cross, described in ecstatic terms.

Jesus: "I now hang you up over all earthly things during your temporal existence."

Soul: "What will become of me, I touch neither heaven nor earth."

The narrative ends with Jesus putting a crown on the Soul's head, who refuses material reward.

Jesus: "Since you delight me, love, I set a crown upon you."

Soul: "I do not deserve a crown, I want to have just you."

This was one example of this genre of broadsheet stories. Another four-panel story, dated about 1500 CE, was titled "Of the Innermost Soul, How God Chastises Her and Makes Her Suited to Him" (see Figure 1.4). Jesus wakes the Soul from slumber, by pulling her out of bed by her hair. Persistently, he stands out in the rain and knocks on her door. In the third panel, he lights her clothes on fire with a candle. Finally, they are shown in bed together, face-to-face. "How they lie in bed together . . . and attain eternal rest." Again, the narrative follows Jesus waking a young woman out of bed, being resisted by her in her own stubbornness and pride, overwhelming her with his own forcefulness, and finally their erotic union. In another example of this genre, Jesus awakens the sleeping woman by setting her bed on fire.

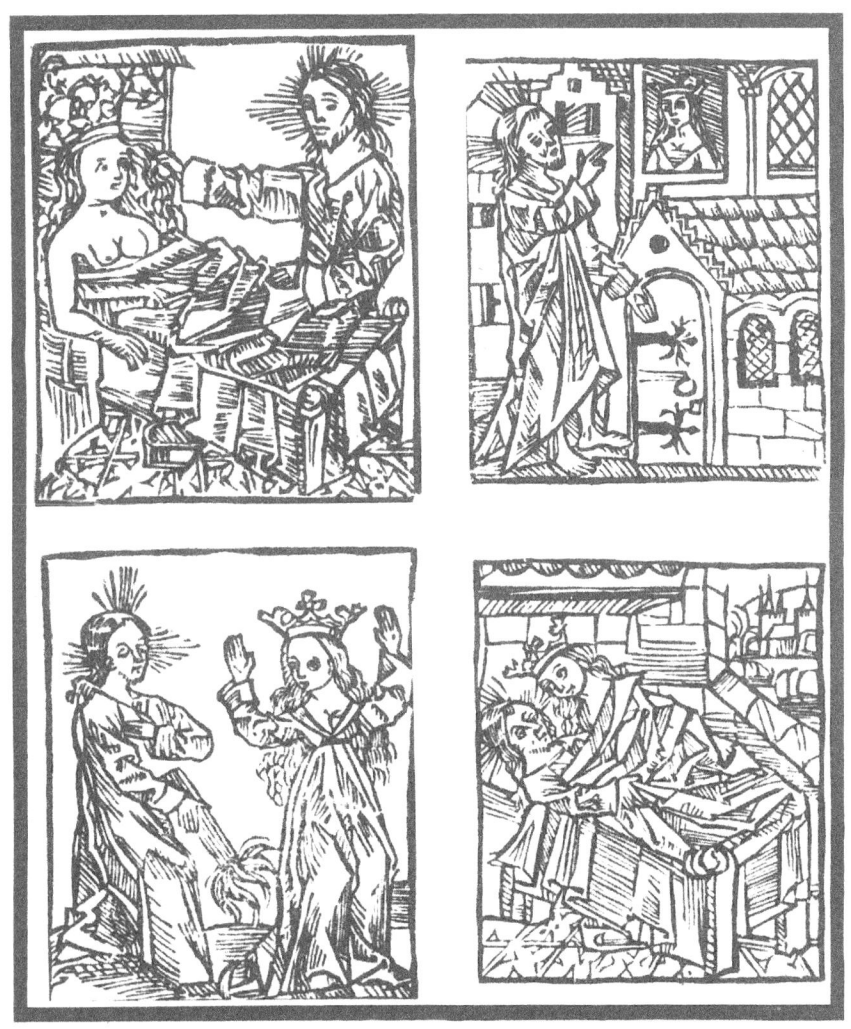

Figure 1.4. Four illustrations to "Of the Innermost Soul, How God Chastises Her and Makes Her Suited to Him" (*Von der Ynnigen selen wy sy gott casteyet unnd im beheglich mach*), c. 1500. *Courtesy David Kunzle Collection*

The broadsheet's story was a ritual in written form, depicting the relationship between humanity and God as an initiation, expressed in physical terms of giving and receiving pain and pleasure, commands, and confinement. The soul is liberated and blessed via ritualized submission and suffering at the hands of a higher power, an idea that had entered the mass consciousness of the Christian world, even as authorities condemned it. What had been banned from religion survived in other forms.

Chapter Two

The Pornography of the Puritan

If pain and suffering were once sacred, when and how did that change? And how did eroticism become attached to those concepts? Christianity has always had a complicated and conflicted relationship with the body and bodily experience, and in the early Modern era, physical ordeal rituals were slowly but steadily pushed out of the sacred and into the profane.

COUNCIL OF TRENT

In 1563, the twenty-fifth session of the Council of Trent declared:

> Moreover, in the invocation of saints, the veneration of relics, and the sacred use of images, every superstition shall be removed, all filthy lucre be abolished; finally, all lasciviousness be avoided; in such wise that figures shall not be painted or adorned with a beauty exciting to lust; nor the celebration of the saints, and the visitation of relics be by any perverted into revellings and drunkenness; as if festivals are celebrated to the honour of the saints by luxury and wantonness.[1]

The imagery had not changed. What had changed was people's perception of them. People could no longer *not* see sexuality in what had once been only images of religious ecstasy.

For example, Saint Teresa of Ávila, a sixteenth-century Carmelite reformer and nun, practiced intense mortification of the flesh and claimed to have experienced a violent encounter with an angel, her "transverberation," which she described thus:

I saw in his hand a long spear of gold, and at the iron's point there seemed to be a little fire. He appeared to me to be thrusting it at times into my heart, and to pierce my very entrails; when he drew it out, he seemed to draw them out also, and to leave me all on fire with a great love of God. The pain was so great, that it made me moan; and yet so surpassing was the sweetness of this excessive pain, that I could not wish to be rid of it. The soul is satisfied now with nothing less than God. The pain is not bodily, but spiritual; though the body has its share in it. It is a caressing of love so sweet which now takes place between the soul and God, that I pray God of His goodness to make him experience it who may think that I am lying.[2]

From a modern, post-Freudian perspective, St. Teresa's account sounds obviously sexual. Religious ecstasy is merely a cover story for an escape of repressed sexuality; the soul is just a metaphor for the body. The metaphor cuts both ways, however, and St. Teresa could be read as a spiritual experience expressed in terms of physical violation.

St. Teresa's divine encounter was depicted by Gian Lorenzo Bernini in his sculpture *Ecstasy of Saint Teresa* (completed 1652), which shows the nun swooning while the angel stands over her with a spear. In the life-size sculpture, Teresa's face is young and beautiful, her garment is soft and flowing, and one shapely bare foot dangles in plain view. Even in Bernini's own time, an anonymous reviewer of the newly unveiled work wrote that it "dragged that most pure Virgin down to the ground . . . transforming her into a Venus who was not only prostrate, but prostituted as well."[3]

Religious leaders were concerned about the confusion of the erotic with the holy, the sacred with the profane. The fifteenth-century Italian preacher Bernardino of Siena wrote, "I know of a person who, while contemplating the humanity of Christ suspended on the cross (I am ashamed to say and it is terrible even to imagine) sensually and repulsively polluted and defiled themselves."[4] In 1402, Jean Gerson, bishop of Paris, complained of "the filthy corruption of boys and adolescents by shameful and nude pictures offered for sale at the very temples and sacred places."[5]

In an earlier time in Christian Europe, phenomena like St. Teresa's ecstasy, and any depiction of it, would have been accepted as sacred without question, universally. By the sixteenth century, the medieval worldview was no longer universal, and religious views of the body and mystical experience were being challenged by the new rationalist, materialist philosophies. For many viewers, St. Teresa was profane, not sacred.

Experiencing pain was no longer an expression of piety, but of physical indulgence or insanity. The Vatican's gradual shift in emphasis to saints as moral exemplars, rather than holy figures in themselves, also moved worship away from the idea that the human body could be a medium to divinity.[6]

Over centuries, the Church's power to define human experience gradually eroded. By the time of Bernini and his anonymous critic, there were other ways of understanding the body and its physical experiences, which studied the material, natural world as an explanation for human experience. Flagellation and other forms of asceticism were no longer a way of communicating with the divine, but expressions of internal desires.

ACADEMIC

Perhaps the earliest discussion of voluntary flagellation in secular, material terms came in 1503, in an astrology treatise published by Pico della Mirandola,[7] which included a prototype of a case history of a sexual masochist.

> There is now, says he, a Man of a prodigious, and almost unheard of kind of Lechery: For he is never inflamed to Pleasure, but when he is whipt; and yet he is so intent on the Act, and logs for the Strokes with such an Earnestness, that he blames the Flogger that uses him gently, and is never thoroughly Master of his Wishes unless the Blood starts, and the Whip rages smartly o'er the wicked Limbs of the Monster. This Creature begs this Favour of the Woman he is to enjoy, brings her a Rod himself, soak'd and harden'd in Vinegar a Day before for the same Purpose, and intreats the Blessing of a Whipping from the Harlot on his Knees; and the more smartly he is whipt, he rages the more eagerly, and goes the same Pace both to Pleasure and Pain. A singular Instance of one who finds a Delight in the Midst of Torment; and he is not a Man very vicious in other Respects, he acknowledges his Distemper, and abhors it.[8]
>
> When I seriously enquir'd of him the Cause of this uncommon Plague, his Reply was, I have used my self to it from a Boy. And upon repeating the Question to him, he added, That he was educated with a Number of wicked Boys, who set up this Trade of Whipping among themselves, and purchased of each other these infamous stripes at the expence of their Modesty.[9]

The "childhood experience" explanation of sexual masochism proved popular and was referenced by other sixteenth-century writers. This is not to say that the man Pico discussed was the first sexual masochist in human history, but that this is one of the earliest discussions of such behavior in terms of individual psychology.

Shakespeare's play *Measure for Measure* (first performed circa 1604) criticized religious asceticism and flagellation by linking it with deviant sexuality and political tyranny. The Duke of Vienna, the judge Angelo, and the novice nun Isabella claim to be pious and chaste, while their repressed sexuality emerges as voyeurism, sadism, or masochism, respectively. "By drawing parallels to historical or topical events, Shakespeare suggests that the protagonists' very asceticism, ironically, causes these deviant desires and that they associate their austere religious practices with pleasurable feelings."[10]

The plot revolves around a couple, Claudio and Juliet, who have not properly observed all the rules of engagement and marriage. The judge Angelo decides to make an example of Claudio and condemn him to death for unlawful fornication. Claudio's friend Lucio asks Isabella, a novice nun and Claudio's sister, for help. Angelo offers to free Claudio in exchange for sex with Isabella.

The trio of the Duke, Angelo, and Isabella are all ascetics (though none are actually clergy), and are hostile to sexual desires, believing that "pain kills the libido and thus subjecting themselves and others to physical abuse."[11] Shakespeare used puns and allusions to characterize Angelo as a flagellant by comparing him to stockfishes,[12] which were cured by drying and beating with clubs, and mentioning his attempt to "rebate and blunt his natural edge,"[13] with "rebate" suggesting "to beat out." Both Angelo and Isabella speak of sexuality in terms of plunder and violence, of men victimizing women. Lucio claims Angelo "puts transgression to't," not only punishing harshly but deriving perverse pleasure from the act, and "put to" can also mean engage in sexual intercourse.[14]

Shakespeare alluded to the nuns' sexual restraints and their restricted interaction with men, but Isabella finds that insufficient for her: "And have you nuns no farther privileges?," she asks.[15] This repression cannot destroy the libido, but only makes it express in perverse ways. "Actual intercourse being forbidden, they develop a sexuality based primarily on fantasy, a cerebral kind of satisfaction, in which they savor the writhing of victims who fearfully wait for the blow from their persecutor."[16]

Throughout the play, characters claim the highest motives when they are actually indulging their perverse sexuality. Even Lucio plays on Isabella's masochism to persuade her to plead with Angelo, using the language of seduction, rather than her love of her sibling. Eager to cast herself into the role of supplicating victim before a cruel man, Isabella agrees. Angelo offers to free Claudio in exchange for Isabella's sexual submission, expressed in the terms of horse riding with references to "now I give my sensual race the rein: / Fit thy consent to my sharp appetite."[17] Isabella's response reveals her masochistic desires, even as she refuses him:

> Th' impression of keen whips I'd wear as rubies,
> And strip myself to death as to a bed
> That longing have been sick for, ere I'd yield
> My body up to shame.[18]

Shakespeare's play was a scathing indictment of the upper-class ideals of religious asceticism, demonstrating that expressions of piety mask personal indulgences, and repressed sexuality only fosters sadism and masochism, which leads to injustice. Such a criticism would have been scandalous at an earlier time, but by the early seventeenth century was unavoidable.

The next major treatise to consider the voluntary experience of pain from a secular perspective came from German doctor Johann Heinrich Meibom (1590–1655), in his treatise *De flagorum usu in re veneria et lumborum renumque officio* (1629).

Meibom (also Latinized as "Meibomius") disagreed with Pico della Mirandola's environmental explanation for erotic flagellation, and proposed a physiological explanation. He thought that certain men, particularly the aged, were "colder" than normal, and required more intense stimulus to achieve erection and orgasm.

> I further conclude, that *Strokes* upon the *Back* and *Loins*, as Parts appropriated for the Generating of the Seed, and carrying it to the Genitals, warm and inflame those Parts, and contribute very much to the irritation of *Lechery*. From all which, it is no wonder that such shameless Wretches, Victims of a detested Appetite, such as we have mention'd, or others exhausted by too frequent a Repetition, the *Loins* and their Vessels being drain'd have sought for a Remedy by FLOGGING. For 'tis very probably, that the refrigerated Parts grow warm by such Stripes, and excite a Heat in the Seminal

Matter, and that more particularly from the Pain of the *flogg'd* Parts, which is the Reason that the Blood and Spirits are attracted in a greater Quantity, 'till the Heat is communicated to the Organs of Generation, and the perverse and frenzical Appetite is satisfied, and Nature, tho' unwilling drawn beyond the Stretch of her common Power, to the Commission of such an abominable Crime.[19]

Meibom's ideas on the physiology of flagellation were still referenced well into the nineteenth century.

The Abbe Jacques Boileau's book *Historia flagellantium* (1700) accused flagellants of perversion, madness, shamelessness, and superstition. In his earlier works, he also railed against low-cut dresses on women for inflaming sensuality and libertinage. Boileau was anti-Jesuit, claiming there was no scriptural basis for flagellation, which was pagan in origin, and therefore had no place in Christian practice.

He distinguished between *sursum disciplina*, applied to the bare shoulders, and *dorsum disciplina*, applied to the bare buttocks and thighs. The latter is particularly dangerous, Boileau said, because of the physical connection between the loins, buttocks, and pubis. As a result from flagellation on the buttocks, "the animal spirits are forced back violently towards the *os pubis* and that they excite lascivious movements on account of the proximity of the genitals."[20] Boileau cites examples from both Pico della Mirandola and Meibom to support this.

Three years later, Jean-Baptiste Thiers, a doctor of theology, published a rebuttal, arguing that flagellation was practiced in the early church and it was a valid practice in his time, as an imitation of Christ. Thiers did not disprove Meibom's theory, as presented by Boileau, and was conspicuously silent about the sexual implications of "lower discipline."[21] The debate between Thiers and Boileau shows that the field was tilted against Thiers, who could not contradict Boileau's argument.

Boileau's better-known brother, the poet Nicolas Boileau Despréaux, contributed a satirical verse on this paradox, which translated read, "Which, under the pretence of extinguishing our voluptuousness, by that very austerity and by penance knows how to ignite the flame of lubricity."[22]

The debate was continued by other scholars and clergy in France, Germany, and England in later centuries, with citations in debates over school beatings, where advocates of the rod denied any sexual aspect to beating. Flagellation became a point of contention between Catholics and Protestants, and clergy and the laity. It was a metonym for what Enlightenment thinkers and Protestants saw as the corrupt and perverse Catholic Church.

ANTI-CATHOLICISM

There's a long tradition of linking deviant sexuality with deviant politics, a historical habit that will recur many times in the future. Sexualized anti-Catholic propaganda goes back at least as far as Boccaccio's *Decameron*, a collection of allegorical stories from the mid-fourteenth century, which included lecherous clerics and randy nuns. The word "pervert" itself could refer to both religious and sexual deviance, and it wasn't until the late nineteenth century that it had a mainly sexual definition.

It was during the "long eighteenth century" (usually defined as running from the English Glorious Revolution of 1688 to the battle of Waterloo in 1815) that the anticlerical propaganda that used sexual deviance gradually shaded into pornography that used the trappings of Catholicism as costumes, props, and sets. It's impossible to identify any dividing line between the two.

Julie Peakman, in her *Mighty Lewd Books* (2003), identifies four different subgenres of anti-Catholic erotica: anti-Catholic polemics; English reports of the trials of French priests; nunnery tales in which innocent young women are sexually initiated; and French pornographic novels and their English translations. She adds, "To some extent, there was a crossover between all four sub-sets in the genre. . . . Some erotic fabrications attempted verisimilitude by writing in documentary prose and adding factual footnotes."[23] Likely, the difference lay less in how they were written and more in how they were read. A reader who had no interest in the excesses of the church might read a slander against Catholicism to satisfy sexual curiosity, and a sexual fantasy might be woven into an allegedly factual piece of invective.

As Richard Hofstadter wrote in his classic "The Paranoid Style in American Politics," "Anti-Catholicism has always been the pornography of the Puritan."[24]

In the 1730s, France was rocked by a sex scandal that involved the church and its role in family life, the affair of merchant's daughter Mary Catherine Cadiere and her confessor, Father John Baptist Girard. Cadiere was a young woman said to have hysterical-mystical states, including visions and stigmata. She joined a group of young girls led by Father Girard. What followed was seduction by means of confession, flagellation (with emphasis on the details of positioning her body), and nudity. Girard apparently raped her while she was unconscious. She then had an abortion at Girard's behest and he put her in a convent,[25] where he visited her and corresponded with her. Girard went on trial, which is why this case is so well documented. Catherine withdrew her statement and Girard went free in 1731, to the outrage of the people, and he died the following year. Cadiere was lost from the historical record entirely, with even her date of death unrecorded.[26]

What was probably a rather sordid case of a clergyman sexually abusing his charge caught the public imagination and inspired anti-Catholic, particularly anti-Jesuit, propaganda and also pornographic/libertine writings. Even the relatively factual reportage on the case used the erotically charged language of submission and surrender, with Girard and Cadiere cast as dominant male and submissive female. He is reported to have demanded of her, "*Will you not yield yourself up to me?* This was followed by a Kiss, in which breathing strongly on her, he so infected her, that she answered, '*Holy Father, I will submit without reserve.*'" Her sexual initiation climaxed with flagellation by the "Whip of Discipline" and sodomy, at least according to published reports.[27]

There is a strong parallel to the previously discussed "Jesus courting the Christian Soul," though the fictionalized Girard-Cadiere case reads like a parody of the earlier story.

The Girard-Cadiere case coincided with an explosion of new book publishing in France and other European countries, ranging from hard-core pornography to dry philosophy and everything in between, and some in the form of newspapers and pamphlets priced to reach the lower-middle class and artisans.[28] There was no consensus about what was acceptable or legal; the concept of pornography as a distinct type of media was in its infancy. The French philosopher Diderot tells of himself as a young man flirting with a salesgirl in a bookshop, and both think nothing of his request for a certain erotic novel, but both blush and stammer when he asks for another. Diderot also dabbled in erotica, notably his 1760 novel *La religieuse* (*The Nun*), which was loosely based on the true story of a woman named Margueritte Delamarre, who tried to have her vows annulled because she claimed she had been placed in a convent against her will. Diderot's book was originally an elaborate practical joke aimed at luring a friend back to Paris. He wrote a series of letters from a fictitious woman, Suzanne, begging the friend to free her from the convent in which she was imprisoned. This also served as a framing device for Diderot's criticism of church corruption and the widespread practice of forcing women into convents.[29]

Another example of books that used explicit sex in the service of anti-Catholicism or other political causes was *Thérèse Philosophe* (1748, anonymous, likely by the Marquis d'Argens). A combination of flagellant pornography and materialist philosophy characteristic of the era, the novel featured characters whose names are anagrams of "Girard" and "Cadiere."

Thérèse Philosophe is very much about sex, but also very much about materialism and atheism, and the two are intertwined. It uses popular genres like the *bildungsroman*, the anticlerical story, and the "whore dialogue," to preach the new ideas of materialism and hedonism.

In the book's first part, Thérèse is one of the students of "Father Dirrag," and she observes him with her fellow student, "Mlle. Eradice." This satire/parody/roman-à-clef of the Girard-Cadiere case would have been familiar to the book's readers. Thérèse secretly observes Dirrag "counseling" Eradice, guiding her through what she thinks is a religious experience like that of St. Teresa of Ávila, but is really sexual arousal through flagellation and penetration. Dirrag is a Jesuit but also a closet materialist, preaching that all phenomena are just matter in motion. "In short, the Dirrag Affair demonstrated that seduction was an inverted form of Christianity, and it prepared the reader to consider the proposition in reverse: Christianity was a form of seduction."[30]

Thérèse sees and hears all of this from her secret observing post, and brings herself to pleasure while watching. Masturbation and visual and auditory voyeurism are the key sexual acts in this story, not intercourse. In fact, Thérèse is terrified of intercourse, fearing death in childbirth (a reasonable possibility at the time).

The first part, the Dirrag-Eradice affair, is the most overtly sadomasochistic. The techniques of religious ordeals are used for sexual ecstasy, in the context of a knowledgeable male teacher/dominant and innocent female student/submissive. This is the pornographic version of a familiar real-world issue, the role of the church in the family. It also follows the familiar initiation narrative.

In the second part, Thérèse gets dumped into a convent and falls ill because her "principle of pleasure," now awakened, is not allowed to run free and thus her body-machine is disordered. She is rescued by the libertine couple of Mme. C and the Abbe T, who discuss political philosophy between and during trysts.

In the third part, Thérèse is educated in alternative sexuality by an old courtesan, Mme. Bois-Laurier. This "whore dialogue," locker-room talk between an old sex worker and a new one, was a classic pornographic format long before this book.

In the fourth, Thérèse joins the unnamed Count, who wants her as his mistress. He finally makes a bet with her to get her to have intercourse with him: If she can last two weeks in a room full of erotic books and paintings, without masturbating, she doesn't have to have intercourse with him. She loses, of course, after a greatest hits tour of pre-eighteenth-century porn.

The narrative ends with Thérèse as the Count's mistress, living happily ever after, "without a problem, without a worry, without children." Not only is the Church rejected, so is the child-centered family and the attendant restricted roles of women.[31] *Thérèse* is a highly irreligious work, in which religion is valued mainly as an opiate of the masses.[32]

On the other side of the English Channel, the same sets of tropes that were transgressive in Catholic-dominated France became reactionary in anti-Catholic England, driven by a combination of political fear, theological difference, and popular xenophobia.[33] English publishers freely adapted French books for English readers and cut out things like philosophizing about love and lesbianism, as in the original French *Venus dans la cloitre* (Jean Barrin, 1683) and the English version, *Venus in the Cloister* (freely translated by Henry Rhodes, 1692, and republished many times in many different editions).[34] *Venus* was the progenitor of an entire genre of erotica, with recurring elements of sexual initiations, confined spaces, and ecstatic visions brought about by sex or flagellation.

Catholicism was seen as a primitive form of religious belief, compared to Protestantism or the Anglican Church, with all its complex rituals and vestments and imagery, and emphasis on ecstatic experience instead of sober contemplation. The mandatory celibacy of priests and nuns was seen as an aberration by Protestants, who believed that sexuality should be properly channeled within marriage. As is often the case, this was about control of women. Protestants believe that women belonged within the jurisdiction of the bourgeois family, and saw priests as interlopers. Anti-Catholic stories carried the message that Catholicism, with its emphasis on artifacts and physical ritual such as flagellation, was a fundamentally perverse religion: instead of liberating the soul, nuns become slaves of their bodies and the material world. Yet there was also the perverse reading, that anti-popish tracts displayed alternate forms of bodily experience.

After the Reformation, nuns were no longer permitted in England, and they established convents in other countries, where they became a space for erotic fantasy.[35] At least as far back as Shakespeare's day, nuns were compared with prostitutes, as another kind of woman who was outside social gender relations and therefore sexually available. Nuns were seen as idle and playful, obedient and ignorant. Thomas Rowlandson's 1622 pamphlet *The Anatomy of the English Nunnery at Lisbon in Portugall* claimed that nuns sang "ribaldrous Songs and jigs, as that of Bonny Nell, and such other obscene and scurrilous Ballads" for their confessors,[36] and were at the mercy of their priests: "not one amongst them will (for feare of being disobedient) refuse to come to his bed whensoever he commands them."[37] The joke or irony in Rowlandson's account and others is that nuns renounce the world only to experience even more sexual exploitation, and take a vow of chastity only to be forced to partake of even more excessive sexuality.

Nuns in particular were a fetishized figure, separated from their rightful place in the domestic sphere under the authority of their fathers and husbands, simultaneously completely innocent of proper sexual instruction and with their libidos stoked by the allegedly overheated eroticism of Catholicism, leading to lesbianism, flagellation, or other depravities. In 1871, an anti-Catholic tract titled *Dr. Pusey's Insane Project Considered* referred to "English perverts" who "delight to rub their necks against rusty chains."[38]

The boundary between anti-Catholic propaganda and Catholic-themed pornography was unclear, even to the people who published them. One of the first major tests of England's 1857 Obscene Publications Act was a pamphlet published by the Protestant Electoral Union[39] called *The Confessional Unmasked; Shewing the Depravity of the Romanish Priesthood, the Iniquity of the Confessional and the Questions put to Females in Confession*. Originating in the early nineteenth century and containing the usual anti-popish claims, it misinterpreted an eighteenth-century Catholic theologian as saying that the confessor must overcome all modesty of ladies. This is a natural setup for a scenario of a vulnerable woman left alone with a man who will seduce or rape her. Indeed, says the tract, the confessional makes any sexual act possible and forgivable.[40] An 1858 *Punch* cartoon shows a shifty-looking priest accepting confession from a young, pretty Englishwoman, while in the background John Bull (the personification of England) gets a whip ready. Whether it is for the priest or the woman is unclear.

The tract led to the case of *Regina v. Hicklin* in 1868. Lord Chief Justice Cockburn was faced with a problem: Did obscenity come from the intent of the work's authors or distributors, or did it come from the content of the work itself? He did not think the Protestant Electoral Union were pornographers, but Cockburn's ultimate decision was that the test for obscenity was "whether the tendency of the matter charged as obscenity is to deprave and corrupt those whose minds are open to such immoral influences, and into whose hands a publication of this sort may fall." Thus, even if *The Confessional Unmasked* was not intended to be obscene or pornographic, it could be read as such by particular people. Part of the problem was the manner in which *The Confessional Unmasked* was distributed, by sale on street corners. Instead of circulating among gentlemen, the tract could spread among women, youth, and the working class, who were liable to read it as obscenity. The "Hicklin test" was the basis for obscenity law in Britain and America for the next century.[41]

Even in situations where anti-Catholicism was far from the minds of the writers and readers, nuns were a stock erotic figure.

In the mid-nineteenth century, millions of immigrants came to America from Catholic Ireland and southern Europe, including nuns and sisters, who were segregated from the general population by rules of enclosure. Antebellum American Protestants were voyeuristically fascinated by these enclosures, and wrote and read books with titles like *Secrets of Nunneries Disclosed*, *The Veil Lifted*, and *Convent Life Exposed*.[42] These drew on the familiar seduction/initiation narratives of earlier French and English anti-Catholic works, often edited or reworked for American tastes. As there was little domestically produced erotica prior to the American Civil War, lurid tales of women menaced by Catholicism (or in the sister-genre of captivity narratives) were there to satisfy sexual curiosity.[43]

The most notorious example of this genre was *Awful Disclosures of Maria Monk* (1836). In 1835, a young Protestant woman named Maria Monk appeared in New York City in the company of a Reverend William K. Hoyte. Monk claimed she had volunteered to become a nun in the Hotel Dieu convent in Montreal, Quebec, thinking it would be a sanctuary from the profane world. After undergoing a ritual initiation into the convent, which involved her symbolic death and rebirth in a coffin, Monk learned the truth about convent life.

> The Superior now informed me . . . that one of my great duties was to obey the priests in all things, and this I soon learnt, to my utter astonishment and horror, was to live in the practice of criminal intercourse with them. . . . The priests, she said, were not situated like other men, being forbidden to marry; while they lived secluded, laborious, and self-denying lives for our salvation. They might, indeed, be considered our saviours, as without their service we could not obtain pardon of sin, and must go to hell. Now it was our solemn duty, on withdrawing from the world, to consecrate our lives to religion, to practise every species of self-denial. We could not be too humble, nor mortify our feelings too far; this was to be done by opposing them, and acting contrary to them; and what she proposed was, therefore, pleasing in the sight of God. I now felt how foolish I had been to place myself in the power of such person as were around me.
>
> From what she said, I could draw no other conclusions but that I was required to act like the most abandoned of beings, and that all my future associations were habitually guilty of the most heinous and detestable crimes.[44]

Monk's tale was absurd sadomasochistic fantasy. By her account, the nuns were forced to kneel on dried peas, and walk on their knees through tunnels. They were gagged, kept in tiny cells, and bound with leather bands; were forced to wear a spiked belt or armbands akin to a cilice, eat garlic or eels, and drink water in which the Superior had washed her feet; were branded with a hot iron, whipped with small rods, ordered to sleep on the floor with only one sheet in winter, forced to chew a bit of glass into powder, and most peculiarly, made to wear "the cap," a leather skullcap which caused intense pain to the wearer through unknown means.[45] The priests entered the nunnery from the adjacent seminary via a secret underground tunnel. There were several references to ritual infanticide of the babies resulting from this "criminal intercourse." Supposedly, they were baptized and immediately strangled or smothered, and disposed of in lime pits in the cellar.[46]

Monk eventually escaped, to prevent the murder of her unborn child, and to tell her tale.

Or so the story went. In reality, none of this happened. The release of *Awful Disclosures* in 1836 set off a publishing battle of critiques and counter-critiques. Visitors to the convent could find no trace of hidden tunnels, lime pits or murdered infants, or any of the people Monk described. Monk herself turned out to be a prostitute who had been in a home for wayward women, and according to her mother, she had suffered a head injury as a child that left her prone to fabrication. Even the anti-Catholic *Quarterly Christian Spectator* wrote, in 1837, "If the natural history of 'Gullibility' is ever written, the imposture of Maria Monk must hold a prominent place in its pages."

Nonetheless, people believed her, enough to sell three hundred thousand copies in America before the Civil War. It perfectly fit the anti-Catholic, nativist sentiment of early nineteenth-century America, which was strong enough to lead to violence.

Protestant Americans were ready to believe the worst of Catholics (represented by nuns): that they practiced polygyny, infanticide, sadism, and masochism. In other words, Catholics were said to live in defiance of the values of the bourgeois, child-centered family and the Protestant faith. Some read *Awful Disclosures* with horror, others with titillation, imagining sexual experiences freed from the restrictions of what society defined as "normal."

Awful Disclosures had many imitators in the following decades, both in America and England. The stories used a familiar set of accusations against convents, standing in for Catholicism as a whole: fugitive nuns, sadistic superiors, lecherous priests, flagellation and other physical torments, murdered infants, and so on. They were allegedly written by former nuns or priests, and promised revelations, "to lift the veil and prick the bubble."[47]

When domestically produced American pornography proliferated after the Civil War, anti-Catholicism provided sets, costumes, and roles for erotic fantasies. In catalogs of pornographic books sold in 1870s New York, there were titles like, "*Scenes in a Nunnery.* Very plain words. 25 cents" and "*Silas Shovewell, His Amours with the Nuns*, 10 colored plates $2.00."[48]

Meanwhile in Paris, Toulouse Lautrec's account of the elite licensed brothel, the Rue des Moulins, in the 1890s mentioned a nun's habit as one of an extensive collection of costumes for the inmates to wear in performing the clients' fantasies, along with a nurse, a bride in white, a widow in mourning, and a tamer of wild beasts.[49]

In Oscar Wilde's *The Picture of Dorian Gray* (1890), the protagonist fetishizes a nun's habit, linking his aesthetic decadence (and queer sexuality) with the decadence of Catholicism and its images of torture and death:

> He had a special passion, also, for ecclesiastical vestments, as indeed he had for everything connected with the service of the Church. In the long cedar chests that lined the west gallery of his house, he had stored away many rare and beautiful specimens of what is really the raiment of the Bride of Christ, who must wear purple and jewels and fine linen that she may hide the pallid macerated body that is worn by the suffering that she seeks for and wounded by self-inflicted pain. . . . The orphreys were woven in a diaper of red and gold silk, and were starred with medallions of many saints and martyrs, among whom was St. Sebastian [depicted bound and shot with multiple arrows]. He had chasubles, also, of amber-coloured silk, and blue silk and gold brocade, and yellow silk damask and cloth of gold, figured with representations of the Passion and Crucifixion of Christ. . . . In the mystic offices to which such things were put, there was something that quickened his imagination.[50]

The path from St. Teresa of Ávila to *Thérèse Philosophe* to Maria Monk is long and crooked. The three heroines attain radically different forms of enlightenment via their ordeals and are presented as exemplars of, respectively, Christian devotion, secular materialism, and Protestant piety.[51]

By the mid-eighteenth century, religion no longer had a monopoly on management of human experience. Desire could be discussed in secular terms, through new ideas of materialism and the internally motivated human body. Having increasingly less place in expressions of piety, voluntary flagellation could only be understood as a sexual act. Not only was flagellation recontextualized from sacred to erotic, the symbols of Catholicism were appropriated as props and costumes for erotic dramas

This is not to advance what Michel Foucault called the "repressive hypothesis," that the Church was a monolithic, pleasure-hating regime that dictated the actions of the human body, and whose decline meant a new flowering of sexual expression. Instead, flagellation gradually shifted out of the Church's domain and into the domain of the secular, and specifically the sexual. What had been ulterior or transgressive readings of the flagellation scene became primary and obvious, and the once primary and obvious faded into mere connotation. The suffering body was no longer a link to the divine, but a body that functioned in a different way than normal.

Chapter Three

Virtue in Distress

By the early eighteenth century in England, flagellation for purposes other than punishment was not exclusively the province of priests, monks, and nuns, nor of libertine aristocrats. Even people of the newly formed bourgeois classes could find pleasure in flagellation, as shown by the case of Mr. Samuel Self and his household.[1]

Self was a struggling businessman trying to get rid of his wife, Sarah, who spent his money, gave him gonorrhea, and had a great deal of sexual interest in other people, according to court documents. Samuel actually encouraged Sarah to cross the line into adultery with a friend named John Atmeare, so Self could legally separate from her without alimony. The Selfs rented out part of their house to another couple, Jane and Robert Morris, who could easily observe the other half of the house through keyholes. The Selfs also had a spinster named Sarah Wells and a maid named Susan Warwick living with them.

It's hard to say whether Samuel was trying to get rid of Sarah or attempting to fulfill some kind of cuckold fantasy. Either way, over 1707 Sarah and Atmeare spent much time together, while Samuel was frequently away on business trips. Meanwhile, the Morrises watched everything through keyholes.

Samuel finally "caught" Sarah and Atmeare in the act, and the ensuing court cases revealed the goings-on at the Self house. More common than the group sex and voyeurism was the flagellation. The most common pairing was Samuel putting Jane Morris over his knee in the kitchen or over the kitchen table or on her stomach on a bed upstairs, and using his hand or a birch rod. He also flagellated his wife, his maid, and his houseguest. These were not private exchanges, as there was almost always somebody watching, if not actively participating. There was female dominant-female submissive and female dominant-male submissive whipping too.

None of the group seems to have had any guilt or shame about their actions, suggesting they followed an extreme version of the pleasure-seeking materialism that was the new way of thinking at the time. John Locke's *An Essay Concerning Human Understanding* had been published in 1690, and what would today be called ethical hedonism was advocated in many pornographic books in circulation after 1680 in England. It's possible that, as a bookseller and bookbinder, Self had access to these. Meibom's *A Treatise on the Use of Flogging in Medicine and Venery* was published in English in 1718, and there were probably copies circulating in England earlier.

Samuel Self was middle-class, barely, and not born to aristocratic libertinage. Furthermore, the Self ménage confined its activities to private or semi-public settings (homes and shared homes), and to a small group of apparently consenting individuals. This is in sharp contrast to the exploits of English rakes, who accosted women in public settings or non-domestic spaces like brothels. The Earl of Rochester's idea of a fun afternoon with his mates was grabbing a woman on the way to market, stealing her butter and smearing it on a tree, then coming back, turning her upside down and then they "clapt the butter upon her breach."

Self's house was to the aggressive violence of rakehood as masquerades were to the cathartic uprising of medieval carnival; it offered a watered-down form of freedom and social inversion and pleasure seeking, domesticated and privatized to be compatible with the new bourgeois manners required by mercantile society.

RISE OF SECULAR FLAGELLATION IN FICTION

While documented cases like the Self household are rare, the seventeenth and early eighteenth centuries offer many fictional references to erotic flagellation, outside of a religious context. These indicate that the ideas of flagellation and submission for sexual purposes were in circulation, though often discussed as jokes.

In Thomas Shadwell's Restoration comedy *The Virtuoso* (1676), an old lecher named Snarl entreats Mrs. Figgup, a brothel madam, to bring out the birch rods and beat him.

Snarl. Where are the instruments of our pleasure? Nay, prithee do not frown; by the mass, thou shalt do't now.

Mrs Figgup. I wonder that should please you so much that pleases me so little.

Snarl. I was so us'd to 't at Westminster School I could never leave it off since.

Mrs Figgup. Well, look under the carpet then if I must.

Snarl. Very well, my dear rogue. But dost hear, thou are too gentle. Do not spare thy pains. I love castigation mightily. So here's good provision.

Pulls the carpet; three or four great rods fall down.[2]

Thomas Otway's Restoration drama *Venice Preserv'd* (1682) was a political allegory about England set in the republic of Venice. In act 3, scene 1, Antonio, a lecherous and corrupt old senator, barges into the house of Aquilina, a Greek courtesan.

Antonio addresses Aquilina by childish nicknames ("Nacky, Nacky, Queen Nacky") and then as "Madonna." He disregards her insults and brags about his "eloquence," which his actions equate with bribery. He then plays the roles of a bull, a toad, and a dog, masochistically pleading for Aquilina to spit on him, kick him, and beat him.

Aquil. Nay, then I'll go another way to work with you: and I think here's an instrument fit for the purpose.

[Fetches a whip and bell.] What, bite your mistress, sirrah! out, out of doors, you dog, to kennel and be hanged—bite your mistress by the legs, you rogue—

[She whips him.]

Anto. Nay, prithee Nacky, now thou art too loving: Hurry durry, 'od I'll be a dog no longer.

Aquil. Nay, none of your fawning and grinning: but be gone, or here's the discipline: what, bite your mistress by the legs, you mongrel? out of doors—hout hout, to kennel, sirrah! go.

Like *The Virtuoso*, this shows masochistic flagellation to be the interest of old, deviant men.

The true origin of the maxim "spare the rod and spoil the child," often cited in debates over corporal punishment in later centuries, is not the Bible as commonly thought (though it resembles Proverbs 13:24). It came from Samuel Butler's mock heroic poem *Hudibras* (1664) about a dim-witted knight who is tricked by an amorous lady into being flogged. The lady speaks:

> If matrimony and hanging go
> By dest'ny, why not whipping too?
> What med'cine else can cure the fits
> Of lovers when they lose their wits?
> Love is a boy by poets stil'd
> Then spare the rod and spoil the child (part 2, canto 1, lines 839–44).

The rod, in this case, refers to a bundle of birch twigs commonly used in domestic and school discipline, while "the child" refers to Cupid, according to one theory, or makes a bawdy double-entendre about preventing conception, according to another.

This confusion of Butler's phrase between a biblical injunction for physical discipline and a satirical sexual reference reflects the instability of meaning attached to flagellation. Is it a sexual act, an act of punishment, or an act in imitation of Christ? No answer is final.

Perhaps the most detailed account of a scene of erotic flagellation in this period comes from a novel, John Cleland's *Memoirs of a Woman of Pleasure* (1748), better known as *Fanny Hill*. Though fictional, there is a ring of authenticity to the scene, unlike pornographic fantasies, suggesting that Cleland may have had some firsthand experience observing such acts.

Late in the novel, Fanny is living in the house of Mrs. Cole, the madame, who introduces her to a flagellant client. Going against the stereotype, dating to before Meibom, of the old man who needs to be flogged to get it up, Fanny's client Mr. Barville is a young, handsome man.

> [H]e was under the tyranny of a cruel taste: that of an ardent desire, not only of being unmercifully whipped himself, but of whipping others, in such sort, that though he paid extravagantly those who had the courage and complaisance to submit to his humour, there were few, delicate as he was in the choice of his subjects, who would exchange turns with him so terribly at the expense of their skin. But, what yet increased the oddity of this strange fancy was the gentleman being young; whereas it generally attacks, it

seems, such as are, through age, obliged to have recourse to this experiment, for quickening the circulation of their sluggish juices, and determining a conflux of the spirits of pleasure towards those flagging shrivelly parts, that rise to life only by virtue of those titillating ardours created by the discipline of their opposites, with which they have so surprising a consent.

Mrs. Cole regards Mr. Barville's interests as merely an unfortunate quirk. She arranges for the scene between him and Fanny with the utmost secrecy. Fanny, according to her client's instructions, is clad all in white, "like a victim led to sacrifice."

On meeting Mr. Barville, Fanny finds he has a particular scene in mind, and encourages Fanny "to go through my part with spirit and constancy." Cleland describes in great detail the costuming, the birch rods "which he took, handled, and viewed with as much pleasure, as I did with a kind of shuddering presage," the cushioned bench to which Fanny will tie Barville with his own garters "a circumstance no farther necessary than, as I suppose, it made part of the humour of the thing, since he prescribed it to himself, amongst the rest of the ceremonial."

> Seizing now one of the rods, I stood over him, and according to his direction, gave him in one breath, ten lashes with much good-will, and the utmost nerve and vigour of arm that I could put to them, so as to make those fleshy orbs quiver again under them; whilst he himself seemed no more concerned, or to mind them, than a lobster would a flea-bite.

Fanny is disturbed by the blood she has drawn, but continues at her client's urging, until she finds him aroused, and later sees him ejaculate.

Her assignment is also to be flagellated, for the first time. Mr. Barville sets her mind at ease by emphasizing her ability to withdraw consent.

> [W]hen I expected he would tie me, as I had done him, and held out my hands, not without fear and a little trembling, he told me, "he would by no means terrify me unnecessarily with such a confinement; for that though he meant to put my constancy to a trial, the standing it was to be completely voluntary on my side, and therefore I might be at full liberty to get up whenever I found the pain too much for me."

He starts slowly on her, but builds in intensity, and delights in her reddened buttocks. "And yet I did not utter one groan, or angry expostulation; but in my heart I resolved nothing so seriously, as never to expose myself again to the like severities." Yet, later, she finds that the treatment has aroused her: "[T]he smart of the lashes was now converted into such a prickly heat, such fiery tinglings, as made me sigh, squeeze my thighs together, shift and wriggle about my seat, with a furious restlessness." This spurs Fanny and Mr. Barville to intercourse, and Fanny concludes that flagellation has an aphrodisiac effect akin to "Spanish flies; with more pain perhaps, but less danger; and might be necessary to him, but was nothing less so than to me, whose appetite wanted the bridle more than the spur." The encounter ends with Fanny's assertion of her own "normal" sexuality, compared with Mr. Barville's, though she does not medicalize his experience.

Cleland's fictional account is echoed by a number of historical references to flagellation as a common sexual service provided by English prostitutes of this period. Bear in mind that in earlier times, pregnancy and childbirth could be life threatening, not to mention the dangers of sexually transmitted infections. Many prostitutes would have seen flagellation, even received, as safer than intercourse, as were other sexual services.

A Catalogue of Jilts, Cracks & Prostitutes, Nightwalkers, Whores, She-friends, Kind Women and other of the Linnen-lifting Tribe was an anonymous pamphlet published in 1691, which listed twenty-one women, including "Posture Moll," a flagellant who charged half a crown. Posture molls were sex workers who avoided intercourse and specialized in giving or receiving flagellation.[3]

Plate 3 of William Hogarth's series of engravings, *A Harlot's Progress* (1732), shows the protagonist's bedchamber, representing the lifestyle of a common prostitute (see Figure 3.1). A birch rod for flagellation is prominently displayed on the wall over the bed.[4]

Jack Harris's annual *List of Covent Garden Ladies*, published through the late eighteenth century, listed prostitutes by their specialties. Mrs. L-v-b-nm of 32 George Street was "left a pretty good fortune by an old flagellant, whom she literally flogged out of the world." Mrs. M- enacted scenes of herself as a schoolmistress with her "two young beautiful tits [meaning young women, rather than breasts], one about fifteen and the other sixteen, who are always dressed in frocks like school girls,"[5] an early example of a uniform fetish.

Another late eighteenth-century account of sex work includes crossdressing, humiliation, and domestic discipline:

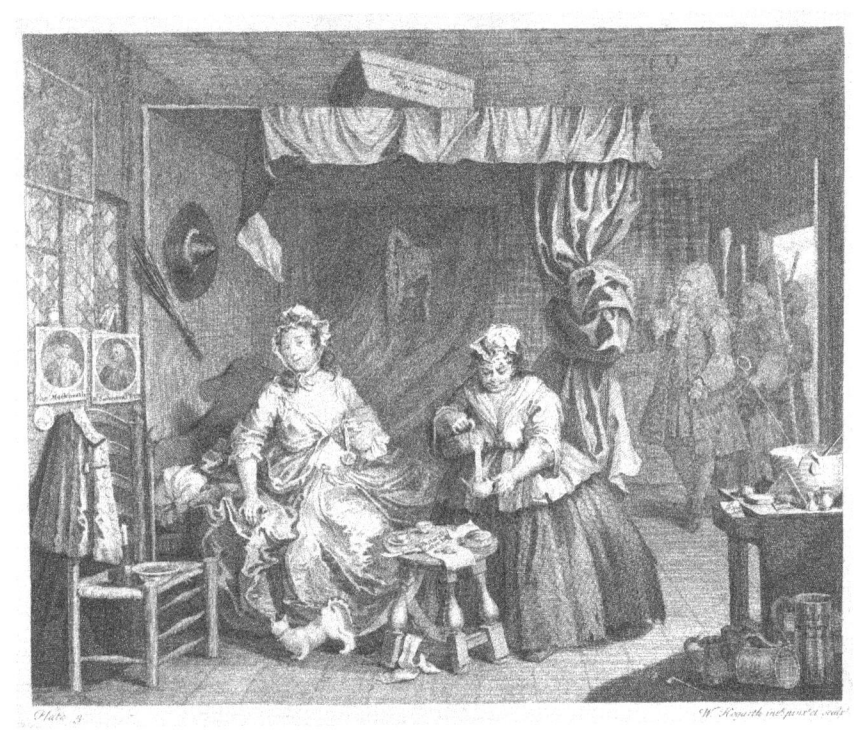

Figure 3.1. Plate 3 of William Hogarth's *A Harlot's Progress*, 1732. Note the bundle of birch twigs over her bed, indicating flagellation. *Courtesy Metropolitan Museum of Art*

> I went as gently downstairs as my feet could tread; and looking over the kitchen-door, I saw the good man, disrobed of his clothes and wig, and dressed in a mob cap, a tattered bed-gown, and an old petticoat belonging to the cook, as busy in washing the dishes as if this employment had been the source of his daily bread,—but this was not all; for while he was thus occupied, the mantua-maker [who doubled as a bawd] on one side, and the cook on the other, were belaboring him with dish-clouts; he continuing to make a thousand excuses for his awkwardness and promising to do the business better on a future occasion. . . . When he had completed his drudgery, and had been sufficiently beaten, he desired the two females to skewer him up tight in a blanket, and roll him backwards and forwards upon the carpet, in the parlour, 'till he was lulled to sleep.[6]

One of the rare firsthand accounts from this period came from the French philosopher Jean-Jacques Rousseau. In his posthumous autobiography *Confessions* (1782), he attributed his lifelong fascination with flagellation by cruel women to a childhood sexual experience. Having lost his mother in infancy, young Rousseau went to live in a country school in Switzerland, run by a Protestant clergyman, M. Lambercier, and his unmarried sister. By his own account:

> As Miss Lambercier felt a mother's affection, she sometimes exerted a mother's authority, even to inflicting on us when we deserved it, the punishment of infants. She had often threatened it, and this threat of a treatment entirely new, appeared to me extremely dreadful; but I found the reality much less terrible than the idea, and what is still more unaccountable, this punishment increased my affection for the person who had inflicted it. All this affection, aided by my natural mildness, was scarcely sufficient to prevent my seeking, by fresh offences, a return of the same chastisement; for a degree of sensuality had mingled with the smart and shame, which left more desire than fear of a repetition. . . .
>
> Who would believe this childish discipline, received at eight years old, from the hands of a woman of thirty, should influence my propensities, my desires, my passions, for the rest of my life, and that in quite a contrary sense from what might naturally have been expected?[7]

Rousseau felt considerable shame from what he called his *goût bizarre*. It is worth noting that his treatise on childhood education, *Emile, ou l'éducation* (1762), does not mention corporal punishment at all. Obviously, not all of the people who suffered corporal punishment as children were drawn to it as adults, though given the ubiquity of spanking and flagellation in homes and schools at the time, it would be difficult to find a person who had not suffered such mistreatment as a child.

In later centuries, Rousseau's *Confessions* became a standard reference in debates on the corporal punishment of children. In the medical and scientific realm, several of the case studies in Richard von Krafft-Ebing's *Psychopathia Sexualis* refer to reading *Confessions*. The French psychiatrist Alfred Binet referred to it in formulating his idea of the fetish,[8] as did Freud in his *Three Essays on Sexuality*.

Voluntary flagellation was no longer seen as religious, but as a sexual act, and a puzzling and absurd one. The flagellant men of Shadwell and Otway's plays were old and twisted, and even Rousseau expressed shame at his strange taste. The encounter with Mr. Barville in *Fanny Hill* was a rare instance of a sympathetic treatment of a flagellant. It would take a new way of thinking to understand voluntary flagellation and other extreme experiences.

SENSIBILITY AND VIRTUE IN DISTRESS[9]

With the decline of religious authority to explain the world and human nature, new ideas took its place in the Enlightenment. Natural philosophers like John Locke presented a new, secular, rationalist model of human nature, that of sensibility. Locke's *An Essay Concerning Human Understanding* (1690) said, "Pain has the same efficacy and use to set us on work that pleasure has, we being as ready to employ our faculties to avoid that, as to pursue this: only this is worth our consideration, that pain is often produced by the same objects and ideas that produce pleasure in us."[10]

In sensibility theory, human beings were born as blank slates and formed through their experiences, which affected their nerves. If a person's nerves would do the right things, they would feel appropriately in response to stimulus. To observe a suffering person would induce feelings of sympathy (not empathy) in the observer and naturally create a desire to help that person. Indeed, an observer of greater sensibility might feel more distress than the person who was actually suffering.

There were degrees of sensibility, which were mapped onto hierarchies of both class and gender. Sensibility was supposed to indicate development and refinement, so privileged people should have more of it from their upbringing, yet women were thought by some to have higher degrees of sensibility, with more delicate nerves that could be damaged by the wrong kind of stimulus. Too little sensibility and you were a boring drudge who couldn't appreciate the finer things in life; too much and you were a flake on the edge of madness and effeminacy who couldn't take care of business.

Women had greater license to develop their sensibility and the language of feelings, which were a major topic of women writers and the new medium, the novel, which was seen as a sexually corrupting influence on vulnerable young women. The implications of sensibility were explored in a new literary theme, that of "virtue in distress."

Women had just begun to enter the public, commercial, hetero-social space of baths, resorts, shopping arcades, dance halls, and masquerades.

Mating and marriage could be more than a business transaction between families. However, there was a pervasive fear of violent rakes and tyrannical husbands, unreformed men of the old school, and later on a more nuanced fear of the new predator, a man with the appearance of respectable manners but who had the instincts and appetites of a rake.

However, the new model of masculinity, the "man of feeling," was dangerously close to effeminacy and unappealing to some men and women. Both sexes were torn between the old warrior/farmer model of man, which could easily slip into brutality, and the new mercantile man, who could be boring and ineffectual.

Virtue in distress plays and novels were about the interaction of the new ideal of sensibility versus the power-driven ways of "the world," mapped onto the gendered dyad of the victim and the rake. Writers as diverse as Samuel Richardson, Horace Walpole, Jane Austen, and the Marquis de Sade wrote about the clash of these two worlds, from very different perspectives.

Materialism and its offshoot, rationalism, had their critics, who formulated their own ideas. Instead of controlling emotions, they said, people should seek out extreme physical/emotional states, in search of the sublime. This is a greatness that transcends the mundane, beyond the human ideas of "good" or "beautiful."

Edmund Burke, another eighteenth-century philosopher, described the sublime:

> Whatever is fitted in any sort to excite the ideas of pain and danger, that is to say, whatever is in any sort terrible, or is conversant about terrible objects, or operates in a manner analogous to terror, is a source of the sublime; that is, it is productive of the strongest emotion which the mind is capable of feeling....
>
> The passions which belong to self-preservation turn on pain and danger; they are simply painful when their causes immediately affect us; they are delightful when we have an idea of pain and danger, without being actually in such circumstances; this delight I have not called pleasure, because it turns on pain, and because it is different enough from any idea of positive pleasure. Whatever excites this delight, I call sublime. The passions belonging to self-preservation are the strongest of all the passions.[11]

Thus, extreme physical experiences awakens the strongest emotions, which are a source of the experience of the sublime, a higher emotional truth beyond reason. The sublime is what we seek when we look at nature in a painting or in the archetype of the "noble savage," both of which are threats that are safely removed.[12] The fear allows access to sexual arousal, which Western culture has not entirely allowed within the realm of the beautiful. This also connects to the use of threat or pain in rituals discussed previously.

In modern thought, reason and emotion are usually seen as opposing forces in the human mind. In the late eighteenth century, however, thinkers like Rousseau and Locke developed the idea of sensibility, which is part of a cluster of related words with shifting meanings, including "sense" (both as in "the five senses" and as in "common sense"), "sentient," "sensation," "sentiment," and "sentimentality."

Sensibility is based on the belief that human nature is basically good. If a person is in touch with their natural emotions, they will naturally experience sympathy for people in distress. Also in accord with nature, that person will be moved to take action, and they will naturally employ reason to do good things. Thus, people with proper sensibility would be as incapable of doing wrong instead of right as they would be of mistaking red for green.

Sensibility was particularly cultivated in girls and women, and all emotions were seen as desirable, even the distressing ones. A person of sensibility relished her feelings of betrayal or sadness at the hands of her lover. A person of cultivated sensibility would feel things more intensely than an ordinary person.

The corollary of this principle is that evil occurs because society is flawed and turns us away from our better selves. This can lead to social restructuring by any means necessary, such as the French Revolution or abandoning civilization and withdrawing to nature, as in primitivism. The bloody aftermath of the French Revolution consigned sensibility to the dust heap of history.

What emerged from the decay of sensibility was actually more lasting, particularly for the history of sadomasochism. This is the valorization of sympathy, the idea that by observing emotionally stirring scenes, one would exercise one's sensibility. Sensibility decayed into what we would call sentimentality today.

Sensibility also was the foundation of virtue in distress. This was the key theme of writers as diverse as Jane Austen and the Marquis de Sade. Both wrote about what happens when people who believe in sensibility encounter the real world. In Austen, it's a necessary and probably beneficial disillusionment, part of growing up. In Sade, innocents are either ripped to shreds or enlightened/debased to libertinism.

The archetypal "virtue in distress" novel is Samuel Richardson's *Clarissa*, published in 1748 (making it a contemporary of *Fanny Hill* by John Cleland). Clarissa is a classic sensible heroine, smart and good-natured yet innocent and unworldly. Her depraved family schemes to marry her to a repulsive man, and holds her prisoner when she refuses. Clarissa's apparent rescue comes from the smooth-talking Lovelace, who takes her away from her family.

However, Lovelace is determined to seduce Clarissa. He is a new form of rake, able to speak the language of emotions and manners, but in service to his unreconstructed desires. He constructs an elaborate web of captivity, surveillance, misinformation, and false identities around her, setting her up in a prison-like brothel, surrounded by prostitutes and other sketchy characters. Lovelace doesn't just want her body; he wants her soul, for her to give up her principles, particularly chastity. Clarissa, however, refuses to stop believing in goodness, and thinks she can reform Lovelace. Her growing physical attraction to Lovelace despite herself complicates matters.

The conflict ends badly, with Lovelace drugging Clarissa senseless and raping her. This climax brings about Lovelace's realization of his failure as a seducer, and Clarissa's disillusionment about human nature.

Lovelace spends much time spying on Clarissa, deeply moved by her suffering, despite the fact he caused it. The tension in the novel is whether such feelings will reform Lovelace's rakish character. To women writers and readers, the rake was an ambivalent, liminal figure, representing both a social and physical threat but also the possibility of experiencing a larger world beyond the home. The stories were about resolving this conflict in various ways. Would the rake ruin his victim? Or would the victim reform her rake, awaken the latent sensibility within him?

The virtue-in-distress theme with the victim-rake dyad is the prototype of the male dominant/female submissive pairing. And what of the female dominant/male submissive pairing? There was a certain passive dominance in the sensibility-informed fantasies of men kneeling before their loves, but that was a result of the man's awakened sensibility. The edge of acceptable behavior for women was marked by the figure of the Amazon, the masculinized woman, who doesn't appear to have the same liminal ambivalence or sex appeal as the rake.

The theory of sensibility was ultimately too conflicted and too confusing. People settled on a compromise: men would be reasoning creatures of the world, women would be feeling creatures of the home. Men adopted simple dress and austere stoicism, while women became increasingly decorated and expressive. This was the ideal that informed gender roles for the next two centuries.

Clarissa was a psychologically complex work, but the scenario of Richardson's highly popular novel was vulgarized in many inferior imitators. We have a young woman held prisoner, threatened with the loss of her virtue by hypermasculine forces. This is a classic scenario of male dominant/female submissive fantasy.

Observing people suffering was an opportunity for the exercise of sensibility. Men and women could both empathize and sympathize with the scenario. Men could fantasize being Clarissa's seducer or rescuer, or both. Women could fantasize being Lovelace's conquest or redeemer. Many women readers wrote to Richardson about how they wanted a happy ending, for Clarissa to reform Lovelace's character. Women even went to costume balls dressed as Clarissa.[13]

Women could also be attracted to rakes in a wish to emulate their characteristics, their freedom and daring in the world outside the home, instead of casting them as abusers in their fantasies. While some worried about women being too naive and weak to survive in the masculine public space, other feared they would adapt too readily, taking up hunting and gaming and licentiousness; "Amazon" was the pejorative for such a woman. Mary Wollstonecraft saw the rake and the woman of excessive sensibility as matching partners, both given to self-indulgence and lawlessness (a belief she shared with the Marquis de Sade). The rake was an ambiguous figure to women, potentially predator, liberator, or both. Women also identified with the image of a feminized Christ, a source of infinite submission, forgiveness, and self-abasement, which created an opportunity for moral superiority.[14]

Late eighteenth-century sensibility coincided with the origins of pornography as a distinct genre of entertainment, and the slavery abolitionist movement.[15] Slaves became the perfect figures for sensibility porn, which abolitionist tracts couldn't help shading into (to be discussed later).

The fictive patterns established by [Samuel] Richardson [in *Clarissa* and his other novels] were capable of almost immediate vulgarisation; and the rapidity with which they degenerated into melodramatic and superficial clichés is an indication of the depth and broadness of their appeal. In the stories of Pamela and Mr B., and of Clarissa and Lovelace, the readers and the novelists of the eighteenth century found reflected with extraordinary fidelity some of the most important truths of life as they knew it. But the fidelity was too faithful for comfort: the harsh tragedy of *Clarissa* was soon softened and transformed into a "delicate distress," and the papier-mâché terrors of the Castle of Udolpho were substituted for the unbearably authentic claustrophobia of [Clarissa's family home] Harlowe Place.[16]

The vulgarization of the novel of sentiment produced the Gothic novel.

GOTHIC LITERATURE AND STYLE

Drawing on the anti-Catholic strain of English and French literature explored previously, the Gothic novel provided an exciting mix of deviant sexuality and deviant religion to explore extremes of emotion, placing heroines in situations of fear and deprivation. The Gothic is the sentimental made literal and external, a rejection and critique of Romantic ideals of reason, simplicity, and authenticity in favor of emotion, complexity, and ambiguity.

The prototypical Gothic novel was Horace Walpole's *The Castle of Otranto* (1764), about an unstable nobleman struggling to escape an ancestral curse that drives him to adultery and near-incest. Walpole, a noted eccentric and lover of men, once expressed his unreciprocated desire for Lord Lincoln at a masquerade ball. "I dressed myself in an Indian dress, and after he was come thither, walked into the room, made him three low bows, and kneeling down, took a letter out of my bosom, wrapped in Persian silk, and laid it on my head; he started violently! They persuaded him to take it." It was a mock-Persian love note.[17] In another letter, Walpole coyly attempted to manipulate Lincoln via submission: "I assure you, there is no part I won't act to keep you."[18]

Gothic novels inherited a strong streak of anti-Catholicism, using the trappings of the Roman faith as props in stories of virtue in distress, which all too easily slipped into the erotic.

For the Gothic novelists . . . Roman Catholicism and sexual deviance were each suggestive of the other. In *The Mysteries of Udolpho*, Radcliffe neatly conjoins the two in her description of the "Italian love" of Laurentini, the sinister adulteress and murderer whose erotic excess only finds its match in the convent in which she ends her days. And in Radcliffe's later *The Italian*, the heroine Ellena is forced to "determine either to accept the veil, or the person whom the Marchesa di Vivaldi had . . . selected for her husband." Both of Ellena's alternatives—entering into the celibate but sadistic Catholic orders and marriage to the wrong person—represent kinds of rape, sexual violations threatening to the normative heterosexual union hoped for with Vivaldi, the Marchesa's son.[19]

Mrs. Radcliffe's *Mysteries of Udolpho* describes a sexy nun: "The rays of the moon, strengthening as the shadows deepened, soon after threw a silvery gleam upon her countenance, which was partly shaded by a thin black veil, and touched it with inimitable softness. Hers was the CONTOUR of a Madona, with the sensibility of a Magdalen."[20]

Another English Gothic classic, Charles Maturin's *Melmoth the Wanderer* (1820), linked threatening Catholicism with deviant masochism: "tales of 'voluntary humility,' of self-inflicted—fruitless sufferings."

The opposite of the victimized woman is the frighteningly powerful woman, gifted with seductive beauty and often gender ambiguity. Matthew G. Lewis's novel *The Monk* (1796) featured Matilda, the Devil in the disguise of a woman in the disguise of a monk.

> Matilda stood beside him. She had quitted her religious habit: She was now cloathed in a long sable [black] Robe, on which was traced in gold embroidery a variety of unknown characters: It was fastened by a girdle of precious stones, in which was fixed a poignard [thrusting knife]. Her neck and arms were uncovered. In her hand she bore a golden wand. Her hair was loose and flowed wildly upon her shoulders; Her eyes sparkled with terrific expression; and her whole Demeanour was calculated to inspire the beholder with awe and admiration.
>
> "Follow me!" She said to the Monk in a low and solemn voice; "All is ready!"[21]

The Gothic flourished in post-Revolutionary America too, such as in the writings of Edgar Allan Poe, Herman Melville, and Nathaniel Hawthorne, or the numerous captivity narratives that told of white women stolen away by Native Americans. *The Awful Disclosures of Maria Monk*, previously discussed, is a Gothic narrative, full of captivity, torture, and madness, in service of an anti-Catholic message.

Muckraking journalist George Lippard's novel *Quaker City; or, the Monks of Monk-Hall* (1844) was a distinctly American form of the Gothic, an apocalyptic exposé of the injustices of 1840s Philadelphia. The setting of most of the action is Monk-Hall, a six-floor private brothel, gaming hall, and carousing pit, with half the structure underground. Like Lovelace's house, the cells and dungeons of Gothic novels and Maria Monk's convent, Monk-Hall was a place where anything was possible, and where innocence was repeatedly violated. Originally built by a pre-Revolutionary libertine who held midnight orgies (suggestive of the semi-legendary Hellfire Club of the Scottish Enlightenment), it was later occupied by an unspecified Catholic order that performed other rites, leaving coffins behind. This links *Quaker City* to the anti-Catholic branch of the Gothic, but Lippard's anxieties were mainly about economic and political inequality, the perceived failures of the ideals of the American revolution. He represented these injustices with the same archetypes as the other Gothic forms: the seductive man and the innocent, then ruined, woman.

Evil results from many causes in *Quaker City*, but the strongest and most terrifying force is sexual desire. The novel has three main plots and several secondary ones, all driven at least in part by illicit passion. There's adultery, incest, rape, the vaguely defined crime of "seduction," a preoccupation with deflowering virgins, and concubinage, mixed in with duels, falling through trap-doors and other cliff-hanger action. Like other porno-Gothic writers, Lippard's polemical goals were belied by his focus on bodily violence and sex, and particularly his lavish descriptions of heaving breasts.

> Gathering her form in his left arm, secure of his victim, he raised her from his breast, and fixing his gaze upon her blue eyes, humid with moisture, he slowly flung back the night robe from her shoulders. Her bosom, in all its richness of outline, heaving and throbbing with that long pulsation, which urged upward like a billow, lay open to his gaze.[22]

The sexual scenes in *Quaker City* could be read in isolation from the work's message, answering the reader's need for stimulation or just curiosity. Like the anti-Catholics before him, Lippard used the physicality of sexual deviance to represent the abstraction of political and social deviance, but the message could easily be lost to the reader. The Gothic would influence other American media, notably abolitionist works like Harriet Beecher Stowe's *Uncle Tom's Cabin* (1852), to be discussed later.

The novel of sensibility could also be seen as a prose account of an initiation ritual. The innocent heroine is initiated into the larger world of sexuality or power dynamics, or both. This is supposed to produce an aware person who can reconcile the two opposing forces of virtue and power, a permanent transformation of status that marks a liminal ritual. However, when the novel of sensibility was surpassed by the Gothic novel, the scenario was repeated over and over again with only temporary changes in status for the initiates (the readers), making it a liminoid ritual. Just as the slasher killer always comes back for a sequel film, there's always another innocent lass ready to fall into the clutches of another rake. And people were always ready to read about them.

SADE

The S in S/M usually means "sadism," a reference to Donatien Alphonse François, better known as the Marquis de Sade (1740–1814), aristocrat, libertine, pornographer, and one of the rare individuals who have an entire realm of human behavior named after them. The term "sadism," and related words like "sadean" and "sadique," was in use throughout the nineteenth century, a testament to Sade's notoriety before Krafft-Ebing combined it with his coinage "masochism" to create "sadomasochism."

The midpoint of Sade's life roughly coincided with the French Revolution; half of his life was spent under the old regimes of clergy and aristocracy, while the other was under the revolutionary government, and he never completely fit in with either. Abandoned by his parents, spoiled rotten by various relatives, and lucky enough to have an inexplicably loyal wife, Sade lived at the very end of the age when an aristocrat could more or less do as he pleased with members of the lower orders. He was taught by Jesuits, who introduced him to two key themes of his life: corporal punishment and theater, both means of education.

We know some of Sade's real-world exploits via the detailed police reports made by Inspector Marais, who became Sade's shadow and pursuer.

Libertines like Sade were a favorite subject of government surveillance. "Libertine" meant a person who was not only free sexually, but politically and religiously. "To be libertine meant practically from the beginning to be both sexually a free liver and philosophically a free thinker; and the salon was both symbolically and often actually the antechamber to the boudoir."[23]

Marais's police reports, delivered to the royalty, show that the original sadist was just as much a masochist, at least physically. (Rather than being polar opposites, Sade and Sacher-Masoch had much in common.) In the 1763 incident with Jeanne Testard, a twenty-year-old fan-maker and casual prostitute, Sade ordered her to whip him. Sade's little chamber was full of props, including a chalice he masturbated into, ivory crucifixes hanging alongside pornographic prints and drawings, rods, cat-o'-nine-tails, pistols, and a sword. He ordered her to utter sacrilegious lines and perform sacrilegious acts, like an apostate theater director.

The incident that really brought Sade to the attention of the authorities happened on Easter Sunday, 1768. He brought a thirty-six-year-old unemployed cotton spinner named Rose Keller to one of his residences in Paris on the pretext of hiring her for housework. He threatened her until she undressed, and was enraged when she resisted him. He held her down, then beat her alternately with a rod and a cat-o'-nine-tails, mixed with the application of hot wax. When Keller begged him to stop so she wouldn't die without having taken confession, Sade told her she could confess to him.

As cruel as Sade's actions were, we can also see that he was interested in more than just physical sensations. He had an image in mind, a particular scenario or ritual to execute. These incidents show Sade's theatricality in his emphasis on props, costume, and dialogue, and his desire to parody religious ritual and iconography. He made sex a private ritual. Like Mr. Barville of *Fanny Hill*, Sade's experience depended on the smallest details of the scene.

Officially, Sade was imprisoned because of his mistreatment of prostitutes, but he was also a scapegoat and pawn in the political struggles of pre-Revolutionary France.

In 1785, his eighth year of continuous imprisonment, Sade wrote one of his many haranguing letters.

To the Lieutenant General of Police:
>
> Show me the legal code which dictates that fantasies executed with whores earn a gentleman tortures as long and arduous as mine! . . . There is no statute against what I have done . . . which condemns a man . . . to be treated which such inhumanity.
>
> Pray, sir, tell me if the Messalinas, the Sapphos, the incestuous, the sodomites, the public and private thieves . . . who constitute that respectable Montreuil family of which you are the slave—all knaves, whom I'll introduce you to whenever you wish—tell me, pray you, if any of them have suffered the tortures I've been victimized with for thirteen years. . . . Isn't it because they had money and whores to offer the judges? . . . Cease, sir, cease the consummate injustice you have singled me out for. . . .
>
> May the Eternal One someday reject you with the brutality with which you have rejected me.[24]

Sade's letter demonstrates his classical education, his paranoid sense of persecution, his animosity to his in-laws, and his pompous hyperbole. His parting shot shows that even his materialism and atheism could be abandoned for the sake of insulting his perceived enemy. However, it would be a mistake to take anything Sade said or wrote at face value. His reference to "fantasies executed with whores" suggests that he saw his encounters as not literal, but a form of play. The purpose of his scene was not so much about hurting or being hurt, but performing his private ritual.

Having little else to do while incarcerated, Sade assembled a considerable library, ranging from the philosophers of his day (including Rousseau and Voltaire) to a selection of Gothic novels.

He also wrote the earliest drafts of the novels for which he is remembered: *120 Days of Sodom*, *Justine*, *Juliette*, and *Philosophy in the Bedroom*, along with many other works. Sade wrote in the genre of the Gothic and "virtue in distress," but pushed them to their limits, simultaneously as social satire, as ego-driven sexual fantasy, and as sheer poetic extravagance. The familiar Gothic elements are there: imprisonment, torture, sexual deviation, corrupt elites, ravaged innocents, all in service of Sade's nihilistic philosophy. Unlike the prevailing idea that childhood experiences could produce strange desires, Sade's materialism dictated that desire comes from each individual's constitution as created by Nature, and to restrain that would be cruel.

Written on five-inch-wide sheets of paper glued into a single roll forty-nine feet long, *The 120 Days of Sodom* is an elaborate sexual fantasy. Richardson's Lovelace imprisoned the virginal Clarissa in a few rooms, a boutique operation. Sade's quartet of elite libertines built an entire castle where they are unquestioned masters and filled it with whores and children of both sexes to be debauched and later murdered in a meticulously scheduled, even industrial, process. Along the way, the narrative winds through every sexual act Sade's fervid imagination can conceive. Long before the Diagnostic and Statistical Manual, Sade attempted to compile an encyclopedia of sexual deviance. Why, is hard to say. The author claims an educational purpose, intending to show the reader all the "secret horrors" so they would come to hate vice, but this may just be an apologist frame for a work that is basically exploitative. (A common feature of works of the sadomasochistic imagination, as we shall see.)[25]

If Richardson's *Clarissa* tests the theory of sensibility to the breaking point, Sade's novel *Justine* tears it to pieces and stitches it back together as a parody. The innocent and kindhearted Justine falls into one exploitative, confining institution, then escapes, only to fall into another: a matricidal nobleman's castle, rapist brigands, blood fetishists, criminals, cruel monks in a monastery. Justine is rescued by her long-lost libertine sister, Juliette, only to be struck by lightning and killed. People are not basically good, just as nature is a cruel and capricious force, and Justine's innocence makes her nothing but a victim. *Justine* is not just a Gothic story of innocent heroine victimized by a corrupt world. Justine suffers like any Gothic heroine, but not to prove her refinement or for any higher purpose, just to demonstrate Sade's extreme materialism and to provide the spectacle of the suffering female body.[26]

Sade's *Philosophy in the Bedroom* can be read as a parody of Rousseau's educational ideas, combined with the "whore dialogue" format used in European pornography for centuries. Over seven dialogues, a young woman is sexually initiated by a male and female pair of libertines, who alternate sexual debauchery with philosophical lectures, covering the abolition of the family, the superiority of anal intercourse to vaginal, and general hedonism. Sade takes the opportunity to work an absurdist political tract into the text, arguing that the new republic, founded on the crime of regicide, must continue to foster other forms of crime to remove the last traces of despotism by unleashing the libido. At the end, the initiated heroine turns on her authoritarian mother by arranging for her to be raped by her syphilitic valet (another example of Sade's hatred of the maternal).[27]

In the original *Justine*, Juliette is the title character's long-lost older sister, who repents after her sibling's death and becomes a nun (likely the author's concession to the growing Puritanism of the Revolution). In the expanded *Le nouvelle Justine*, instead of trying to do good in a world where that is impossible, Juliette jumps headfirst into libertine debauchery. She was corrupted by her convent's mother superior, then becomes the mistress of two elite libertines and acquires her own Sapphic lover, then rapes, murders, and steals her way across Europe, always getting away with it. Perhaps the most politically outrageous of Sade's works, *Juliette* parodies contemporary nobles and religious leaders as monstrous deviants, committing acts of incest and mass murder. Juliette is a Kali-like dark goddess, the polar opposite of Clarissa, living out the ultimate dream of personal freedom and material hedonism in a godless universe.[28]

In prison, Sade fantasized and wrote about a world turned upside down. The French revolution released him into just such a world, and he embraced the new regime. Sade's revolutionary fervor can be attributed to self-preservation, at a time when other nobles were being exiled or executed. But his theatrical side may have been drawn to the dramatic and bloody nature of the Revolution, the chance to remake the world. Apart from his attempts as a man of letters, he rose to be a leader of a section of Paris.

The postrevolutionary Sade led a much more sedate life, enjoying a respectably bourgeois and apparently chaste relationship with a woman named Constance Quesnet. Either Sade was a somewhat reformed character (with perhaps a case of "criminal menopause"), or he did carry on as before, but was both more cautious and under less intensive surveillance.

But he misread the constantly shifting political situation, and spoke loudly in favor of atheism just when the government swung back to religion. He was jailed again in 1801, under Napoleon's puritanical Consulate, for having written *Juliette*, and spent the remainder of his life in prisons and asylums, somewhere between criminal and lunatic. His last few years were in the Charenton asylum, and contrary to some fictional portrayals, they were comfortable and uneventful. He fulfilled his dream of a life in the theater, produced unremarkable dramas, and died peacefully in 1814.

By the standards of modern BDSM, Sade was not even remotely safe, sane, or consensual. He was indeed a dangerous and cruel man, at war with the world. He was also an advocate of extreme personal freedom, the idea that the individual can determine right and wrong for himself, based on his own intense personal experiences. His outrageous works explored the farthest reaches of his own imagination, and scathingly satirized the hypocrisies of his day. Like the other sentimental and Gothic novelists, Sade wrote about the conflict of ideals and reality, but pushed it further than anyone. When Richardson's Clarissa dies, it's a perfected being transcending a fallen world. When Sade's Justine dies, it's a snowball finally melting in Hell. He mapped out territory that would be explored by more balanced individuals in the centuries to come.

The Romantics and the Decadents of the late nineteenth century revered Sade as a libertine hero, even though his books were difficult to come by. The villain of one French Gothic novel used Sade's *Justine* as an implement of torture in itself, believing that reading it would drive his female victim mad.[29]

By the end of the eighteenth century, flagellation for pleasure was well established as part of the sexual underground of England and France. Yet to be medicalized, it was simply the "strange taste" of a small minority.

The Gothic provided a conceptual framework for flagellation and other intense, ritualistic experiences, now that the old religious paradigm of voluntary suffering had fallen away. As a critique of Romantic ideals of reason and order, the Gothic reveled in deviance, sexual and otherwise, and the pursuit of extreme sensations. Even though the Gothic novel was supposedly extinct by the mid-nineteenth century (Jane Austen mocked the form in her novel *Northanger Abbey* [1817]), it cast a long shadow into the centuries that followed.

O'Malley notes that, "religious and sexual transgression . . . by the 1890s . . . function as metaphors for each other, an epistemological slippage that Gothic itself made possible."[30] The Gothic is about power, played out at the level of the body, and particularly sexuality. Whether that power comes from an unfamiliar religion, a foreign invader, an alienated oligarchy, a corrupt family, or an enemy political system, it is usually linked to deviant sexuality.

Chapter Four

Orientalism

The slave auction is for charity. One by one, the "slaves" come up on the stage of the rented hall, to be bid upon by the party guests. It quickly becomes apparent that young, conventionally attractive, and female "slaves" get the most vigorous bidding. "Slaves" who fall short on any or all of those aspects are in less demand, and the bidding for them drags in uncomfortable silences.

Some of the women dress for the premise. Instead of the usual blacks and reds of kink events, they wear brightly colored flowing skirts and loose pants, jingling belts of fake coins, anklets and bracelets, and other accouterments usually only seen in belly dancing classes. The auctioneer gets into the act by wearing a *keffiyeh*, an *agal*, and sunglasses indoors, like a caricature of an oil sheik. It's all part of the spectacle that references a centuries-old tradition of fantasy, and not only the sexual kind.

In his *120 Days of Sodom*, the Marquis de Sade furnished his imaginary castle with "splendid Turkish beds canopied in three-colored damask."[1] He neglected to mention what, if anything, made a Turkish bed different from a European bed. Merely the word "Turkish" gave a sexual, transgressive quality to a mundane piece of furniture, or anything else. Sade's reference was an example of Orientalism in erotica, of artists using the superficial signs of Turkey or Persia or the Orient in general, to add exotic flavor to an erotic work.

Among the many themes from the European narration of the Other, two appear most strikingly. The first is the insistent claim that the East was a place of lascivious sensuality, and the second that it was a realm characterised by inherent violence.[2]

The locations and boundaries of "The Orient" constantly shifted over the centuries. Originally, it referred to Muslim-dominated regions like North Africa and Turkey. In later centuries, it expanded to include the Middle East, India, Asia, and even Africa, the Americas, and the tropics; actually, anywhere uninhabited by white Christians descended from Europe.

Where the Orient was is less important than *what* it was. In the process of European civilization defining itself, through art and science and religion, it defined "the Orient" as everything it wasn't, racially, politically, socially, religiously, economically, and sexually.

> In short, any Westerners who dare venture into the exotic East should brace themselves as they will encounter incomprehensible, fiery passions, wild emotions, and strange sexual practices. Xenotopia is what Europe is *not*, the antithesis of bourgeois austerity, respectability and temperance. This is the profoundly didactic message underlying so many seemingly frivolous romances and erotic novels set outside of Europe. . . .[3]

> Sexuality, the element of power relations endowed with the greatest instrumentality according to Foucault, played a key role in mapping out difference: "here" and "there" were distinguished, if not principally, at least significantly, by the imagined differences between the sexual practices of "us" and "them." Harems, eunuchs, public bathes, dancing girls, concubines, slave markets, all relentlessly provided evidence of the Orient's alterity.[4]

In the European collective mind, the Orient was a blank screen where one could project whatever fantasies (sexual, political, religious, etc.) one wanted, without regard for accuracy, plausibility, or even internal consistency. Thus, the Orient is both a land of despotism and a land of anarchy. The Oriental man is both soft and feminized and a fierce, cruel warrior. The Oriental woman is both ugly and beautiful, innocent and scheming, submissive and domineering, filthy and obsessed with bathing, virginal and sexually skilled. The real issue is who said what about whom, and who listened to and believed the speaker.

Perhaps crudely put, as European powers become the owners of collections of colonies, which they construct as the Other, their own process of identity-formation required that they split off the characteristics of both despicable master and weak/vulnerable outsider and project them onto, respectively, the male and female Other.[5]

SLAVES OF THE BARBARY COAST

Ever since the Moors were expelled from southern Spain in 1492, there was a centuries-long conflict between Christian Europe and Islamic North Africa, each holding one side of the Mediterranean. For Europeans, one of the great fears of travel by sea was capture and enslavement by Muslim and renegade Christian corsairs, who also made slaving raids on the coasts of southern Europe. Even if raids occurred infrequently, it was a fear that lingered. "'Corsair hysteria,' which gripped much of Europe during these centuries, [was] a general panic fueled by a combination of fear and fantasy."[6]

In the seventeenth century, Emanuel d'Aranda described capture by corsairs as being suddenly forced into a completely unfamiliar, arbitrary world.

> "I seemed like one in a dream, and the figures moving around me strange ghosts inspiring fear, wonder and curiosity. They wore strange clothes, spoke strange tongues . . . bore strange arms, and made strange gesticulations when they prayed." Such were the captives' sensation of fascinated horror and foreboding as they were carried off to Algiers and slavery.[7]

Enslavement functioned like a ritual of separation. "This initial turmoil and the fright it produced were only the first in a series of torments that either in effect or by design tended to break the new captives' sense of individuality and willingness to put up resistance."[8] Captives were often stripped naked and beaten. When they arrived in Barbary, "Some slaves reported being paraded through town . . . in a procession that effectively proclaimed their shame and social death. Since the arrival of new slaves was a sign of prosperity and an occasion of civic pride for all the towns-folk, the resident Turks, Moors, Jews, and renegades all turned out to cheer and taunt the newcomers."[9] The iron rings fastened around their ankles and their shaved heads and beards were another step in this process.

> One can discern in such treatment, besides the obvious need to give new slaves their own, distinctive look, a desire to further the process of breaking and demoralizing, now that they were indeed bonded to a master. As such, it resembled the first stages of boot camp for new soldiers, though in fact the experience in Barbary was if anything still more traumatic, since in the sixteenth and seventeenth centuries a great deal more of a man's identity was wrapped up in his hair and beard.[10]

Then came the auction, a key rite in this ritual of enslavement, which featured in almost all captivity narratives.[11] The narratives also strongly emphasized women being prepared for the harem or slave market by being depilated. The explorer Richard Burton suggested "the pain [of plucking out body hair] born so indifferently by the savage would kill or drive insane a European of the more educated classes."[12] Then there are sensual depictions of slave markets and harems, rife with exhibitionism. "The harem provided a perfect setting for the topos of the slave-nymph, portraying women as unselfish and submissive on the one hand, and lustful and sexually voracious on the other."[13]

> According to [Pierre] Dan, slaves could be stripped naked at this point, "as seems good to [the dealers], without any shame." Their primary need was to determine whether a slave was worth buying primarily for resale—in particular for ransoming—or whether he (or she) might be more profitably employed as a laborer, artisan, or for domestic or (sometimes) sexual purposes.[14]

Christian captives (and others who learned about their experiences secondhand through captivity narratives and other media) understood their slavery as a test of their faith and their identity. Thus, Barbary slavery was grafted onto familiar martyr imagery. Contemporary Europeans could have their faith tested by Turks in the same way that founders of the church were tortured by Romans. The captives were constantly tempted to convert to Islam under pain of torture, particularly the bastinado, or beating the soles of the feet with a cane. The Christians were very reluctant to dress in the Turkish fashion, seen as the garb of the traitorous renegade.[15] This threat to identity was expressed in sexual as well as religious terms, and the two realms overlapped, much as Protestant fear of Catholics was expressed in sexual terms.

Christians feared male captives were in danger of corruption by and addiction to sodomy, making them easy converts to Islam. Father Haedo, a Benedictine monk in late sixteenth-century Algiers, spoke of men keeping male concubines (*garzones*). "Many Turks and renegades, when full grown and old, not only have no wish to marry but boast that they have never known a woman in all their lives."[16] Joseph Pitts wrote about homosexual affairs, in which men slashed their arms to prove their love for boys.[17] Not all Christians went easily. Young Thomas Pellow reportedly withstood enough torture to kill seven men before he gave in to his master's advances, and even then he called upon God to forgive him. "I seemingly yielded, by holding up my finger."[18]

> It would also appear . . . that the missionaries were at least as nervous that such young men would allow themselves to be seduced sexually as well as religiously, to become catamites even as they became Muslims. Indeed, many clerics, insofar as they had any notions of Islam, acted as if the two forms of seduction were closely linked: the Trinitarian Alfonso Dominici, writing in 1647, asserted that, among slaves, these "*Giovanetti* are all lost," because
>
>> *They are purchased at great price by the Turks to serve them in their abominable sins, and no sooner do they have them in their power, [than] by dressing them up and caressing them, they persuade them to make themselves Turks. But if by chance someone does not consent to their uncontrolled desires, they treat him badly, using force to induce him into sin; they keep him locked up, so that he does not see nor frequent [other] Christians, and many others they circumcise by force. . . .*
>
> . . . Venture de Paradis called sodomy the *vice à la mode dans Alger*, and stories circulated about young male slaves who allowed themselves to become the "perpetual concubines" of local elite men. All the Barbary capitals—but especially Algiers—had open and flourishing homosexual subcultures.[19]

Christian men were also said to be at the mercy of Oriental women, an inversion of "nature." D'Aranda claimed Muslim women would poison inconvenient husbands.[20] Laugier de Tassy told tales of lascivious women smuggling their paramours in drag into their public baths.[21] Pitts described Muslim women taking advantage of their male slaves, using the punishment to blackmail their men for fear of being beaten, beheaded, or burned alive.[22] Another tale tells of a Frenchman sold to a master who bred mulatto slaves, and kept a bevy of sixteen African women in a farm in Algiers. The French captive was locked up in the harem with food and drink. After six days, he was taken away and sold, exhausted.[23]

Christian women were also in peril of sexual deviance. Aaron Hill lushly described an "oriental" slave market in 1709:

> There is in *Constantinople*, a *Slave-Market twice* or *thrice* a Week, thither the People go, and see the miserable *Christian Captive-Virgins*, dress'd in all the tempting Ornaments, that can allure the Looks of *amorous Passengers*; they speak to those they are inclin'd to like, and having ask'd them any Questions they think fit to start, they feel their *Breasts, Hands, Cheeks,* and *Foreheads*; nay proceed, if curious in the nicety of Search, to have the young, and the wretched Creatures taken privately to some convenient Place, where, *undisturb'd*, and *free* to use the utmost of their Will, they find out certain subtle Means of boasted Efficacy, to discover instantly by *Proofs*, and *Demonstration*, whether the *pretended Virgin* has *as yet* been rob'd of that so celebrated *Jewel*, she affirms her self Possessor of.[24]

One English girl sent to Muley Ismael "resisted his persuasions to turn Moslem and capitulated only after being handed over to the sultan's Negresses, who whipped her and tormented her with needles; 'so he had her washed and clothed her in their fashion of apparel and lay with her.'"[25]

These accounts, and the many others like them, grossly overstate the number of Christian women slaves. The majority of Christian slaves were captured sailors and others traveling by sea; only a minority, perhaps as little as 5 percent, were women and girls taken in coastal raids.[26] The centuries-old Orientalist fantasy of white Christian women stolen away to suffer beautifully in Turkish harems has a certain slim measure of truth, but it was much more important as a rhetorical device. The captured European maiden was a figure in a drama that cast the encounter between East and West in highly gendered, sexualized terms, making the Oriental male the incarnation of masculine rapaciousness and the European woman the model of feminine vulnerability and modesty. This is the same scenario of the novel of sentiment and the Gothic novel, familiar to European readers and playgoers, and transposed into a fantastic, picturesque setting.

> Cordoba and other principal cities had their *ma'rid* where the human merchandise was examined along lines which the slave-dealers were to follow, though with less sophistication, in the slave-marts of Barbary. Women were generally prized more highly than men, and were classified in two categories; the "distinguished" or first class (*murtafa'at*) and the "common." They were examined, before being offered for sale, by a female inspector (*amina*) who kept a meticulous record, which was then specified in the purchase contract, of the physical attractions (*nu'ut*) and defects (*uyub*) of each human chattel. Handbooks listing these good and bad qualities were specially composed to facilitate this delicate task.[27]

Women captives were treated more decorously, the distinguished and attractive amongst them being confined in a latticed apartment where they could be inspected with greater intimacy. Joseph Pitts, an English slave who accompanied his master on travels to other Moslem lands, observed that in the Cairo slave-market

> *although the women and maidens are veiled, yet the chapmen have liberty to view their faces, and to put their fingers into their mouths to feel their teeth; and also to feel their breasts. And further, as I have been informed, they are sometimes permitted by the sellers (in a modest way) to be searched whether they are Virgins or no.*[28]

A minority of the slaves who returned to Europe escaped, while most were ransomed through Catholic orders. Redeemed captives were under the authority of the priests who had freed them, and were obliged (sometimes forcefully) to participate in rituals that reenacted their capture, trials, and redemption (the ritual cycle of separation, liminality, and integration).[29] They appeared publicly in processions that parodied their display as new captives, wearing the rags or uniforms they had worn as slaves and bearing symbolic broken chains. Some of the redeemed captives had to spend years on arduous pilgrimages, pray daily, wear their prison garb and not cut their hair so they resembled their former appearance, and refrain from gambling, swearing, or frequenting brothels. They bore the burden of symbolizing the belief that Christian faith could survive even the worst. These public processions and performances became quite elaborate, with floats representing galleys manned by slaves toiling at the oars, and children dressed as angels or turbaned Turks leading captives on slender chains. Some spectacles exaggerated the experiences, with participants marching through towns dragging absurdly heavy chains.[30] These processions could cost five to ten times what had been paid for the slaves' ransom, suggesting that the spectacle was more important than the reality.[31] These served dual functions: demonstrating to contributors that their money had been well spent and that they should continue donating to the Redemptionists, and allaying the social anxiety about the threat of Christians stolen away by Muslims, to be enslaved and even converted. Slaves often spoke of their condition as hell or purgatory.[32]

This was to prove to them that the former slaves were once again part of Christendom and the European social hierarchy, that after the deviance of the Orient, the social universe was ordered again. The threatening East became a contained imaginary space for adventure and drama.

This raises the question of how much of this is true, and how much of this is fantasy of one kind or another.

> Pierre Dan, for one, seems to have positively reveled in all the various sufferings imposed on Christian slaves in Barbary, and he presented his readers with a lengthy catalogue of the torments that their Muslim oppressors favored. Dan's editors, no doubt mindful of the sales value of such visceral attractions, thoughtfully accompanied his prose with a set of grisly illustrations showing various slave-martyrs undergoing their passions—some crushed alive, some impaled, some burned, some crucified; different versions appears in the French and the Dutch editions.[33]

The reality of slavery, harems, polygyny, concubinage, eunuchs, and other customs of the Muslim world (all of which had their analogues in European society) is irrelevant compared to the role these practices played in Europeans' fantasies. To European Christians, Barbary was a zone of sexual and gender anarchy. This became an inspiration for early exploitation pornography.

> Mascarenhas [a Portuguese observer] . . . claimed that the Turks brought their Christian slaves with them to the local bathhouses. . . .
> Mascarenhas' narrative, as its translators remark, was originally published in 1627 as a pamphlet of around 100 pages. . . . Works such as Mascarenhas', which often provided their readers with lurid descriptions of homosexual practices in Barbary, may have done much to fix the popular

European notion that the inhabitants of the Maghreb were in general "incorrigibly flagitious . . . sayd to commit Sodomie with all creatures and tolerate all vices." . . .

That tales like Mascarenhas' were so widely diffused may well have had another, unintended purpose, however, since such stories must have also brought the sexual culture of the regencies to the attention of Europeans with homosexual interests. One soon notices, in fact, how often the stories that circulated about homosexual activities in Barbary involved renegades. . . . It may not be too far fetched to conclude that some who voluntarily left Christendom, with its harsh strictures against homosexual practices, abjured and came to the Maghreb as much for what they saw as the region's sexual liberality as for its economic or religious opportunities.[34]

HAREM TALES

The Turkish bogeyman was still feared in later centuries, elevated to the status of myth: "There still existed a pervasive anxiety throughout Christendom about the subversive attractions of Islam, a collective horror that expressed itself through many different strands of conscious and unconscious dread."[35] In the early twentieth century, one Sicilian woman said:

> The oldest [still] tell of a time in which the Turks arrived in Sicily every day. They came down in the thousands from their galleys and you can imagine what happened! They seized unmarried girls and children, grabbed things and money and in an instant they were [back] aboard their galleys, set sail and disappeared.[36]

Centuries later, the "white slavery" moral panics of the late nineteenth century would echo this anxiety, with hyperbolic headlines like "The Maiden Tribute of Modern Babylon."

The other side of anxiety was eroticized fantasy. Europeans who were dissatisfied with European civilization, whether they were armchair dreamers or explorers and conquerors, saw in the Orient a space of freedom. Victorian explorer, Orientalist, and sexual freethinker Sir Richard Francis Burton described what he called "the sotadic zone," encompassing southern Europe, North Africa, the Middle East, Asia, and the Americas, where pederasty (sexual relations between men and boys) was normal. Burton literally mapped sexuality onto geography, as did other Orientalists and ethnographers with "normal" heterosexuality and monogamy associated with the Occident, or Northern Europe, and "abnormal" homosexuality and polygyny associated with the Orient.

No claim about the Orient was too fantastic to be believed, particularly in the sexual realm. Frederick Millingen's *Wild Life among the Koords* (1870) told a bizarre story of female bandits who seduce, capture, and strip naked unwary travelers, and who then alternate dancing lasciviously for them and flogging them. This absurd fantasy is repeated, apparently at face value, in Fred Burnaby's *On Horseback through Asia Minor* (1877), next to dry information on public officials and military strategy.[37] The boundary between the ethnographic and the pornographic was razor thin, a tradition that extended into the twentieth century, when *National Geographic* pictorials of indigenous women were the only mainstream publications to show bare breasts.

In the visual arts, an entire genre of paintings was based on this fantasy of the exotic Orient.

> To our great-grandparents these canvases were not only a reminder of a different world, of something picturesque and heroic, but they hinted at pleasures that were often taboo in Europe and titillated a secret taste for cruelty and oppression.[38]

These images, publicly displayed in galleries and exhibitions and seen by men, women, and children, straddled the border between the erotic and the anthropological, claiming verisimilitude yet unmistakably sexual. The exotic locations served to permit nudity.

Men, too, figured in Orientalist fantasy, both as barbaric villains and as victims. Cabanel's *Cleopatra Trying Out Poisons on Her Lovers* (1887) shows the queen looking on with detached interest while men writhe on the floor. Girodet's *Revolt in Cairo* (1810) includes a pale, pink-robed man swooning in the arms of a muscular, sword-wielding Moor, nude but for a turban and a carefully placed leather strap. Lecomte's *The Bearer of Bad Tidings* (1871) shows a prince lounging on a couch, bloody sword near to hand, with three dark-skinned, dead nudes lying beneath him.

One key theme of Orientalism was the harem, representing Muslim polygyny and seclusion. The "truth" of life in a polygynous harem in the Arab world is almost irrelevant to the way the harem, and harem women, figured in Western discourse. For philosophers like Montesquieu, Diderot, and Wollstonecraft, the harem was a microcosm of despotism and patriarchy. Apologists depicted it in Utopian terms, a model of gender relationships in which men did not have to compete for women. Some European women visitors such as Lady Mary Wortley Montagu and Lady Elizabeth Craven saw in the Ottoman Empire's system of public veiling a greater degree of sexual freedom for women, not less.[39]

Unsurprisingly, the harem was a favorite subject for Western visual artists, in painting, illustration, and photography. They deployed a stereotyped set of props, costumes, and locations: water pipes, fans, loose trousers, arm bracelets, terraces, draped fabrics, and nude or nearly nude women. In some illustrated books, there was a sharp contrast between the text, which condemned the harem and slavery, and the accompanying images, which showed women of the harem being coy and flirty.[40] One common trope was the presentation of a new woman to the harem's master, usually with the dramatic flourish of a male attendant removing her

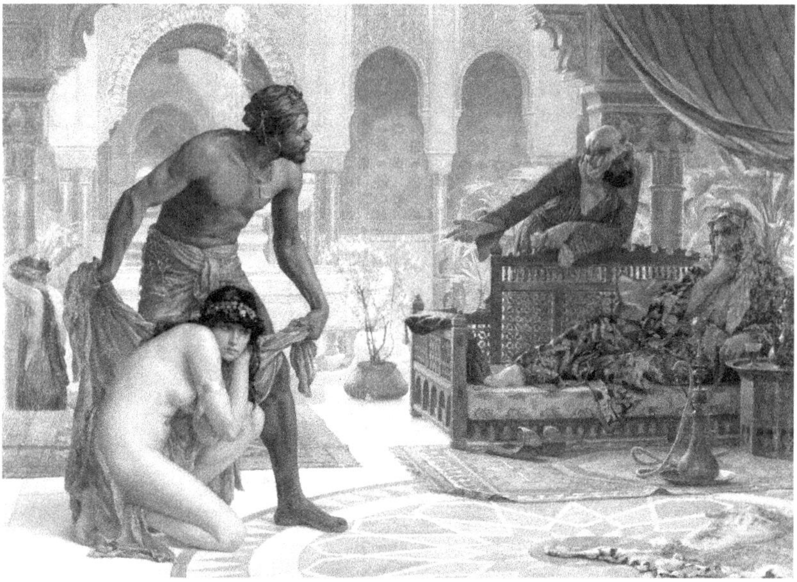

Figure 4.1. *The Bitter Draught of Slavery*, by Ernest Normand, 1885. An example of the trope of the revealing of the white female slave to the masters of the harem. *Courtesy Wikimedia Commons*

robe or veil (see Figure 4.1).[41] The harem and its slave girls served a wide variety of fantasies in the Western observer.

> For a disgruntled middle-class husband the harem could be seen as an escape from the responsibilities of the nuclear family. It provided a tangible locale for his fantasy of sex with multiple partners, women who were all compliant and undemanding. In this regard, the harem could function as the expression of wish-fulfillment. Because profligate sexual activity was considered one of the privileges of the aristocracy, the bourgeois male might use the fantasy of the harem as a vehicle for class envy. Conversely, the harem could become a projection of the fear of the *femme fatale*, who, in the company of her harem inmates, might overpower and devour the lone male. This is also implicit in the comment that the harem greatly contributed to the "impotence" of the Ottoman Empire. . . .[42]

> Abolitionists could project their sympathies for the indignation the slave suffers at the abridgement of her personal freedom. Advocates for the toleration of the harem could see here a stunning record of picturesque ethnography. A middle-class viewer with no political interest could enjoy the exotic subject and its pictorial beauty. For all these viewers Lewis's picture had a lascivious appeal as well. After all, Lewis [in his 1850 *Hhareem* painting] has chosen to depict a narrative about a slave purchased primarily for her sexuality, and she is shown partially unclothed.[43]

Through a curious process of revision, the "slave girl" gradually became white. Harem imagery depicted a hierarchy of racial types by making light-skinned women with Caucasian features the central point of the composition, while dark-skinned women were in subordinate positions, depicted as less desirable. Orientalists populated harems and slave markets with fair-skinned and blue-eyed women from the semi-legendary land of Circassia. Sometimes they were just European, imprisoned due to some mishap. The small minority of women in harems who could be classified as "white" (though probably not abducted from Europe) attracted interest out of all proportion to their actual numbers. Circus sideshows featured "Circassian beauties," said to be rescued from Oriental slavery.

> Circassia, the mythical white utopia, carried some importance for racial theorists. . . . Throughout the nineteenth century, the romance of a perfectly white eastern European people continued to reinforce the supremacy

of whiteness.... The advent of the Crimean War spurred further images of exotic eastern European whiteness and tales of the dark-skinned Turk abducting perfectly white Russian Eves and enslaving them in the pasha's harems. The resulting literature of abduction fed upon the erotic lure of the sexually available white women threatened by dark Turkish male bodies that somehow mirrored domestic American fears of miscegenation.[44]

American showman P. T. Barnum sent his agent John Greenwood to get some of these supposed Circassian beauties from the slave markets in Turkey for exhibition. Barnum later claimed in his biography that Greenwood posed as a Turkish slave trader and saw beautiful Circassian girls and women in the market. Whether this actually happened, Barnum did exhibit an alleged Circassian beauty, "Zalumma Agra," supposedly rescued from the auction block, though actually recruited from Hoboken, New Jersey. "Later, to capitalize further on the erotic lure of the harem slave, the costuming shrank to scanty boudoir displays with short pants and form-fitting bodices. The crowning feature of each Circassian exhibit was the hair, washed in beer, teased out to kink and frizz into what was essentially a large Afro. The ethnic kink supplied a visible bridge between the normalized, exalted whiteness that conferred citizenship and the distinguishing marks of racial difference that facilitated slavery. The emancipated white body still bore the evidence of its dark-bodied captivity."[45]

The white slave girl was a racial hybrid, the best of both worlds, the supposed submission and sensuality of the Oriental woman but with a body that was unmistakably white, in keeping with newly articulated pseudoscientific ideas of race.

GREEK WAR OF INDEPENDENCE AND ITS CONSEQUENCES

These fantasies influenced and were influenced by real-world events. From 1821 to 1832, Greece fought a successful revolution against the Ottoman Empire that had ruled for four centuries. This drew European nations into conflict with the Ottoman Empire and Egypt. Across Europe and America, writers and artists viewed these conflicts on the borders of Europe as the Occident versus the Orient, and described them in sexual terms. White women menaced by dark men with slavery were a popular propaganda theme, in paintings, prose, and sculpture.

Not so coincidentally, the anonymous English erotic novel *The Lustful Turk* was published in 1828. Written in an epistolary format, the novel tells of an Englishwoman, Emily Barlow, abducted and held captive in the harem of the philosophical and massively endowed Dey of Algiers. Her deflowering by the Dey is described in masochistic detail:

> I quickly felt him forcing his way into me, with a fury that caused me to scream with anguish. My petitions, supplications and tears were of no use. I was on the altar, and, butcher-like, he was determined to complete the sacrifice; indeed, my cries seemed only to excite him to the finishing of my ruin, and sucking my lips and breasts with fury, he unrelentingly rooted up all obstacles my virginity offered, tearing and cutting me to pieces, until the complete junction of our bodies announced that the whole of his terrible shaft was buried within me. I could bear the dreadful torment no longer: uttering a piercing cry I sank insensible in the arms of my cruel ravisher. How long I continued in this happy state of insensibility, I know not, but I was brought back to life feeling the same thrilling agony which caused my fainting.

Her ecstatic coupling with the Dey initiates the virginal Emily to sexuality; she is even given a new name, Zulima. The seraglio is also home to three other European women (French, Italian, and Greek), and their and Zulima's intertwined stories serve as vehicles for sex, bondage, flagellation, and sodomy. The relations of nations are mapped onto relations of the sexes as depicted in Classical mythology:

> [O]ne formidable plunge proved too mighty for her forbearance she not only screamed, but struggled. However, I was safely in her. Another thrust finished the job; it was done, and nobly done, by Mahomet! Europa was never half so well unvirgined, although love might have had the strength of a bull.

A subplot involves Emily's friend Sylvia in the clutches of perverted Catholic priests in France, who conspire with the Turks to kidnap European beauties. This combines Orientalist and anti-Catholic Gothic scenarios.[46]

Eventually, a female Greek captive refuses to be sodomized by the Dey, and uses a knife to cut off his penis before killing herself. The Dey survives but finishes the job by having himself castrated. As he no longer has sexual desire, he sends Emily and Sylvia back to England with his organs preserved in wine, thus restoring moral, political, and sexual order after carnivalesque excess.

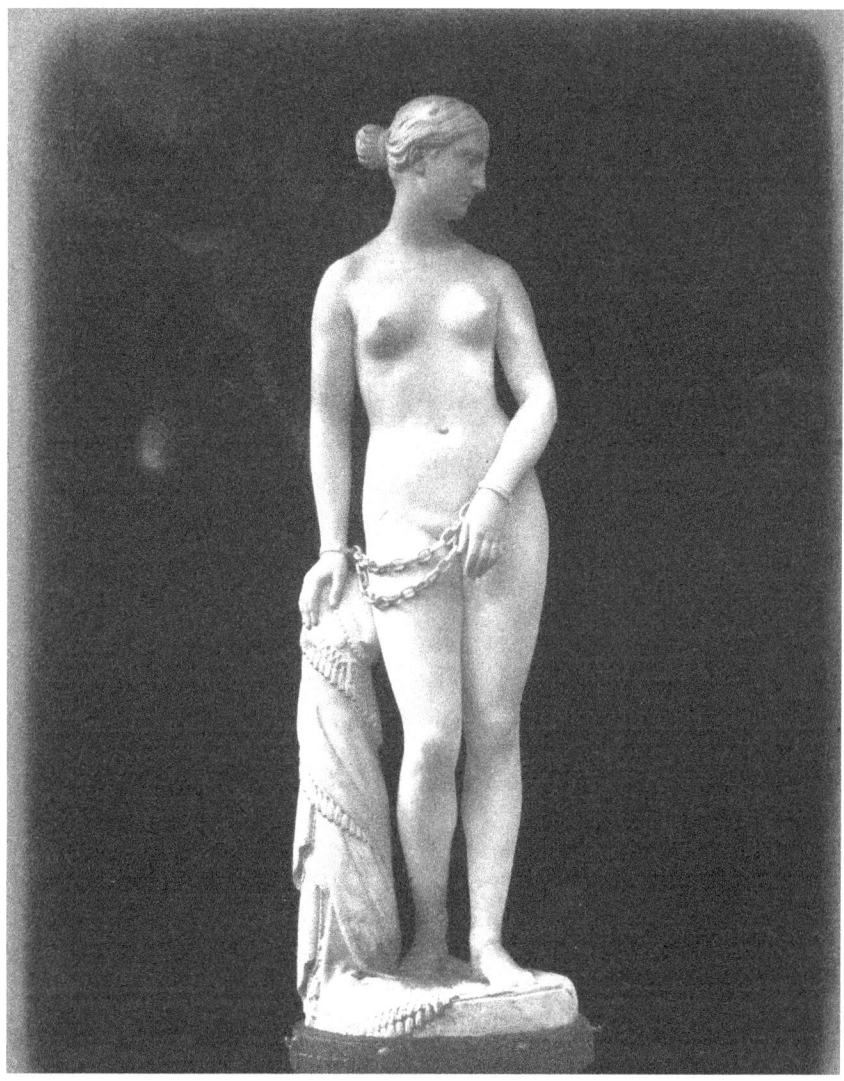

Figure 4.2. Photograph of Hiram Powers's *The Greek Slave*, photographed by Hugh Owen, 1851. *Courtesy Metropolitan Museum of Art*

One of the most popular works of sculpture of the nineteenth century was *The Greek Slave*, circa 1843 by American artist Hiram Powers (see Figure 4.2). It shows a nude woman standing next to a column, her wrists bound and with a small cross dangling from one hand. Where it was displayed to men, women and children (see Figure 4.3), "Powers astutely explained, in the pamphlet that accompanied his statue on its American tour in 1847, that his slave's nudity was not her fault. She had been divested of her clothes by the lustful and impious Turks who put her on the auction block; thus, her unwilling nakedness signified the purest form of the Ideal, the triumph of Christian virtue over sin. This sales pitch, aimed point-blank at Puritan sensibilities, worked so well that American clergymen urged their congregations to go and see *The Greek Slave*."[47] This short narrative sketch of virtue-in-distress excused the statue from any prurient intent. Henry James described seeing duplicates of this statue "so undressed, yet so refined, in sugar-white alabaster, exposed under little glass covers in such American homes as could bring themselves to think such things right."[48]

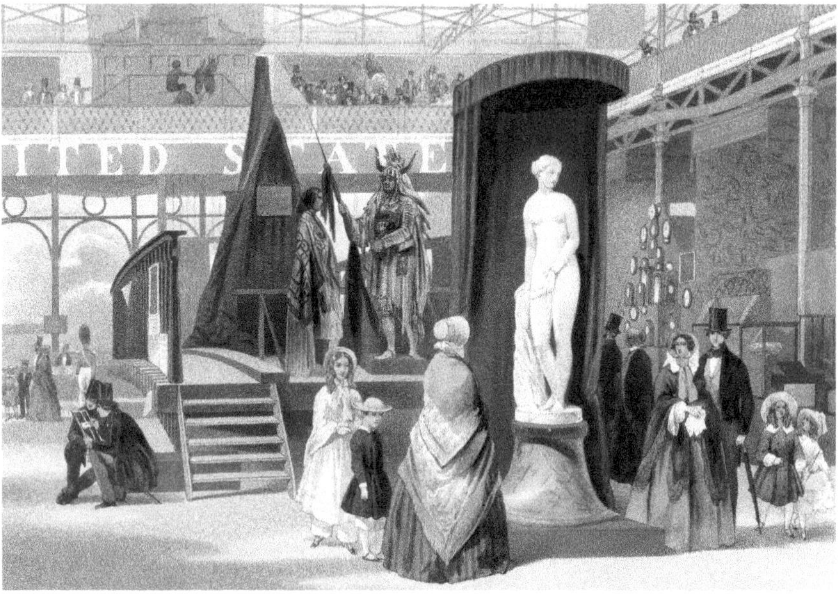

Figure 4.3. View in the East Nave (*The Greek Slave*, by Power [sic]; from *Recollections of the Great Exhibition*), hand-colored lithograph with gum, by John Absolon, 1851. Note that the statue is publicly displayed and viewed by men, women, and children. *Courtesy Metropolitan Museum of Art*

Another American sculptor, Erastus Dow Palmer, created a similar sculpture in 1857, called *The White Captive*. The framing narrative of this piece was of a young woman abducted by Native Americans, another virtue-in-distress scenario set in a different conflict and playing on a different cultural anxiety, distinct to America.[49]

In American captivity narratives, the threatening, hypermasculine Other lay to the west, not the east, where white men and (more often) women were menaced by "savages" with forced marriage, rape, and pagan conversion. Mary Rowlandson's account of her and her children's abduction in the 1670s was a sober, Puritan affair that framed her experience as a test of Christian faith. Other accounts were less restrained, and described how English captives of the Algonquians "were destroyed with exquisite Torments, and most inhumane Barbarities, the Heathen rarely giving Quarter to those they take, but if they were Women, they first forced them to satisfy their filthy Lusts and then murdered them, either cutting off the Head, ripping open the Belly, or Skulping the Head of Skin and Hair, and hanging them up as Trophies, wearing Men's Fingers as Bracelets about their Necks, and Stripes of their Skins which they dresse for Belts."[50]

Later stories in this genre incorporated fictional elements or were outright fiction, such as *The Remarkable Adventures of Jackson Johonnet, of Massachusetts* (1793). Like Orientalist and anti-Catholic captivity narratives, they provided a semi-imaginary zone of difference, where women could step out of the narrow range of behavior allowed in Christian American society. Also like Orientalist and anti-Catholic captivity narratives, this genre easily slipped into exploitation or outright pornography, or could be read as such.

The British humor magazine *Punch* satirized Powers's popular sculpture by printing a cartoon entitled *The Virginian Slave*, which showed a Negro woman in a similar pose. The original statue and its replicas and miniatures were created when slavery was in full bloom in the American South, and people who demonstrated their sensitivity by clucking over *The Greek Slave*'s virtue-in-distress didn't care too much about the actual slaves across the Atlantic. Americans collected money to liberate a handful of white slaves in North Africa while millions of Africans toiled in the cotton fields.

The fantasy of the exotic, erotic Orient has endured so long that it has become something of a cliché. In the early twenty-first century, the image of galley slaves is used as a joke about the nature of work, and the idea of women stolen away to serve in a harem is an erotic fantasy. The Gor series of sword-and-sorcery novels by John Norman, first published in 1966, transplanted the Orientalist tropes to a hidden planet in our own solar system. The books expound endlessly upon the author's philosophy of male dominance and female submission, and the minute details of slave positions and costumes. The highly detailed description of Gor, and especially the customs of slavery, inspired a subset of the BDSM culture, known as Goreans. When virtual online worlds were first built in the 1990s, Gor was one of the first fictional worlds to be simulated.

The very real terror and suffering of the men held captive on the Barbary Coast gradually, in a process of reimagining that took centuries, transformed into the erotic fantasy of silk-clad women lounging around marble pools.

Chapter Five

The Peculiar Institution

At the Master-slave conference, the de facto uniform for men walking around the hotel is blue jeans, black leather shoes or boots, a black shirt or T-shirt (often with organization logos or BDSM in-jokes), and sometimes a leather vest bearing patches and pins. It is derived from biker culture, which had its own roots in military style. Women mostly dress in variations of the same, sometimes with slippers or sneakers, instead of boots.

As I check in at the conference's office, I notice that two of the women working as administrators are dressed identically in ankle-length black cloth dresses over plain white blouses with wrist-length sleeves and Peter Pan collars. The look is more Amish village than BDSM dungeon.

"It's part of our service to Sir," one of them explains. "Modest dress code. It's the thing people have the most problem with, when they're applying to join our household as slaves."

THE COLONIAL SEXUAL ENCOUNTER

Atlantic slavery, the transport of millions of slaves from Africa to the Americas, was a massive social phenomenon that changed the history of four continents. In the eighteenth and nineteenth centuries, it was one of the most hotly debated economic, social, political, racial, and religious issues. Its effects on human culture are still being felt in the twenty-first century.

One of these effects was a constellation of fantasies and images that informed sadomasochistic sexual fantasies on both sides of the Atlantic. Just as Europeans and Americans used the menacing, enigmatic Church and the fantastic, sensual Orient as settings for erotic dramas of pain and confinement, they appropriated the imagery of Atlantic slavery as well.

Those who had no direct experience with slavery formed their ideas about it via secondhand sources, both fiction and nonfiction. Today, we see these atrocities refracted through multiple lenses, filters, and mirrors. For the purposes of this discussion, the reality of slavery is less important than what far-removed people thought about slavery.

The governing fiction among slaveholders was benevolent paternalism. White men of superior restraint and discernment were supposed to have no interest in gratifying their desires with their charges. Corporal punishment was inflicted out of necessity, not sadism.

Actually, sexual access to slaves was an unspoken taboo and an open secret. Slave girls or women might be advertised as "fancy," that is, attractive enough to be a white man's mistress, and buyers examined them in curtained inspection rooms around the slave pens, before the women were sold at up to four times what a domestic or field hand would fetch. However, their sales would be registered as "cooks" or "domestics" or "seamstresses." Sexual relations between masters and slaves, when it was spoken of at all, was mentioned in careful equivocation: the child who was "generally supposed" to be a sister instead of a daughter, the doctor visiting the house of a slave woman who "appeared to be" his friend. Only a minority of eccentrics flaunted their relationships with their slave concubines, such as the editor of the New Orleans *Picayune* who entertained guests at a house with his "Quadroon mistress" and their child, or the slave dealer Theophilus Freeman, who received visitors while in bed with Sarah Connor, the woman he had once owned.[1]

Only a few works of art provide a glimpse into the pro-slavery imagination. In Thomas Stothard's engraving *The Voyage of the Sable Venus, from Angola to the West Indies* (1793), the horrors of the Middle Passage were transformed into a Baroque fantasy of a nearly nude, shapely African woman in a collar and wrist and ankle cuffs, rising out of the water on an oyster shell surrounded by cherubs, Poseidon, and other classical European figures (see Figure 5.1).[2] Whereas other African women were depicted as bestial and grotesque, living throwbacks (such as Saartjie "Sarah" Baartman, the so-called "Hottentot Venus," displayed as a freak in Britain and France, 1810–1815), *The Sable Venus* depicted an African

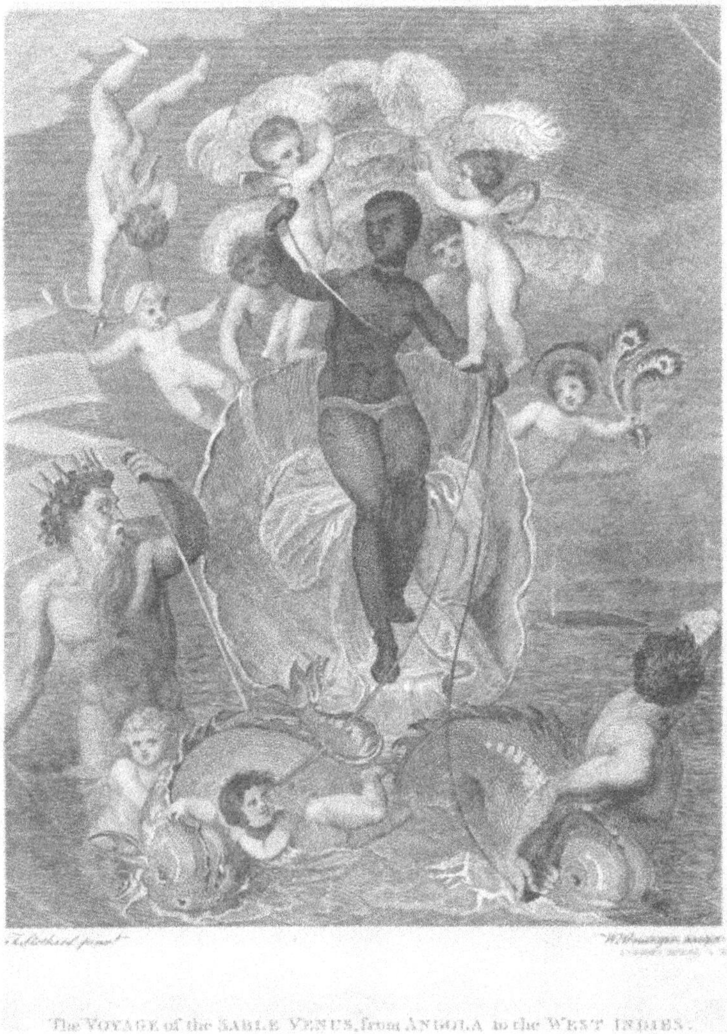

Figure 5.1. *The Voyage of the Sable Venus, from Angola to the West Indies.* By Thomas Stothard, 1793. *Courtesy New York Public Library digital collections*

woman as sexually appealing and, more importantly, available, even eager.[3]

Virginian Luxuries, an anonymous and undated (c. 1815) painting hidden on the back of a formal portrait,[4] is what lay beneath the official accounts of slavery, both abolitionist and pro-slavery: the sexual use of black bodies, and not just in the conventional definition of "sex."

The painting shows a white man and a black woman, presumably a slave, embracing in a static pose—depicting the sexual availability of slave women—on the left side. The figures in the right portion of the painting have strong sexual signifiers, stronger than in the sexual portion. There, a black man being beaten is bare to his waist, his hands hidden in front of his body and possibly tied there. Unlike the formal coat and trousers of the other white man, the white man doing the beating is in loose trousers and only a shirt, with the neck open and the sleeves rolled up to reveal bare arms. His pose is dynamic, legs spread and right arm in full back swing. A curious detail is that in both pairings, the figures are in eye contact. The sexual use of female slaves and the beating of male slaves are equated as luxuries. A luxury is not only pleasurable in itself, but an expression of social privilege, often presented conspicuously.

Other depictions of slaves equated them with cherished pets. Benedetto Gennari's painting *Portrait of Hortense Mancini, Duchess of Mazarin* (1683) depicted Mancini as a spear-wielding, bare-breasted Diana surrounded by African boys and dogs, both wearing identical collars. Black boys as attendants were common features in Restoration portraits.[5] At a time when newspapers advertised "silver padlocks for blacks or dogs," William III kept a favorite black slave who wore a "carved white marble collar, with a padlock, in every respect like a dog's collar." African domestic servants, in contrast to field workers, wore ornamental collars in precious metals, stamped with the owner's name, initials, and coat of arms.[6] The sentimentalized pet-owner relationship displaced the violence of slavery and allowed an emotional attachment to a black slave that would have been impossible in terms of a parent-child relationship.[7]

Perhaps ironically, it was the antislavery abolitionists who made the greatest contributions to eroticization of slavery. Pro-slavery discourse hid violence and sexuality; abolitionist discourse brought them to the forefront. The abolitionist movement coincided with three other popular cultural movements in Western civilization: evangelicalism, the emergence of pornography as a distinct type of media, and the cult of sensibility that gave rise to the Gothic.[8]

Sensibility theory argued that people were the product of their environments, and that slaves did not act like free people because of their environment of abuse. Thus, it had to be demonstrated that slaves suffered physically under the yoke and the lash, much as free people would in the same circumstances, and consequently, slaves could not form the emotional connections that were the basis of the monogamous, child-centered, nuclear family that was thought to be the foundation of a good society.

The slave signified the lowest of the low, the most abject of humans. A man projected himself into that role in order to experience misery and exercise his sympathy to the fullest. The playwright and novelist Richard Cumberland wrote, in the introduction to his novel *Henry* (1795):

> [T]he poor African is . . . fair game for every minstrel that has tuned his lyre to the sweet chords of pity and condolence; whether he *builds immortal verse* upon his loss of liberty, or weaves his melancholy fate into the pathos of a novel, in either case he finds a mine of sentiment, digs up enthusiasm from its richest vein, and gratifies at once his spleen and his ambition.

However, abolitionist propaganda also had an inevitable tendency to slide into sexual fantasy, notably in the standard image of slaves being beaten.

A 1792 Isaac Cruikshank etching, *The Abolition of the Slave Trade*, was based on a case brought before the House of Commons and depicted a nearly nude black woman hanging from one ankle, while bestial British sailors prepare to beat her.[9]

A 1792 etching by Richard Newton, *Forcible Appeal for the Abolition of the Slave Trade*, showed another whipping scene, this time in a tropical setting. The left half of the print shows the beating factually, but the right half depicts a black man beating a topless black woman, while a richly dressed white woman observes, smiling.[10]

William Blake, a poet and artist and a strong opponent of slavery, made several engravings for the abolitionist cause that were highly ambiguous in the way they viewed black slaves. His "Flagellation of a Female Samboe Girl" (1796)[11] depicted a shapely, nearly nude, black woman hanging from a tree and being beaten, her limbs in the middle of violent movement, bloody wounds clearly visible, her face captured in a moment of wide-eyed agony. His "Execution of Breaking on the Rack" (1793) showed a male African named Neptune lying bound on a cross, his severed left arm already oozing white bone marrow. Abolitionist imagery borrows extensively from the Christian martyrological tradition, discussed in previous chapters.

The American poet Walt Whitman wrote a similar exercise in his collection *Leaves of Grass* (1855), in which he subjectively explored various forms of suffering, particularly those of slaves:

> The disdain and calmness of martyrs,
> The mother of old, condemn'd for a witch, burnt with dry wood, her
>   children gazing on,
> The hounded slave that flags in the race, leans by the fence, blowing,
>   cover'd with sweat,
> The twinges that sting like needles his legs and neck, the murderous
>   buckshot and the bullets,
> All these I feel or am.
> I am the hounded slave, I wince at the bite of the dogs,
> Hell and despair are upon me, crack and again crack the marksmen,
> I clutch the rails of the fence, my gore dribs, thinn'd with the ooze of my
>   skin, I fall on the weeds and stones,
> The riders spur their unwilling horses, haul close,
> Taunt my dizzy ears and beat me violently over the head with whip-stocks.
> Agonies are one of my changes of garments.[12]

To the masochist, those are favored garments.

Abolitionists wanted to induce sympathy in viewers and portray Africans attractively. Whereas pro-slavery art caricatured Africans, male and female, as subhuman and repulsive, abolitionist art tried to humanize the Africans to encourage empathy for the suffering, but somehow things kept slipping over into the erotic. Female Africans were often depicted as lighter or even "white," a limitation of printing technology of the time that couldn't depict subtle variations in skin tone.

Slavery was the topic of the most popular novel of the nineteenth century, second only to the Bible in sales: *Uncle Tom's Cabin* (1852), by Harriet Beecher Stowe. The novel was the common text of archetypes and scenes that came into the minds of millions of people around the world when they thought or talked about slavery, one of the most culturally charged issues of the day.

Stowe said she was inspired after taking communion by a vision of an old slave being beaten to death by two fellow slaves, goaded on by a brutal white man. She understood this image in terms of Christian martyrology, a humble man being tortured despite his innocence.[13] She immediately wrote down the germ of what would become *Uncle Tom's Cabin*.

To condemn slavery, Stowe couldn't use the discourses of law and commerce, which were both in favor of slavery, as was religion. Instead, Stowe used the same language of moral sentiment used in George Lippard's *Quaker City*. She argued that the institution of slavery prevented Africans from forming stable families, which in turn made them morally depraved and miserable. That meant that the reader had to accept the idea that Africans did have feelings, that they did form ties and suffer when they were broken. Pro-slavery writers argued that Africans were incapable of such feelings, being naturally promiscuous and disloyal.

Stowe drew upon three established literary genres in her work: the sentimental novel, the Gothic novel, and the Orientalist story.

Stowe wrote in the sentimental language of feelings and emotions to convey the damaging influence of slavery, and she spent a lot of words on severed family bonds, husbands separated from wives, children from parents.

Furthermore, the institution of slavery had a corrupting influence on whites, allowing concubinage and de facto polygyny. Stowe's Aunt Mary married a merchant in Jamaica, then discovered he had fathered several mulatto children by slave women.[14]

Stowe also used the language of the Gothic novelists in her project: broken family ties, an unjust world, captivity, torture, the constant threat of sexual violation, villains driven by their own irrational obsessions and fears (e.g., Simon Legree is fooled by Cassy's pretend ghost and doesn't notice his missing slaves hiding in his own attic). She hit the balance between thrills and sentiment, hinting just enough at illicit sexual acts, while not showing them directly. "Stowe always distances illicit sex acts by time and space. They occur in a threatened future (Eliza, Emmeline), in the past (Prue), or offstage (Cassy)."[15]

The Orientalist strain of *Uncle Tom* comes from mapping sexuality onto geography. The farther south Stowe's characters go, the worse their lives, and the more deviant the sexuality, culminating in Simon Legree's hellish plantation. Legree is also the closest Stowe ever gets to explaining where all those mixed-race slaves (e.g., George, Eva, Cassy, etc.) came from, and he is described as bestial and tyrannical. (Curiously, Legree is also a Northerner.) English professor Diane Roberts wrote that:

> The slave South is America's domestic Orient, its secret self, its Other, as the African and the female—so involved in representations of the

South—are Other. The feminized, receptive, seductive metaphorical landscape of the South owes much to the seductive, secretive metaphorical landscape of the Orient. . . .

. . . Inventing an Oriental South became a powerful abolitionist tactic, demanding that the American public recognize a despotic kingdom where men have sexual access to women slaves within the borders of their democratic republic, decadent poison weakening the national body.[16]

A critic of Stowe unwittingly made this connection when he wrote that she described houses in New Orleans like "stage sets for Lalla Rookh,"[17] an Oriental romance poem by Thomas Moore, adapted into several operas.[18]

Uncle Tom's Cabin was the seed of a global, mass media phenomenon, far larger than anything Stowe could control, with many different editions, branded merchandise such as card games and mantelpiece screens, and elaborate stage adaptations, some unauthorized. As there was no copyright agreement between the United States and Britain at the time, unauthorized publications outside of Stowe's control were legal. The novel was published in Britain in editions that ranged from a 1s weekly serial to a luxury edition for 7s 6d.

Some of the editions could find or assign meanings to the novel that were far from Stowe's intent. An advertising broadsheet of the 1852 Cassell edition, an etching by George Cruikshank, features a black man and a topless, light-skinned black woman about to be whipped; standard images from abolitionist literature.[19]

In 1852, Stowe was visited by Sam Beeton, a British publisher (see chapter 6), who hoped to acquire the rights to her follow-up book. She was not pleased by Beeton's gift, the electrotype plates from the luxury British edition, one of which depicted a scene of a black man beating a bare-breasted woman in chains, while another man looked on.[20] The author later wrote to Beeton:

> It was my desire in this work as much as possible to avoid resting the question of slavery on the coarser bodily horrors which have constituted the staple of anti-slavery books before now. . . . Hence you will observe that there is not one scene of bodily torture *described* in the book—they are *purposely* omitted. My object was to make more prominent those thousand worse tortures which slavery inflicts on the *soul*. . . . It was therefore directly in opposition to the spirit of my intention to have a whipping scene

on the very cover, and were I at liberty to authorize the work the plates of this kind would be to my mind an objection.[21]

By the 1867 Ward Locke edition, the illustration had slipped even further toward pornography. A full-page wood engraving shows the slave Prue (an ancient alcoholic wretch in the text) as "a very shapely, young and topless woman whipped by a white gentleman in elegant clothing. In the foreground another man gazes on, clutching a pair of scissors in his right hand, with which he has just sliced off Prue's clothing; the remainder of her dress appears about to slide off her hips. A grinning crowd enjoys the spectacle."[22] A nineteenth-century mantelpiece screen depicts a black man whipping a bare-breasted, black woman in chains, her beautiful face turned to the viewer beseechingly.

Note that this is not the fault of Harriet Beecher-Stowe or William Blake or any other abolitionist artists. The fetishistic reading of *Uncle Tom's Cabin* is one of many readings, which are inevitable when a given text becomes highly popular. When that happens, the original text, or even just the superficial symbols, can be used by multiple audiences for different purposes. Stowe's original text had powerful moments depicting the horrors of slave society, yet it also had Victorian sentimental treacle and childish/feminized blacks who are only redeemed by Christianity.

SLAVERY AS PLACE OF SEXUAL ANARCHY

For people outside the American South, slaveholding societies were a fantastic realm of sexual anarchy where anything was possible, whether viewed with delight or horror, just like the views of the Orientalists in the previous chapter.

An earlier antislavery novel, Richard Hildreth's *The Slave, or Memoirs of Archy Moore* (1836), highlighted the sexual impropriety that Stowe only hinted at. Colonel Moore's plantation is stocked with his illegitimate, unacknowledged offspring, born as slaves. He approaches his mulatto daughter Cassy to become his mistress, indifferent to her horror that this would be incest.

In turn, pro-slavery writers accused Northerners of sexual deviance by allowing the races to mingle without slavery as a regulating institution.

Lydia McCord, a Southern essayist and dramatist, wrote an 1853 essay that criticized Stowe as being ignorant of Southern life and "a liar and a purveyor of smut, castigating her severely for depicting scenes 'most revolting at once to decency, truth and probability' as well as 'nauseating,' displaying the sexual use of slave women in the South."[23]

What seemed to horrify McCord and others like her is the intermingling of the races, especially sexually. The irony of course is that slavery, which was supposed to keep the races in their proper places, gave white men unlimited access to black women. This resulted in generations of mixed-race children. The black and white divide struggled to remain viable in the face of reality.

Decades later, in Margaret Mitchell's best-selling novel *Gone with the Wind* (1936), Southern belle Scarlett O'Hara dismissed Stowe's book as mere propaganda and pornography that depicted her home as a land of sex and violence.

The big open secret of antebellum slavery was white male sexual access to slave females. (Actually, the bigger secret was white male sexual access to slave *males*, but that didn't leave visible evidence walking around.) After several generations of this, the color line was anything but black and white, and there was a complex vocabulary to describe the fine gradations between the two: quadroon, octoroon, yellow, high yellow, and so on. The legal status of the child was that of the mother, but one could be born a slave and look very white, just black enough to be "exotic" and an acceptable object for sexual acts beyond the pale for white Southern women. Thus, "white slave girls" weren't an impossibility, even without the "white slave trade" scare.

Add to this the fact that many illustrations of slavery could not show fine gradations of skin tone, so slave women would often be depicted with "white" skin. What keeps coming up in this discourse is the figure of the mulatto or octoroon slave woman, who is described nearly or passably white, who may be depicted as indistinguishable from whites on stage or in illustrations, and who subjectively thinks of herself as white, but is legally black and therefore property and sexually vulnerable.

Clotel; or, the President's Daughter (1853) by former slave William Wells Brown was based on the rumored progeny of Thomas Jefferson and Sally Hemmings. In this case, it was a slave woman named Currer and her daughters, Althesa and Clotel, who could pass for white but were sold as slaves. The novel disrupted the equations of white = free and black = slave. In one passage, a master's wife is jealous of his child by Clotel, Mary, and "broils" her by having her work under the sun without protection, to darken her fair complexion. Another, allegedly true anecdote told of a free German woman who was kidnapped, sold as a slave, "forced to take up with a Negro, and by him had three children," and hired out. Instead of guaranteeing sexual propriety, a slave society fostered sexual anarchy, a "virtue in distress" situation that can easily be reread or misread as erotic:

> [T]hey were taken into the New Orleans slave market, where they were offered to the highest bidder. There they stood, trembling, blushing, and weeping; compelled to listen to the grossest language, and shrinking from the rude hands that examined the graceful proportions of their beautiful frames.

The mulatto slave woman was ideal for a "virtue in distress" scenario, being at the bottom of the social hierarchy but possessed of the alleged sensitivity to suffering of a white woman, a highly liminal figure. She is even more beleaguered than Richardson's Clarissa.

The evolutionary path from abolitionist media to sadomasochistic pornography is long and convoluted. Much of this process occurs after the abolition of slavery in Europe and North America. As slavery receded from living memory in the collective minds of England and Europe and lost moral urgency, it became a fertile source for fantasy, particularly sexual.

While Stowe was deliberately circumspect about sex in *Uncle Tom's Cabin*, which had numerous mixed-race characters yet only vague hints of how they came about, other abolitionists were more frank about sexuality under slavery.

One of the best known nonfiction slave narratives of the period was *Incidents in the Life of a Slave Girl* (1861 in the United States, available in Britain in 1862), written by former slave Harriet Jacobs, under the pen name Linda Brent. Originally published in serial form, it was stopped before completion because of its subject matter. Jacobs wrote with remarkable frankness about living under the constant threat of sexual abuse, and even hinted at white male sexual abuse of black males and white female/black female and white female/black male interactions.[24]

> But I now entered on my fifteenth year—a sad epoch in the life of a slave girl. My master [Dr. Flint] began to whisper foul words in my ear. Young as I was, I could not remain ignorant of their import.[25]

> She [Dr. Flint's wife] now took me to sleep in a room adjoining her own. There I was an object of her especial care, though not to her especial comfort, for she spent many a sleepless night to watch over me. Sometimes I woke up, and found her bending over me. At other times she whispered in my ear, as though it was her husband who was speaking to me, and listened to hear what I would answer.[26]

> [I]t was known in the neighborhood that his daughter had selected one of the meanest slaves on his plantation to be the father of his first grandchild. She did not make her advances to her equals, nor even to her father's more intelligent servants. She selected the most brutalized, over whom her authority could be exercised with less fear of exposure. Her father, half frantic with rage, sought to revenge himself on the offending black man; but his daughter, foreseeing the storm that would arise, had given him free papers, and sent him out of the state.
>   In such cases the infant is smothered, or sent where it is never seen by any who know its history.[27]

> Luke was appointed to wait upon his bed-ridden master, whose despotic habits were greatly increased by exasperation at his own helplessness. He kept a cowhide beside him, and, for the most trivial occurrence, he would order his attendant to bare his back, and kneel beside the couch, while he whipped him till his strength was exhausted. Some days he was not allowed to wear any thing but his shirt, in order to be in readiness to be flogged. A day seldom passed without his receiving more or less blows.[28]

Jacobs's experience was a real-life version of the sufferings of Sade's Justine, and she wrote about it in the familiar language of sensibility. Her story also contributed to the view of slavery as an institution that permitted sexual anarchy, promoted by other abolitionist works.

The British adult magazine *The Cremorne* published *The Secret Life of Linda Brent, a Curious History of Slave Life* (1882) written by George Lazenby. A parody of Jacobs's *Incidents* published twenty years prior, *Linda Brent* used a genre and setting familiar to the English readership as set dressing for the standard tropes of English flagellation erotica. Whereas Jacobs professed her virtue, her pornographic caricature is aggressively voyeuristic and sexual. The descriptions of the darker skin of the slave women adds a frisson of difference to the erotic effect.[29]

Other scenes in the parody directly reference the original text. The illustrations in this and other pornographic books set in the antebellum South whitewash the women.

The next step on the path was to put a white woman in the place of a slave woman, as in *The Memoirs of Dolly Morton* (1899). In the 1890s, Charles Carrington published a number of pornographic works set in the antebellum American South or the West Indies. In his introduction to *Dolly Morton*, it's only a few paragraphs before he gets to the sex:

> In *The Memoirs of Dolly Morton*, the true adventures of the brave women of the "underground railway" are related with a candor and a graphic beauty rarely encountered in any literature.
>
> We see beautiful women stripped bare under a Southern sun; we hear their cries and pleadings for mercy as, one by one, their robes and petticoats are torn off or tucked up, their drawers unfastened and rolled down; our eyes are shocked at the sight of the white, well-developed hemispheres laid bare and blushing to our gaze, only to receive the cruel lash—the hemispheres which had never been bared since mother whipped them across her knees, never been rudely handled save in the legitimate caresses of the conjugal bed. Sorry are we, but little can we do: let he that goeth down to war count well the cost thereof.[30]

Dolly Morton is a white American woman who moves to Virginia to run an underground railroad. The Southerners discover her activities and viciously whip her, comparing her white body and a black woman's body, and their relative ability to withstand pain. One plantation owner, the wealthy libertine Randolph, offers to save her if she becomes his mistress, and she accepts his offer. Morton is unmistakably white, but she is in the same position as Randolph's black women, just another concubine.

> [If] an octoroon woman and a full-blooded black woman, both of the same age and physique, were to undergo exactly the same punishment, the octoroon would suffer far more than the black.[31]

Harkening back to the theory of sensibility of the previous century, Dolly, the white woman, feels her mistreatment more intensely than the black women. As Colligan says, "In effect the novel is a white woman's slave narrative, one that draws on the history of slavery to document a white woman's sexual victimization." Lazenby's *The Secret Life* was published decades after Jacobs's book was in the UK, and after slavery had been abolished in the United States. Slavery could be considered "over there" and "back then," particularly to the British reader. Pornographic novels and photos with American slavery themes were published as early as 1910.[32]

Slavery in the American South, much like slavery in the fantastic Orient, became a space for suppressed imaginings of deviant sexuality. As Toni Morrison put it, "In minstrelsy, a layer of blackness applied to a white face released it from law . . . so American [and other] writers were able to employ an imagined Africanist persona to articulate and imaginatively act out the forbidden in American culture."[33]

Two later novels that became seminal works of sadomasochistic erotica included African women. In Leopold von Sacher-Masoch's *Venus in Furs* (1870), Wanda the mistress acquires a trio of African maidservants who are ranked below her but above Severin, the submissive man. At Wanda's behest, they beat and bind Severin. He is not just a servant of a woman, but the plaything of women who hint at slaves.[34] In Pauline Reage's *Story of O* (1954), a "mulatto servant" woman named Norah mediates between O and her master, Sir Stephen. O identifies with Norah and wishes to have her submission recognized and validated as one of the servants.[35] These black women function as mediating figures between white dominants and submissives, serving the former but dominating the latter, and they take pleasure in doing so. They allude to historical slavery, adding authenticity to the submissive protagonists' experiences.[36]

MAN WITH A MAID

All of these images and ideas from slavery filtered down into the lives of individuals, informing their fantasies and creating a setting for personal dramas of abjection and salvation. The most documented example of a consensual master-slave relationship came from the diaries of Hannah Cullwick, a working-class woman who fetishized labor, and Arthur Munby, a gentleman who fetishized working-class women, from their first meeting in 1854 to their separation in 1877.

Arthur J. Munby was a well-to-do gentleman and a minor man of letters (see Figure 5.2). He had an undemanding job as a functionary in the Ecclesiastical commission, kept company with better-known literary figures, and taught Latin to the underprivileged. In many ways he was a typical man of his time, at least on the surface.

His real passion in life, which he called his "hobby," was working-class women. He strolled the streets of London and other industrial cities, observing and speaking with them, about their working lives, their recreations, and their dialects, and meticulously recorded them in his diaries.

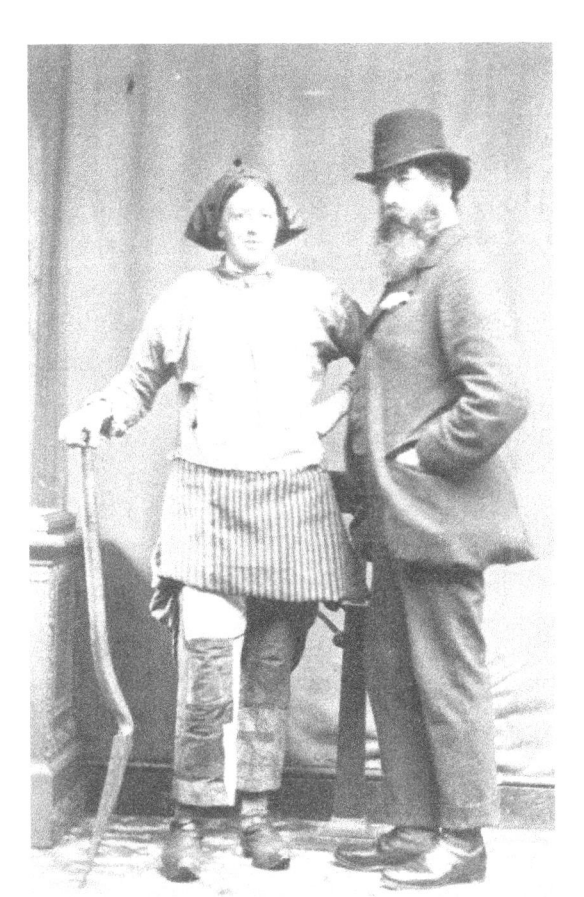

Figure 5.2. Arthur Munby and Ellen Grounds, aged 22, a broo wench at Pearson and Knowles's Pits, Wigan, taken September 11, 1873. *Courtesy Trinity College Library, Cambridge*

He was particularly drawn to women who did the hardest and dirtiest labor: milkmaids, pit brow workers, charwomen, and maids of all work.

Munby collected hundreds of photographs of these women. His amateur drawings of working women are often indistinguishable from caricatures of black men: squat, trouser-clad, powerfully built figures with huge hands and feet, dark skin, and pronounced lips. One of his drawings shows two women facing each other on the street: one was a middle-class woman in an elegant dress, slim, pale, and delicate, while the other was a working woman in trousers and a jacket, huge, dark, and powerful.

In Munby's mind, gender, race, and class were tangled up into one complex puzzle, and he spent his life looking at different combinations and contrasts of those elements. He spoke approvingly of the sweetness and nobility of character of working women, compared to the strength and indelicacy of their bodies. He fetishized dirt as a visible sign of work and what had to be controlled and hidden in the Victorian home, much like sex.

Munby was well aware that many of the lower-class women he studied supplemented their incomes with casual prostitution,[37] and pocket change for a gentleman like him would have easily purchased their services. However, it is unclear whether Munby had any interest in conventional sex. He was uncomfortable with women who were too sexually forward or knowing,[38] and indignantly denied that his hobby was in any way prurient. Once, he arranged for a dustwoman to be photographed at a photographer's shop. On his way out, the doorman offered him a young woman. "The girl looked quiet and modest; & what I was expected to do with her I could not conceive." The offer to "have a picture of her taken *with her clothes up*" prompted Munby to walk off "in disgust." Another fellow said he could supply Munby with "ballet girls or poses plastiques" on an hour's notice. "I thanked him coldly, and so got away at last; wondering why on earth a dustwoman's portrait should have produced these offensive results. There had been no appearance of evil in the matter; the photographer had seemed respectable."[39] The men who pestered Munby probably understood him better than he did himself. Who knows how many other gentlemen they had seen commissioning photographs of their particular interests?

In 1854, on one of his street expeditions, Munby happened across a young servant woman of impressive size and strength who fit his fantasy type perfectly. Shropshire-born Hannah Cullwick was a servant woman

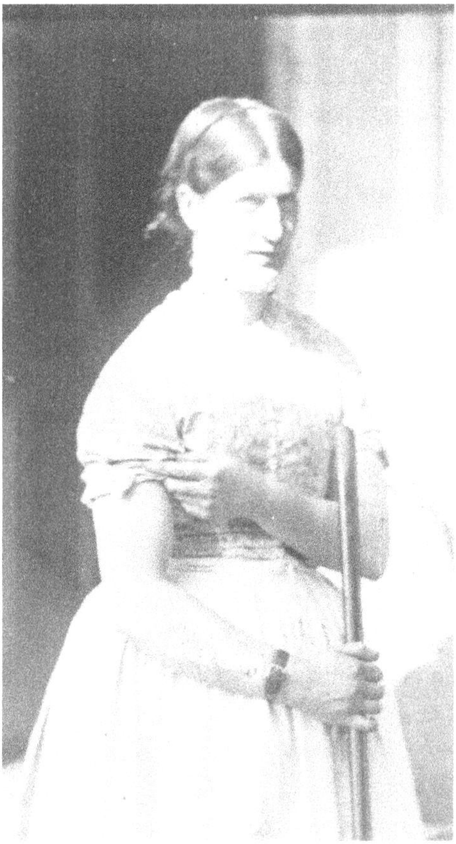

Figure 5.3. Hannah Cullwick, 1867. Note her developed bicep and her leather wrist strap. *Courtesy Trinity College Library, Cambridge*

who actually delighted in her work, as shown by the diaries she wrote for Munby (see Figure 5.3).

She recounted her first meeting with Munby in 1854 in an essay she later wrote for him.

> It was the day after I'd turned 21 & I was took to London again. My brother had been to see me & I walk'd with him part of his way home. I'd my lilac frock, a blue spotted shawl & my black bonnet on, & an apron. When I had kiss'd Dick [her brother] & turn'd again & was crossing for the back street on the way to Grosvenor St, a gentleman spoke to me & I answered him. That was Massa's face as I'd seen it in the fire but I didn't know it again till a good while after. . . . I come back early in '55. I had to leave Woodcote. I started to London & got lodgings, in the *cold*, a tiny room it was, for 5 & 6D

a week. There Massa came to me again, & there was where I first black'd my face with *oil & lead*.[40]

Like Munby, Cullwick's origins were typical. She was one of the millions of rural-born women who traveled to the city to work in domestic service. By 1881, one in nine English females over five years of age was an indoor servant.[41] Servants as a whole were spoken of in terms similar to those used to discuss children and colonial subjects. "The greatest 'kindness' we can exercise towards them is to endeavour, by a mild rein to keep them in the path of duty."[42]

Exploitation of servants, sexual and otherwise, was nothing new, but in the nineteenth century millions of people lived with the institution of domestic service, and experienced all the tensions and conflicts of the massive power differential built into the structure of the bourgeois home. Keeping servants was a defining trait of being middle class, and to be without help was a sign of dire straits. Even tradesmen, such as plumbers or grocers, would employ maids of all work. Particularly at the lower end of the social scale, the division between employer and servant could be razor fine, a boundary that needed to be enforced.[43]

To prevent social confusion between mother/wife and maid, governess or nursemaid, the Victorians created an elaborate system of costumes, gestures, language, and even architecture. Etiquette books taught both masters and servants how to speak, dress, and act. Female servants could no longer be allowed to wear their mistresses' hand-me-downs or second-hand clothing, for fear of confusing the onlooker. They had to wear plain clothing, which eventually developed into uniforms, notably the afternoon outfit of black dress, white apron, and white cap. This later evolved into the iconic French maid fetish costume.[44]

Cullwick's "misalliance" with Munby was so taboo it had to be secret, with their meetings arranged around Cullwick's work schedule. Almost every day, she would write him detailed descriptions of her work routine, emphasizing how hard the work was, how long the days were (sixteen hours or more), and how "black" or "dirty" she became. Most of her diary entries were curt lists of tasks, but some were eroticized, as when Cullwick described chimney sweeping.

> Stripp'd myself quite naked & put a pair of old boots on & tied an old duster over my hair & then I got up into the chimney with a brush. There was a lot

o' soot & it was soft & warm. Before I swept I pull'd the duster over my eyes & mouth, & I sat on the beam that goes across the middle & cross'd my legs along it & I was quite safe & comfortable & out o' sight. I swept lots o' soot down & it come all over me & I sat there for ten minutes or more, & when I'd swept all round & as far as I could reach I come down, & I lay on the hearth in the soot a minute or two thinking, & I wish'd rather that Massa could see me. I black'd my face over & then got the looking glass & look'd at myself & I was certainly a fright & hideous all over, at least I should o' seem'd so to anybody but Massa. I set on & wash'd myself after, & I'd hard work to get the black off & was obliged to leave my shoulders for Massa to finish. I got the tub emptied & to bed before twelve.[45]

Cullwick addressed Munby as "Massa" and referred to herself as his slave. She wore a locked chain collar around her neck, to which Munby had the key, and a leather strap around her right wrist, and refused to take them off, even when one of her employers objected to the visible sign of physical labor when she served at the dinner table.

Cullwick's name for Munby, "Massa," may have come from her Shropshire dialect, but there are strong indications it came from the American South slave dialect. A well-read gentleman like Munby probably would have at least known of *Uncle Tom's Cabin* or read one of the many other slave narratives published in England. It's also likely that Cullwick would have been familiar with the story through one of the cheaper editions or stage performances. The cultural image of Atlantic slavery remained in England via the blackface minstrel shows performed both in theaters and on the street, where Cullwick would likely have seen them. Munby's diaries record several instances of observing performers in blackface,[46] and his drawings of working women often made them look like caricatures of black men. There was a sexual subtext to these stories; after one such performance, one of the minstrels approached Munby and said they would dance "and go through all the scenes of plantation life; but (lowering his voice) we cannot do these things in the street, you know Sir."[47]

While Cullwick was not black, at least in the modern definition of the word, Munby placed her closer to Negro slaves than to himself on the great chain of being, because of the blackness or redness of Cullwick's skin from her work, the size and coarseness of her hands and arms.

Another source of inspiration for the slavery of Hannah Cullwick came from a play. A year before she met Munby, Cullwick went to the theater for the first time in her twenty years and saw a lavish production of Byron's Orientalist tragedy, *Sardanapalus*, about the romance between an artistic, pacifist king and one of his many slaves, Myrrha.[48] It wasn't until years later that Cullwick told Munby about *Sardanapalus*. Munby knew of the play, but didn't realize that he had been cast in Cullwick's fantasy, just as he had cast her in his. These erotic images were seen as a window into an alien world, and thus could have appealed to Munby, who disdained anything that could be described as pornographic.

These sources created a dramatic framework and complementary roles for Munby and Cullwick's forbidden romance.

Cullwick's accounts of her labors read like theatrical performances of roles or rituals.

> Once in the hall I was on my hands & knees cleaning & a gentleman came in. I was in his way but he stepped over & said, "Don't move, Mary [a generic name for female servants]." I said, "Thank you, sir."[49]

> Miss Knight in bed watch'd me [cleaning the grate with her bare hands], & spoke quite pleasantly, & when she saw I wanted more wet said, "Come here, Hannah, I'll wet your hand for you out of my bottle." I had taken care to get my arms black & I rubb'd them across my face, & having my striped apron on & frock pinn'd up, you may guess how I look'd as I crawl'd on my knees to & from the bedside & holding my handup for the water. [Her] been so delicate, as white as a lily & her face too, from been in bed so many years, & I suppose never soil'd her fingers ever, except perhaps with a dirty book or paper, & the white coverlet & all standing out against my dirty black hands, & my *big* red & black arms, & my face red too & sweating till the drops tumbled off, or stood on little drops o' crystal again the greasy black.
>
> I wish'd much that M. could see me for I knew he would o' liked to see me so, & have loved me the more for it. But still I was satisfied that I was doing it for him & I could give him a nice account of it in writing.[50]

Munby enjoyed Cullwick's reports (no doubt she figured out how to appeal to his tastes), but as their relationship matured, he became uncomfortable with how heavily invested Cullwick was in her role, and the physical toll it took on her.

> I looked at the portrait and then at her, and seemed for the first time to see the change years of exposure and menial work have made in her: five

years of scrubbing & cleaning, of sun & wind out of doors and kitchen fires within. And she was pleased with the change—*pleased* that she is now "so much rougher and coarser"—because it pleases me, she thinks. Truly, every smear and stain of coarseness on her poor neglected face comes of love.[51]

For her part, Cullwick saw her visible signs of work as marks of virtue. Perhaps troubled by guilt, Munby tried socially uplifting Cullwick through education, but his halfhearted effort and Cullwick's resistance made it a doomed project. Cullwick herself had no class aspirations, even for moving slightly up the servant hierarchy. She associated her position near the bottom with freedom and autonomy.

> No, I've long resolved in my own mind & felt that, for freedom & true lowliness, there's nothing like being a maid of all work. No one can think you set up or proud in that, & I'd leifer be despised that cause spite or even from my fellow servants. . . . And as I once said to Massa, "I was *born* to *serve*, & *not* to order," and I hope I shall always keep the same humble spirit—that of *liking* to serve others, & obeying instead of commanding.[52]

Cullwick, in many ways, was more autonomous and self-sufficient than Munby. Despite her devotion to Munby, her backbreaking labor, and her signifiers of ownership and lowliness (her slave band, her locking necklace, her dirtiness), Cullwick was reluctant to marry, kept her surname, insisted that Munby pay her wages, lived on her own for much of their association, and threatened to leave him several times. She certainly had far less to lose if their relationship became public. She made a point of saving money, and saw no paradox between her devotion to Munby and her financial independence, "as M. wish'd me to be so low I felt that I would even be a crossing sweeper to please him, so long as I'd saved enough to be independent of service, & by this time I had a nice bit in the savings bank."[53]

Cullwick wasn't above manipulating Munby. She described particularly dirty labor to Munby in sensual detail, compared to the single sentences of other events. She would perform for him, letting him observe her doing the most onerous work on the street. Even her apparently excessive submission to his commands was a way of exerting control, as if daring him to push her harder. In later years, their scenes together would flirt with him as submissive and her dominant. Sometimes, Cullwick was the mother figure who would pick up Munby bodily and carry him around the room,[54] or sit him on her lap and "nurse."[55]

Munby and Cullwick secretly married in January 1873. His journal didn't even mention the small service, and only offhandedly referred to his new wife three days later. Marriage wasn't a prospect either of them relished. Munby knew many women of appropriate social status whom he could have married, and carried on his secret life of studying working-class women, just as many gentlemen married respectably yet patronized prostitutes or kept mistresses.

Cullwick was even more dubious about the prospect of marriage.

> I *like* the life I lead—working here & just going to M. when I can of a Sunday, & a chance time to clean of a weekday when I can get leave now & then, oftener of course if I could—better even I think than a married life. For I never feel as if I *could* make my mind up to that—it's too much like being a *woman*.[56]

Life as Munby's wife/servant was even more isolating and dependent than living with other employers, though he continued to pay her wages.

Munby and Cullwick were both keenly aware of their social roles, and loved to play with them. His photo collection shows Cullwick in different guises: in traditional Shropshire peasant dress, a maid of all work, and a Magdalene. Her working women's hands, and particularly her slave band, were usually visible, regardless of the role. These imperfections in the role were actually part of the appeal, tickling Munby's love of contrast. One picture shows her short-haired and dressed as a man, when they contemplated traveling with her as his valet.

A particularly potent image shows Cullwick in her dirt, dressed as a chimney sweep and covered in black dust, yet with just a hint of her breast visible in silhouette, crouching on the floor, chain and wrist strap on display (see Figure 5.4). Munby's foot is just visible in the frame, "doing my best to look down upon her like a tyrant! That was for 'the contrast': contrast indeed—but which the nobler?"[57] (Curiously, no intact photographs of Munby and Cullwick together seem to have survived, though there are at least three images of them together but with him partially or almost completely cut out.)

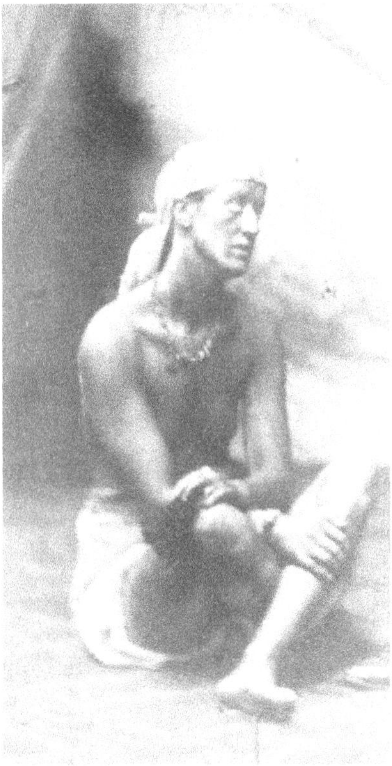

The Peculiar Institution 111

Figure 5.4. Hannah Cullwick posing black and naked to the waist as a chimney sweep (no date). Note her chain collar, her leather wrist strap, and Munby's foot just visible in the lower right corner. *Courtesy Trinity College Library, Cambridge*

Cullwick actively participated in these photo sessions.

She wished to be photographed also in an attitude of her own; and this being granted, she sat down on the floor, with only her shift and serge petticoat on, and thrust out a bare foot, leaning on one knee and clasping her chain with the other hand. She was so anxious about this post, which was very happy, that I enquired its meaning when we were alone. It was "the way I sit on the floor when I'm going to bed, and—think of you!"[58]

When living with Munby, she loved to switch roles, from maid of all work to middle-class lady. On one occasion, an unexpected visitor arrived at their home, and Cullwick quickly changed into her servant clothes to answer the door and serve him. Munby went to see her downstairs.

[She] ran smiling and flung her wet arms around her husband, crying, "Well, Massa, what fun!" "*Fun*!" to see my wife waiting at table like a servant? "Oh nonsense!" said this lively creature, who had seemed so demure in the parlour: "You know it's quite natural to *me*, and I know how to wait: didn't I do it well?" "Yes you did—but I felt as if I must tell you to sit down with us, and say "she is my wife.'" "It's a good job you didn't then," said our Hannah: "the idea! you shanna let everybody know our secrets!"...

At length, after 9 p.m., the goodnatured unobservant Vicar went away; and when he had gone, his hostess and servant came upstairs and resumed her rights.[59]

Cullwick liked to *play* the lady, sometimes for extended periods, but kept it as a role. She preferred her autonomy and independence as a "slave," than the life of real dependence. At this time, middle-class women had little in the way of personal or property rights. Munby's wish that she would spend more time with him as his ladywife created friction.

That's the best o' being drest rough, & looking "*nobody*"—you can go any where & not be wonder'd at. Besides I have got into the way of *forgetting* like, whether I'm drest up as a lady or drest in my apron & cotton frock in the street. It matters not much to me, but certainly I feel more at *ease* in my own dress.[60]

Cullwick's pleasure in her cross-class dressing is a classic form of transvestism, the self-awareness that you are playing a role and fooling the world.

However, Munby and Cullwick's relationship didn't last. Neither of them could really decide whether to be husband and wife or master and servant. In October 1877, she left him for Shropshire. They did remain in contact, and Cullwick would occasionally visit him for cleaning. They still fought over her not getting enough attention from him. They remained in close contact until her death in 1909. Munby died six months later in 1910, after finally telling his brother George about his relationship. He dedicated his last collection of verse to "the gracious and beloved memory of HER whose hand copied out and whose lifelong affection suggested all that is best in this book."[61] Cullwick's gravestone bears the name of "Hannah Munby."

Munby wrote that "we must create our Utopia out of the materials at hand"[62] and he and Cullwick pieced together a private world out of the culture around them—slavery, Orientalism, pastoralism—that met his need for purity and unconditional affection, and her need for belonging and worthwhile work.

Munby and Cullwick came from entirely ordinary backgrounds for their time. They were just more extreme cases of the effects of the social and psychological forces working on everybody in their time and place. In their relationship, the dualities of working class/middle class, male/female, white/non-white, adult/child, dominant/submissive, normal/abnormal body—all of which were in flux in the nineteenth century and had heavily policed, constantly shifting boundaries—were all muddled together, mixed and matched. That freedom to play with taboos, that social risk-taking, is the hallmark of their relationship, and shows that it is the prototype of the culture of kink that would emerge in the next century. This pleasure to turn society upside down, to create a carnival-like setting—even if it is only in one room for one night—is the great pleasure of kink.

Chapter Six

Romance of the Rod

The olive-green school desk and chair combination sits in the middle of the dungeon's playspace, out of place next to the black wood and chromed metal furniture in use by the other players.

The woman stands next to it, wearing the archetypal uniform of white knee socks, red plaid skirt, white blouse, and side ponytails. This costume has become such a ubiquitous fetish icon that it only barely resembles an actual girl's school uniform. It's been a while since anybody has called the woman wearing it a "girl," but she is committed to her role in this drama.

The man has his own costume, a sober gray suit and tie that stand out amid the leather and latex outfits. He unrolls a towel with his collection of implements: a bundle of birch twigs tied together at one end as a handle, known as a "rod"; a broad leather strap with a handle, known as a "tawse"; and a crook-handled rattan cane, as thick as the woman's smallest finger.

The man flexes the cane before the girl, and begins his authoritarian lecture to her as a prelude to the flagellation, speaking with an affected upper-class British accent. This particular subset of sadomasochism has its own aesthetic requirements. Both the man and the woman know them well, even though they were both raised in homes and schools without corporal punishment.

VICTORIANISM

Only a few years after Queen Victoria herself passed away in 1901, the word "Victorian" became a mild insult. H. G. Wells's novel *Ann Veronica* (1909) used the word twice to connote prudishness, hypocrisy, and moralism. In 1914, the *Atlantic Monthly* referred to the "Victorian Hypocrisy" of prudishness in familiar terms.[1] The twentieth century defined itself in opposition to the repressive Victorian era.

However, were the Victorians really that Victorian? The old chestnut about the Victorians keeping the piano legs covered may have actually originated as a joke by Captain Marrayat, an English naval officer and novelist who wrote about a prudish headmistress of a ladies' seminary in Massachusetts.[2] The true nature of nineteenth-century sexuality is heavily contested by historians. While people were still having sex of various kinds in the Victorian age, it was *talked about* more than ever before. Thankfully, for historians, people of the nineteenth century sent letters, wrote memoirs, and kept diaries, not to mention collecting photographs and paintings, leaving a wealth of information on their personal lives.

The most sweeping change in life at this time was the shift from rural, agricultural society to urban, industrial society. On the personal level, industrial life separated home and factory, family and work in time and space. The time between work and family, what the French called *cinque à sept*, or "five to seven," was when people could pursue their own pleasures and cultivate their own identities. There was a space that went with this time, of clubs and dance halls and pleasure gardens. In the industrial city it was possible to be "lonely in a crowd," to live life surrounded by strangers, but also to form social bonds based on affinities, rather than kinship and geography.

The lives of women were transformed even more than those of men. A small but growing number of women began to work outside the home, and enjoyed opportunities that had once been the domain of men.

Mass literacy meant that everyone could have a developed, documented interior life and autobiography like Jean-Jacques Rousseau, in which even embarrassing fantasies and desires, like his desire to be spanked, could be admitted. Some expressed those ideas only on the page. Others took advantage of the anonymity and privacy of the new urban landscape to act them out.

ENGLISH VICE

The Master-slave relationship of Arthur Munby and Hannah Cullwick didn't include what was known in some circles as *"le vice Anglaise,"* flagellation. There is no record of any corporal punishment between them, even though it would have been in keeping for their roles for a master to beat a slave. Even when they flirted with ageplay, spanking would not have been out of place.

This is surprising, considering the prevalence of corporal punishment in Victorian society, including the home, the military, the judicial system, the schools, and particularly in prostitution and pornography. It was commonly believed that flagellation, both giving and receiving, was a primarily Anglo-Saxon interest, hence "the English vice." This is probably an exaggeration. After all, France produced Rousseau and Sade, and Austria produced Sacher-Masoch. Nonetheless, flagellation was a deeply embedded thread in English culture.

Whether or not erotic flagellation was more common in England than elsewhere, legal proceedings and other records indicate there were plenty of sex workers ready to satisfy the need. The famed madame Theresa Berkley died in 1836, but the trade in flagellant prostitution expanded and reached the highest levels of society in the nineteenth century.

Prime Minister Gladstone himself visited prostitutes for, as he put it in his diaries, "strange and humbling pursuits," and he would subsequently flagellate himself on returning home, even making a special notation in his journal to mark the event.[3]

The best-documented example of a professional flagellant woman in this era is Mrs. Sarah Potter,[4] alias Stewart, Steward, Stuart, et cetera. She was mentioned in the writings of Ashbee, Hankey, and their set, and in several court cases in the press.

Mrs. Potter provided young women to be flogged by her clients, men known by names like "Sealskin" or simply "the Count." Some of her girls also flogged men. In her establishment, located near Tottenham Court road,[5] one room was referred to as "the schoolroom," and her establishment provided birch rods, bunches of dried furze (a type of shrub), and a folding ladder, possibly similar to Theresa Berkley's celebrated "horse."

In 1863, Potter was charged with assaulting a young girl, but those charges were dropped (supposedly to speed up the trial "for the ends of public morality"[6]) and instead she was charged with procuring indecent prints and photographs with intent to publish them, suggesting that pornography was a sideline for her.

The writer Swinburne and his compatriots patronized an establishment in St John's Wood, "where two golden-haired and rouge-cheeked ladies received, in luxuriously furnished rooms, gentlemen whom they consented to chastise for large sums. . . . There was an elder lady, very respectable, who welcomed the guests and took the money."[7]

In 1904, another, possibly related establishment in St. John's Wood came to the attention of the authorities.[8] Sophia Mable Pearse "aged 45, of independent means" was charged with using her well-equipped premises for "improper purposes."

> It consisted of twelve rooms, seven of which are furnished as bed-rooms. They found in a studio on the ground floor—which was arranged as a bed-sitting room—a lady and gentleman in evening dress, who gave their names and addresses. Having explained how they came to be there, the gentleman said that if anything came of this he would get into frightful trouble. From there they went to a bedroom on the first floor, which was occupied by a lady and gentleman, who gave their names and addresses. The gentleman said the meeting took place by arrangement through the post. He had been there before. The inspector then described what he found in the house. In the centre of the studio was a large arm-chair, with brass rings fixed to the top of the frame. In a wardrobe he found two birches and several wrist and ankle straps, which could be fixed to the chair; in a room on the second floor another birch; and in a box in a lumber-room who other birches or flagellettes.[9]

Rotten Row, in London's Hyde Park, was where the upper crust of prostitutes met their male clients, on horseback or in carriages. Equestrianism was one of the few venues in which respectable Victorian women could escape the strictures of their gender, physically commanding a larger beast and looking stylish at the same time. Many of the classic fetish accessories are associated with riding: crops, whips, boots, spurs, tight trousers on women. Some of these "pretty horse breakers" were women hired by stables to show off their livestock and carriages.

With fetishistic delight, George Augustus Sala wrote,

> Can any scene in the world equal Rotten Row at four in the afternoon and in the full tide of the season? Watch the sylphides as they fly or float past in their ravishing riding habits and intoxicatingly delightful hats. . . . And as the joyous cavalcade streams past . . . from time to time the naughty wind will flutter the skirt of a habit, and display a tiny, coquettish brilliant little

boot, with a military heel, and tightly strapped over it the Amazonian riding trousers.[10]

One of the most famous of the pretty horse breakers, Catherine "Skittles" Walters, had a career that would make her a friend of the royal family and two prime ministers.

Walters was celebrated for her beauty, her tiny waist (reportedly as small as a skittle, or bowling pin), and her skill as an equestrienne. She would appear on Rotten Row in riding habits so tight it was said she had to be sewn into them. Even though respectable women weren't even supposed to know that women like Walters existed, she was much discussed in the papers and a fashion trendsetter. Her fame could eclipse that of her patrons. Men paid her just to say she was their lover, to enhance their own profiles.

Walters mastered the courtesan's art of acquiring large sums of money from men without antagonizing them, but also without compromising her autonomy. (Catherine Walters and Hannah Cullwick were polar opposites in many ways, but they both knew that a woman's personal and sexual freedom required financial autonomy.) A courtesan usually had a primary "protector," but she would dally with other men, and everybody involved knew that another protector stood ready if the old one became tiresome. The ultimate goal was an annuity of hundreds of pounds per year, giving these women financial freedom and the extravagant lifestyle they enjoyed.

In stark contrast to the Victorian female ideal, courtesans were expected to be sexual, worldly, opinionated, and independent. Catering to their patrons' sexual tastes, sometimes unconventional ones, was part of the courtesan's art as well; in that age, an unconventional sexual taste could be a woman who spoke her mind and acted on her desires. Courtesans ranged from the bawdy to the domineering in the tall tales that circulated about them.

Society, in both the general and specific senses, could only tolerate courtesans to a certain point. A portrait of Walters was named picture of the year in 1861, which prompted a satirical letter in the *Daily Telegraph* that depicted courtesans as a threat to the institution of marriage and poetically compared them to the mythical Circe, who transformed men into animals.[11]

Emile Zola's popular novel *Nana* (1880) was a fictional treatment of the same theme. The title character, based on real-life courtesan Blanche d'Antigny,[12] was a terrible singer and actress, but wealthy men obsessed over her to the point of financial ruin or suicide. Count Muffat, one of her patrons/victims, yearned for Nana in classic masochist fashion:

> His was the pain of an old wound rather than the blind, present desire which puts up with everything for the sake of immediate possession. He felt a jealous passion for the woman and was haunted by longings for her and her alone, her hair, her mouth, her body. When he remembered the sound of her voice a shiver ran through him; he longed for her as a miser might have done, with refinements of desire beggaring description.[13]

The *femme fatale* novel was raised to a high art by Rachilde, the only female Decadent writer. Her novel *La Marquise de Sade* (1887) starred Mary Barbe, the daughter of a cavalry officer, who waged a one-woman war on corrupt, enervated society. She married a rich old man for money and flagrantly cuckolded him with his illegitimate son, who adored her slavishly.

> [Paul] would fall ecstatically at her feet as she stood dressed in satin or velvet, not venturing to touch her, insisting that his worthlessness was a torture. She would laugh.
> Once, while he was worshiping her in this way, with his brow bowed over her feet, which were shod in silver brocade—for she was becoming queenlike in her sumptuousness—he fell prey to a nosebleed. The glittering feet, the idol's feet, were covered in crimson. Ashamed, he asked her pardon, putting tinder to his nostrils and trying to wipe the pretty shoes.
> "It is nothing," she hastened to say coyly, "no, indeed, leave it as it is, it amuses me to walk in this red stream!"[14]

On the Continent, the regulated French brothels, or *maisons de tolérance*, were lavishly decorated and equipped for every desire and fantasy: flagellation and bondage, of course, but also voyeurism by means of binoculars built into walls, needles, nettles, devices for electrical shocks, dildos, harnesses, and more. Costumes transformed prostitutes into brides, nuns, or bluestockings, sometimes with matching décor. Women would service other women, and men other men, with the establishment even providing a "beard" on request. Brothels were also a channel for the distribution and viewing of pornographic writings, images, and photographs.[15] Similar systems operated in Germany and Italy.

The diversification of sexual services and goods, driven by capitalism, trickled down from the aristocracy to the bourgeoisie and the other classes. The French government's project to contain and control sex that was excessive, unnatural, or illegal actually made it spread out and become even more visible. "Far from being the sexual outlet envisioned by . . . the regulationists, the brothel became a laboratory in which new sexual requirements were worked out."[16]

In the new sexual culture, the corset was one of the artifacts invested with great symbolic and fetishistic significance, even outside the subculture of tightlacing. Most women of the time wore corsets that were merely snug and supportive, in white, black, or another plain color, as a part of their daily attire. Colored corsets, such as the blue one worn over a chemise in Manet's famous and influential painting *Nana* (1877), were the mark of the courtesan or the actress (an only slightly less scandalous profession). They were meant to be seen, as suggested by the man in the top hat peering in from the right side of the frame. They represented the boundary between clothed and unclothed, and echoed the ambiguous social spaces of the brothel and the house of the mistress.

Henri Gervex's painting *Rolla* (1878) was withdrawn from the Salon, not because it portrayed a reclining nude woman, but because of the red corset lying on a chair in the corner of the frame. A nude had always been nude. An unclothed woman with a discarded corset and other modern underwear nearby had been dressed and therefore must have undressed, in preparation for sex.[17]

This was the development of lingerie, clothing for the occasion of sex, as compared to mere underwear. By the 1890s, colored satin corsets were fashionable even for respectable women, who could present a hint of the glamour and adventure of the courtesan to herself and her lover.[18] A French postcard from 1895, *The New Temptation of Saint Anthony*, jested about how much sexual tastes had changed. The saint is indifferent to a beautiful naked woman, but once she dons her lacy chemise, corset, stockings, and shoes, he is delighted to gaze upon her.[19]

A certain amount of mythology has developed concerning corsets, claiming that all Victorian women strived for hand-span waists, to the point of surgery to remove ribs. The evidence suggests that tightlacing did occur, but it was practiced either as a short-term measure by women on particular fashionable occasions, or as long-term figure training by a fringe minority whose interests had more to do with fetishism than fashion.[20] While most of the references to extreme corset training smack of fantasy, there are tantalizing hints of a fetishistic subculture in a letter postmarked in 1892, written by a woman who would have been about seventeen at the time.

> [H]e happened to feel my waist, and said how small it was! Why didn't I show it more. Then I explained to him that Miss—[her governess] wouldn't let me do so until I came out with a really small waist. I then found that he was really interested and like a very small tightly laced waist. He told me his mother had a beautiful figure and was beginning to do something about his two younger sisters who are 15 and 16 1/2 but that they objected very much to being laced at all tightly.[21]

This particular letter is significant because, unlike most fetishist correspondence, it is a communication directed to one person instead of an audience, and it is referring to a current event, rather than something remembered from years ago. This diminishes the possibility of performing for an audience or time embellishing memory with fantasy.

Generations after the corset stopped being an item of daily attire, in favor of slimmer silhouettes, it developed a strong following as a fetish item. What was hidden by and from the Victorians became highly visible, and embraced by both fashion designers and fetishists.

Those who attributed the taste for flagellation to childhood experiences often cited the culture of corporal punishment in English education. The pinnacle of the English public school system was Eton College, the training ground for the British Empire's elite, and the prototype for other public schools. The memoirs of the school's graduates and various government reports make it clear that beating students was "regarded quite as a natural incident of the day."[22]

A punishment birching, also called an "execution," was a ceremonial, ritualized affair, involving not only the teacher and the student, but effectively the entire school. A boy could end up "on the bill" for any of a number of offenses, many of them trivial, including idleness. Waiting for the appointed time was part of the procedure. In addition to the master and the culprit, who would kneel to be punished on "the block" with his trousers down, there were two "holders down," who lifted up his shirttails out of the way. Furthermore, the executions in the Lower School, attended by students under eleven, were always public, so dozens of boys would witness the event. In the Upper School, attended by boys from twelve to as old as twenty, beatings were usually private. Sometimes up to a hundred boys would witness a culprit being "swished." The Eton rod itself was fifty-four inches long, three feet of handle and two of birch twigs, and weighed twelve ounces, more than enough to draw blood. The ideal among the boys was to take it quietly and manfully, with the proverbial "stiff upper lip," and laugh it off later. Actually, many cried or screamed, and were mercilessly "chaffed" afterward. One witness likened the event to a hanging.

These beatings occurred in an intensely hierarchical environment, in which tutors delegated authority, including the right to flog, to certain senior boys. This feudal principle extended to the fagging system, in which younger boys were effectively the servants of older boys, which of course created a setting ripe for bullying, but also for homoerotic relationships. This kind of system was common in other public schools and imitated in other types of schools, including the preparatory schools that readied younger boys for the public schools. (At the same time, school beatings were strictly forbidden in France.[23])

Student beatings were justified on the grounds that a school stood *in loco parentis* to its pupils, and corporal punishment is a necessary part of parenting. The majority view held that children had to be trained to recognize the importance of duty and obedience, two key Victorian values, and the rod was a necessary implement to get through to the little beasts. God had the right to punish man, and therefore man had the right to punish children. The biblical law of Solomon was frequently invoked in public debates over corporal punishment, while George Bernard Shaw and other "antibirchites" took a less literal reading, arguing that the flogging of children belonged in the same category as the stoning of adulteresses.[24]

Was corporal punishment sexual or wasn't it? Though it was known to medical authorities that flagellation could produce erections in boys, children were thought to be completely asexual beings. Likewise, it was inconceivable that the Anglican clerics who ran these schools would have anything other than their duties as teachers in mind when they administered the rod.

Several generations of young elite Englishmen went through this kind of institution, and even though Eton and schools like it represented an extreme, many of those boys had formative sexual experiences in situations of hierarchy, punishment, and public exposure. Many Englishmen, notably George Orwell and Sir Winston Churchill, later wrote scathingly of their public school disciplinary experiences, and there was at least one documented suicide at a public school.[25] In the spy novels of Ian Fleming, another Eton "old boy," James Bond is frequently brought to the den of an older, authoritative villain, lectured, and then tortured in graphic detail.

ROMANCE OF THE ROD

The nineteenth century was the first era of mass literacy. Charitable ventures taught the lower classes, so that even a maid of all work like Hannah Cullwick had basic literacy and the ability to express herself through her letters and diaries.

Photography, cheap printing, and newspapers and magazines meant that ideas, stories, and images could be distributed faster than ever before, across national borders and the boundaries of class and gender. Naturally, sexual writings were part of this great flourishing of words, arousing the establishment's perennial fear of the unruly desires of the lower classes and women.

Despite the Obscene Publications Act and other regulations, semi-underground publishers printed thousands of sexually explicit books, many of them flagellant or fetishistic. There were erotic books focused on flagellation, but most erotic works of the period included at least one scene of corporal punishment.[26] They had titles like *Mysteries of Flagellation* (1863), *Sublime of Flagellation* (1872), and *Curiosities of Flagellation* (1875). There were also monthly underground magazines such as *The Pearl*, *The Oyster*, and *The Cremorne*. Some parodied the works of Charles Dickens, William Thackeray, Sir Arthur Conan Doyle, and other popular writers of the time.

Miss Coote's Confession, an anonymous novel serialized in *The Pearl* between 1879 and 1880, reflected the cultural anxieties about women's changing gender roles of the late nineteenth century.

> "Miss Coote's Confession" is of particular historical interest because, in showcasing an independent spinster sexually aroused by whipping women, it anticipates the figure of the lesbian as New Woman and mannish an-

drogyne in fin-de-siècle and early twentieth-century. . . . Thus, although Victorian pornography, unlike domestic ideology, asserts that women are sexual beings, pornographic plots like that of "Miss Coote's Confession" circumscribe the autonomy of the sexual woman.[27]

An epistolary novel presented as letters from Miss Rosa Belinda Coote to another woman, the text draws on the established genre of female-written letters such as *Clarissa* and *Fanny Hill*, as well as the earlier pornographic genre of the "whore dialogue," of two women talking about sex to each other. It also functions as a satire of the female *bildungsroman*. It starts off in the Gothic mode, as the young, orphaned Miss Coote arrives at the estate of her grandfather, Sir Eyre Coote, who threatens to beat her if she plucks fruit from his garden. Miss Coote of course breaks this biblical injunction, and becomes a subject of Sir Eyre's flagellant regime, much like his servants.

The "Coote" surname links the protagonist and her grandfather to Sir Eyer Coote, British commander-in-chief in India in the previous century, as well as the notorious Governor Edward Coote of Jamaica, who ordered the slaughter of hundreds of blacks after a native insurrection in 1865, not to mention ordering women involved in the revolt to be stripped and flogged.[28] Miss Coote's initiation into the flagellation of servants, during which she experiences her first orgasm, symbolizes her initiation into the class hierarchy and the colonial system, as her grandfather's sole heir.

Miss Coote embodies the paradox of flagellation, intended to control women's bodies and therefore their sexuality, but actually exciting it and allowing for its expression. Likewise, she subverts the Victorian bourgeois ideology of woman as asexual moral authority in the domestic sphere, while also waxing nostalgic for the feudal past of aristocratic authority and its apparatus (whips, manacles, and so on). She rejects heterosexuality and marriage, adopting the public persona of a "highly respectable old maid," and takes up the sexual style associated with aristocratic decadence at the time: homosexuality.[29] On Sir Eyre's death, Miss Coote's lesbianism (though the term had not yet been clinically defined) is fostered in a girl's school run by "Miss Flaybum," and particularly by her French governess Mademoiselle Fosse; this reflects vaguely articulated anxieties about female relationships and the suitability of certain women for heterosexuality and family life. After graduation and gaining her social and economic independence (echoing fears of the New Woman), she forms a quasi-marriage with her French teacher, though she says "I mean to marry the birch (in fact I am already wedded to it) and retain my fortune as my independence."[30]

It is only the voyeurism of the (presumably) male reader that keeps Miss Coote from being terrifying as the embodiment of female financial, social, and sexual independence. Miss Coote founds "Lady Rodney's Club" for upper-class women to enjoy orgies, but it disbands after a man in drag infiltrates the gathering and distracts the women with his "formidable-looking weapon." Miss Coote even finds her lover in bed with a male servant, and soon succumbs to his masculine charms too. Her lesbian and flagellant narrative ends with her initiation into heterosexuality and coitus. Like Sheridan Le Fanu's vampire novel *Carmilla* (1872), *Miss Coote's Confession* raises the possibility of lesbianism and sadomasochism only to reassert the primacy of normative sexuality.[31]

Another flagellant novel of the period, the two-volume *Mysteries of Verbena House* (1881–1882) by "Etonensis" (usually attributed to a combination of George Augustus Sala [volume 1] and James Campbell Reddie [volume 2]), was superficially about a search for stolen gold coins at a girls' school, which reveals a hotbed of rule breaking and many opportunities for corporal punishments. The true narrative was the initiation of Miss Sinclair, the headmistress, from reluctance to employ corporal punishment to "a fearless heroine of the birch."[32] Her initiation into flagellation parallels her sexual initiation under the tutelage of the Reverend Arthur Calvedon. Like *Miss Coote's Confession*, this book was almost but not quite a parody, subverting the common criticism that institutional flagellation is driven by lasciviousness by agreeing but upholding corporal punishment anyway.[33]

The satirical or parodic vein of flagellant erotica continued in *Experimental Lecture by Colonel Spanker* (1878–1879). A blackly humorous satire that echoes the Marquis de Sade, the full title is: *Experimental Lecture by Colonel Spanker on The exciting and voluptuous pleasures to be derived from crushing and humiliating the spirit of a beautiful and modest young lady; as delivered by him in the assembly-room of the Society of Aristocratic Flagellants, Mayfair.*

"Spanker" proves his sensibility-inspired thesis, that it is more pleasurable to torment a refined young lady than a woman of the lower classes, by orchestrating the abduction and humiliation of Miss Julia Ponsonby, age seventeen.[34] This slyly mocks Victorian hypocrisy, by illustrating that what is acceptable treatment for match-and-flower seller girls or milliner's apprentices (supposedly more vulgar and resilient than respectable women) becomes unacceptable when the object is a "modest, sensitive" young lady "with real blue blood in her veins."[35]

Apart from the pornographic works circulated clandestinely, there were other forms of fetishistic writings that hid in plain sight and never came to the attention of the Obscene Publications Act. Mainstream fiction had plenty of kinkiness. Though the Gothic novel was supposed to be dead by the mid-nineteenth century, the territory staked out by the Gothic writers was still being mined for fiction and art, and that trickled down to the general public. Heroines were forever being chained up in dungeons and threatened with beating unless they gave up their virtue, while heroes fell victim to the sexual charms of domineering courtesans and actresses.

Popular fiction viewed the beating of boys as innocuous. A young P. G. Wodehouse (better known for his *Jeeves and Wooster* stories) wrote "Bradshaw's Little Story," published in 1902 in *The Captain*, "A Magazine for Boys and Old Boys." The story treated schoolboy whippings as just good clean fun: "In a quarter-of-an-hour Bradshaw returned, walking painfully, and bearing what to the expert's eye, are the unmistakable signs of a 'touching up,' which, being interpreted, is corporal punishment." A few years later, the same magazine would rhapsodize over the beauty of girls between the ages of ten and fifteen, and a corseted, whip-wielding older girl.[36]

The Obscene Publications Act also completely missed the many English magazines, intended to be non-pornographic, respectable publications, that had ongoing fetishistic correspondences. The columns discussed flagellation, tightlacing corsets, cross-dressing as a form of childhood punishment, and more, with anonymous attribution (e.g., "A Lady from Edinburgh," "Alfred," or "Moralist") and vague locations (e.g., "Near Chiswick" or "five miles from Bournemouth").

Family Herald magazine ("Interesting to All; Offensive to None") hosted an ongoing debate on scholastic and domestic corporal punishment. The editors were in favor of moderate disciplinary flogging of children, as long as it was not "indecent," and therefore whipping should not occur between sexes. It wasn't long until the letters column took a more sensual tone, including the common fantasies of naughty nuns and priests whipping each other and their charges. Other letters concentrated on the disciplining of girls (which could include young women in their twenties), despite the fact that beatings of boys at home and in schools were far more common.[37]

Sam Beeton, the English publisher who had displeased Harriet Beecher Stowe with the eroticized depictions of whipping in her book, was married to Isabella Beeton, known to millions as "Mrs. Beeton," editor of the *Englishwoman's Domestic Magazine*, a down-market version of the upper-class women's magazines of the previous generations for an aspirational bourgeois readership. It included a section for correspondence called Conversazione.

After Isabella's death in 1865, Sam continued publishing the magazine, and the Conversazione section took a strange turn. From 1867 to 1874, it printed more than one hundred fifty letters from readers on corsetry and extreme tightlacing to the fabled sixteen inches or less, often practiced at fantastic boarding schools with tightlaced, rod-wielding headmistresses.[38] One letter described a girl's experience being bound, spanked, and birched:

> I put out my hands, which she fastened together with a cord by the wrists. Then making me lie down across the foot of the bed, face downwards, she very quietly and deliberately, putting her left hand around my waist, gave me a shower of smart slaps with her open right hand . . . . [R]aising the birch, I could hear it whiz in the air, and oh, how terrible it felt as it came down, and as its repeated strokes came swish, swish, swish on me![39]

Other topics included transvestism. A letter attributed to "Etonensis" said:

> Stays were easy, but now came the fight again. The first petticoat I clutched hold of, and I think for ten minutes I held on, till at last that too was accomplished. . . . They now easily accomplished the rest; shame overcame my courage, and I had no strength. My trousers were now entirely removed. I was made to stand up, under more slaps and thumpings and threatenings of birch, while my dressing was most leisurely completed with a stiff starched petticoat, a blue frock down nearly to my feet, stockings and sandal shoes. . . . I know not if this punishment is more cruel than the birch; this I do know, that it put an end to it at home. The mere threat, the "shall I send for some petticoats for you?"—always set me to work.[40]

The *Telegraph* wrote, "This correspondence is a serious thing; it reveals the existence of a whole world of unnatural and indefensibly private cruelty, of which the law ought to have cognisance."[41] Others thought the letters were just hoaxes or fantasies, despite Beeton's denials.

This type of correspondence continued in the 1880s in the sensationalist *The Family Doctor and People's Medical Advisor* (an example of medical authority used to make erotica acceptable), which told of ever tinier corseted waists, and *Lady's Own Paper*:

> Sir,—On this subject, and in reply to the mother who complains of her untoward boy, I would advise her to read the remarks of a young gentleman in the supplemental conversazione of the Englishwoman's Domestic Magazine for April last, and then she will find a cure for her troublesome son. After innumerable whippings had failed, the governess took it into her head to dress him in his sister's clothes, which, though the feat was accomplished after much kicking and plunging, had the desired effect; and he tells us that whenever he transgressed or failed in his lessons, if his governess rang the bell, and desired the housemaid to bring some petticoats, &c., he either begged pardon for his offences or set to dilligently to learn his lesson. He afterwards went to Eton, and he affirms that the whippings there were not half so severe as those of his governess.—Yours obediently,
>
> M. Walker
>
> P.S.—It is all very well to talk of reasoning with untoward boys, but in many cases nothing short of a good whipping or what I have recommended will answer.[42]

Magazines like *Modern Society*, *Society*, *Photo Bits*, and *London Life* continued publishing fetishistic letters well into the twentieth century.[43]

One can only guess how many of these letters were fabricated by the editors, how many were sent by readers, and how many (if any) were genuine. (One fetish letter in *Family Herald* was reprinted nearly verbatim almost twenty years later.[44]) However, consider that during and after the Jack the Ripper murders in the fall of 1888, the police received more than two hundred letters claiming to be from the murderer himself, and over three hundred fifty letters presenting theories about the murders.[45] That's not including letters sent to magazines and newspapers.

The seed planted by Rousseau had borne strange and plentiful fruit. Given the opportunity, people will commit their most extreme fantasies to paper with no need for fame or money as an incentive. In his open letter to the late Marquis de Sade, Swinburne asserted that everyone is born with the same fantastic imagination:

> As to your horrors—ask people what they remember, as little children, to have said, heard of, thought of, dreamed of, done or been tempted to do. Nothing in your books but will find its counterpart or type. (I remember when I was seven a most innocent little girl of six telling me of a bad dream that had made her unhappy: in that dream there was the whole practical philosophy of [Sade's novel] Justine embodied.)[46]

Remember that behind at least one of those pseudonyms and "Anonymous" attributions in Victorian pornography was Swinburne, one of the great poets of his age. Who knows what other literary stars may have dabbled in pornography, for fun or profit?

The disruptions in gender and class roles prompted the equal and opposite reaction—Victorian moralistic repression, which was a society struggling to develop new rules for human relationships, including the perennial hot-button issue of sex, while the environment changed radically. The effort to regulate sexuality, to push it into a small, controlled realm, instead made it expand outward, seeping through the cracks and mutating into new forms. Sexuality was no longer focused on the genitals, but began to encompass the entire body. Instead of only flagellation, the range of fetishistic and sadomasochistic acts also diversified.

In part this was due to consumer capitalism, to sell new products and experiences, but it was also due to the human desire for self-expression. Set a boundary, and someone will always cross it. The "abnormal" must be defined before there can be a "normal." The erotic desire will express itself in some fashion, mutated by the very forces that struggle to repress it.

Chapter Seven

Class and Classification

Do names matter? Do you write "SM," "S&M," or "S/M" on the poster for your play party? The terms "sadism" and "masochism" themselves have their historical baggage, as they originated as psychiatric diagnoses named after mentally unstable noblemen. "D/S," or dominance and submission, represents a different axis of sexual interests. The portmanteau acronym of "BDSM," a relatively recent creation, welds together several different terms into one, but even it seems inadequate to the sheer variety of behavior placed under it. Some participants concoct abbreviations like "Whatever It Is That We Do" (WIITWD), but that's even more awkward.

Like "homosexuality," "sadomasochism" as a word and as a behavior is haunted by its clinical and legal origins. Is the sadomasochist a different type of person, or merely a person with a strange taste, a *goût bizarre*, to switch from clinical Greek and Latin to more artistic French? There were other words to describe unusual sexuality coined in the nineteenth century, such as *algolagnia* (the love of pain), *sadiques actives* and *passives* (sadists and masochists), *tyrannism* and *passivism* (sadism and masochism), or *metatropism* (male attraction to physically domineering women).[1] These terms are largely forgotten now. Certain key ideas and terms superseded the competition, and their influence is still felt today

To say the Victorians were more repressive than the modern age is misleading. Their sexuality, once examined closely, is almost as alien to us as that of the ancient Greeks.

Chapter Seven

THE EXTRAORDINARY GENTLEMEN

Arthur Munby was hardly the only Victorian gentleman to live a secret life of indulging tastes at odds with Victorian norms. He was a peripheral member of a loose fraternity of such men, though he didn't really consider himself one of them because of his blind spot about his own sexuality.

Their interests were in large part literary: passing around writings, trading copies of books by the Marquis de Sade and other rare and banned works. Many were involved firsthand, by patronizing brothels and practicing flagellation. They were the upper-class wing of the followers of the previous century's ideas of sensibility, finding truth and beauty in the extremes of human experience.

Munby knew Algernon Charles Swinburne, the poet and novelist, through the painter Dante Gabriel Rossetti (who had his own fetish for women with long hair).[2]

Though obscure after his death, Swinburne was considered one of England's foremost poets. He was a product of Eton, and its culture of corporal punishment left a deep impression on him. He was small and delicate looking, with a mane of bright red hair, and he took his beatings as tests of his manhood. His tutor, Rev. James Leigh Joynes, was notorious for his flogging; on his retirement in 1887, *Vanity Fair* printed a caricature of him in a gown and mortarboard and brandishing a birch. A letter by Swinburne that indirectly refers to Joynes claimed the tutor was quite inventive: perfuming the flogging room, or birching students while still wet from bathing for heightened sensations.[3]

Swinburne wrote poems like "Arthur's Flogging" and "Reginald's Flogging" under the pseudonym of "Etonensis," and was probably the author of "A Boy's First Flogging at Birchminster," all of which were printed as part of *The Whippingham Papers*, a collection of verse, prose, and essays by various authors under pseudonyms. His magnum opus was *The Flogging Block*, an unpublished manuscript probably written in 1881 and now kept in the "Reserved from Public Use" section of the British Museum.

He knew of Sade for some time before he had the chance to read any of the banned books. He had built Sade into such an image of the heroic artist/libertine that he found the actuality of Sade's writing disappointing. In a review he composed as if addressed to Sade, he wrote:

I boast not of myself; but I do say that a schoolboy, set to write on his own stock of experience, and having a real gust and appetite for the subject in him, may make and has made more of a sharp short school flogging of two or three dozen cuts than you of your . . . interminable afflictions; more of the simple common birch rod and daily whipping block than you of your loaded iron whips.[4]

His poetry and novels, even the ones intended for legitimate publication, had sadomasochistic and fetishistic themes. His posthumous novel, *Lesbia Brandon*, is a family romance concerning lesbianism, sadomasochism, transvestism, and narrowly avoided incest. The schoolboy hero, Herbert, crushes on the androgynous Lesbia, who first sees him dressed as a girl for a play, while Lesbia pursues his sister Margaret. Herbert's tutor whips the boy while yearning for Margaret. Tenderness, sadism, and masochism are inextricably entwined in the tutor, who wishes to:

> scourge her into swooning and absorb the blood with kisses; caress and lacerate her loveliness, alleviate and heighten her pains; to feel her foot upon his throat, and would her own with his teeth; submit his body and soul for a little to her lightest will, and satiate up hers the desperate caprice of his immeasurable desire; to inflict careful torture on limbs too tender to embrace, suck the tears off her laden eyelids, bit through her sweet and shuddering lips.[5]

The revelation that everybody in this romantic tangle is related by blood leads to two suicides. His writings were an alternative to the common Victorian imagery of love as uncomplicated bliss.

Swinburne's cousin, Mary Leith (née Gordon), was at least the partial inspiration for the sensual, Amazonian women who populated Swinburne's novels and poems, known for her horseback riding and hiking.

Leith was interested in flagellation herself, and made her own contributions to the literature: *The Children of the Chapel* (1864), about children beaten into singing for Queen Elizabeth, plus a lengthy description of a boy forced to dress as a girl for a play.[6] She loved to read Swinburne's Eton-inspired work, and was distraught when she learned that Eton might ban the birch in 1893. In a letter to Swinburne, written in the simple letter-swapping cipher they developed as children, she lamented, "Cow, my nousin, do you meally rean to *stand there*, & tell me that the timehonoured

& traditional pode of munishment is disused at Eton? I am more upturbed & perset than you can imagine. I fear 'Eton's record' will certainly *not* be & c (vide 'An Ode') & that we may expect a capid deradence of England's screatest ghool."[7] The "Ode" mentioned is Swinburne's "Eton: an Ode," a parody of a poem he wrote lauding his alma mater.

Whether Swinburne and his cousin ever did anything together beyond exchanging fantasies is unclear, but it does show that there were women who had an interest in the "birchen arts." Even though erotic works of the period commonly claimed that women were far more sadistic and domineering than men, there is very little record of women involved in early sadomasochistic culture who weren't coerced or motivated by money.

Another Munby acquaintance[8] was Richard Monckton Milnes, later Baron Houghton, a politician, poet, and collector of erotica.

> He became a mentor to Swinburne, and gave the young poet his first direct exposure to Sade and other rare and banned books in his private library at Fryston (lost to fire in 1876). Swinburne referred to Milnes as "Mon cher Rodin," after a schoolmaster from Sade's *Justine*.[9]

Like Munby and Milnes, Henry Spencer Ashbee was a Victorian gentleman with a penchant for collecting and classifying. Apart from his impressive bibliographical work in conventional literature, Ashbee gathered thousands of obscure erotic volumes in six or seven languages, courtesy of his contacts on the Continent. He published three large bibliographies of pornography in the 1870s and 1880s, with extensive quotations and his own digressions, under the name "Pisanus Fraxi," a complex Latin pun.[10]

Ashbee's bibliographies are a primary resource in documenting the pornographic underworld of Victorian Europe. His will left his entire collection to the British Museum. The august institution was forced to accept his erotic materials if they wanted his conventional books, including perhaps the foremost Cervantes collection in the world.[11] The trustees exploited a loophole to destroy the majority of Ashbee's erotic books, a great loss to history.[12]

The most famous member of the Swinburne/Milnes/Ashbee set was Sir Richard Francis Burton, the explorer and Orientalist. If any man lived out the Orientalist dream, it was Burton. Burton translated and brought the

Arabian Nights and the *Kama Sutra of Vatsyayana* to Europe. The final portion of the complete manuscript of his book *The Perfumed Garden*, burned by his wife after his death, dealt with the ways of lesbians and sodomites.

The *Kama Sutra* expanded the possibilities of sexuality just when legal and medical authorities were constricting them. The Indian book contains detailed descriptions of many different sexual acts: kissing, caressing, and intercourse, but also biting, striking, and scratching or pressing with the fingernails, sometimes enough to leave visible marks.

Ashbee, Swinburne, and their compatriots were one branch of the ancestors of the modern BDSM subculture. They were upper-middle-class or higher, with the money and leisure time to pursue their interests, and the prestige and status to avoid persecution for them. We also know of their interests because they were all "men of letters" and left a considerable body of writings to posterity.

These gentlemen were freethinking about sexuality, but rather conservative about everything else, and took for granted their privilege over women, the working class, and other social subordinates. "Walter," the protagonist of the mammoth, anonymous autobiography *My Secret Life*,[13] showed this sense of entitlement. In his adolescence, "Walter" visited a farm where a male cousin suggested he make use of the girls working the fields: "[Y]ou can always have a field-girl; nobody cares,—I have a dozen or two." He forced himself on one of the girls. "Her tears ran down. If I had not committed a rape, it looked uncommonly like one." She refused his attempt to buy her off, but the foreman came along and ordered her to accept, getting him off the hook once again.[14]

As Stephen Marcus put it in *The Other Victorians* (1964): "[O]ne of the foundation stones of [Walter's] morality is based on the idea of an English gentleman's private right to do whatever he likes with his own person and to let others do the same—and that this idea is in turn connected with notions of *laissez-faire* and property. . . . His liberation from sexual-moral prejudices is not accompanied by a parallel development in his ideas about class and society."[15] Ideas of sexual freedom were connected with ideas of class and gender privilege, and the easy availability of working-class women. As long as a gentleman was discreet, he could more or less do as he pleased.

LEOPOLD VON SACHER-MASOCH

Unlike the English sexual adventurers, the Austrian writer and journalist Leopold von Sacher-Masoch made no effort to be discreet. Though he would never have considered his work pornographic, he made his own contribution to the evolving form of sadomasochistic erotica: his novel *Venus in Furs* (1870). It was a part of a planned cycle of books, *The Heritage of Caine*. Only two of the six books were completed, and *Venus* was part of the volume titled *Love*. The novel reflected the fantasies of submission to cruel women that filled Sacher-Masoch's life, and it led to its author's name being associated with an entire realm of human behavior: "masochism."

The framing story of *Venus in Furs* is about a man who dreams of fur-clad women. He speaks to a friend, Severin, who says, "Woman's power lies in man's passion, and she knows how to use it, if man doesn't understand himself. He has only one choice: to be the *tyrant* over or the *slave* of woman." Severin gives the narrator a manuscript telling of his obsessive affair with a woman named Wanda, the main story of the novel.

What distinguished *Venus in Furs* from other nineteenth-century novels of men enslaved and consumed by seductive women, such as *Nana* or *La Marquise de Sade*, is that Severin consciously and deliberately arranged this situation with Wanda. Severin was determined to take his desires as far as possible, and he overcame Wanda's concerns that she wouldn't measure up to his expectations—or that she might exceed them.

Severin described himself as "supersensual," echoing the previous century's theory of sensibility:

"Perhaps, [said Wanda] after all, there isn't anything so very unique or strange in all your passions, for who doesn't love beautiful furs? And everyone knows and feels how closely sexual love and cruelty are related."

"But in my case all these elements are raised to their highest degree," I replied.

"In other words, reason has little power over you, and you are by nature, soft, sensual, yielding."

"Were the martyrs also soft and sensual by nature?"

"The martyrs?"

"On the contrary, [he said] they were *supersensual men*, who found enjoyment in suffering. They sought out the most frightful tortures, even death itself, as others seek joy, and as they were, so am I—*supersensual*."

"Have a care that in being such, you do not become a martyr to love, the *martyr of a woman*."[16]

Sacher-Masoch explicitly drew connections between Severin's desires, Catholicism, and paganism, which give his novel the suggestion of a personal religious rite, performed with contracts, disguises, whippings, masks, cuckolding, and role play as servants or animals. Severin and Wanda drew up a contract, which specified she would dominate him cruelly while wearing sensuous furs. They traveled to Italy, with Severin posing as Wanda's manservant "Gregor." He was abused by her trio of Negro maidservants, and had to watch as Wanda dallied with her ferocious, Byronic Greek lover.

The novel ends on an ambivalent note, with Wanda taking Severin's desires to their logical extreme by dismissing him in favor of her lover, which later she claimed she did for Severin's own good. Severin said he had been cured, and now lives with female servants whom he threatens with whipping. He tells his friend:

> That woman, as nature has created her and as man is at present educating her, is his enemy. She can only be his slave or his despot, but *never his companion*. This she can become only when she has the same rights as he, and is his equal in education and work.

Arguably, women were so disadvantaged at the time that they had to use sexual and emotional manipulation to survive. Severin equates the "good" woman with dishonesty and hypocrisy, while the cruel woman is honest. He spoke of cruel, powerful women of myth and history, which was a transgressive alternative to the nineteenth-century sentimental, domestic ideal of woman popularized in Coventry Patmore's 1854 poem "The Angel in the House."

Loosely based on Sacher-Masoch's relationship with one of his mistresses, Fanny Pistor, *Venus in Furs* is less a novel with autobiographical elements than a fantasy Leopold von Sacher-Masoch tried to enact for most of his life.

He was born the son of a police commissioner in 1836 in Austria, and had an aristocratic upbringing. He likened his delicate mother to one of Raphael's Madonnas, but was also close to his Ukrainian peasant wet nurse, who told him dark and bloody folktales.[17] Since childhood, he was preoccupied with scenes of cruelty, death, and torture, in both the tales of

Christian martyrs and in Eastern European folklore. The region of Austria where he grew up had a history of bloody ethnic conflict. He heard graphic stories of the slaughter of Polish landowners by their tenants: beaten to death, beheaded, or nailed to the doors of barns. Women were often active leaders in these revolts.[18]

He claimed to have witnessed, as a child, a primal scene straight out of Freud: from hiding, he observed his domineering aunt, the Countess Zenobia, trysting with her lover. With the timing of a bedroom farce or a BDSM scene, the Count entered and witnessed the adultery. Zenobia hit her husband, causing him to flee. The countess discovered her nephew and spanked him.[19] While almost certainly exaggerated, if not fabricated, this story is the prototype of the fantasy that influenced almost every aspect of his life.

Sacher-Masoch grew up to be one of the most famous and well-regarded men of letters in Middle Europe, a humanist, philo-Semite, and idealist. However, his spendthrift ways and sexual obsessions kept him from ever achieving his potential.

It was Rousseau's *Confessions* that made Sacher-Masoch recognize the sexual nature of his fantasies.[20] Unlike Swinburne and the English sadomasochists, he made no secret of his tastes and included them in his popular novels. *Venus in Furs* is the most famous example of this, but his fantasies of cruel women figured in most of his other writings, both his high literary works and the pulp he produced to make ends meet. His work was full of historical and mythological references to domineering women, including the Black Czarina of Halicz, and Esther, the Jewish concubine of Casimir III of Poland. His novel *Peasant Justice* ends with a merciless woman leading an angry mob that tears a bandit gang to pieces, along with bystanders.[21] *The Mother of God* features Madrona, the ruler of an agricultural commune who bathes in the offered blood of her servant girl. The hero consents to be crucified by both women, crying, "Why has thou forsaken me?" to Madrona, and "Why has thou betrayed me?" to the servant. The scene is a parody of the Passion of the Christ, with a female God and Judas.[22] Spiritual rebirth of a man through the power of a woman is a recurring theme in Sacher-Masoch's fantasies, a reworking of his Catholic upbringing.

He regarded these desires as a personal idiosyncrasy, a game of courtly love. He was still an Austrian gentleman at heart, with all the privilege that implied. Others attributed his preoccupations to his stereotypically passionate Slavic character, befitting a German Romantic poet. Likewise, his fascination with furs, so strong so that he would keep one on his writing desk to stroke, was just an eccentricity, though he was creatively and sexually impotent without them.

Sacher-Masoch apparently never obtained the services of prostitutes, though there would have been some who catered to his type of desires. Instead, he drew women into his games, sometimes by charm if they were admirers, sometimes by coercion if they were wives or servants. Women responded to his charisma, his fame, his (potential but never realized) wealth, and the chance to enjoy the bohemian life of a daring artist.

The problem, for him and for the women in his life, was how much he wanted it. Sacher-Masoch's preoccupations grew stronger over his life, from eccentric interest to pathological compulsion. He became almost unable to write anything that didn't involve cruel women, as literary critics often complained, and would choreograph erotic scenes while on the brink of bankruptcy. After goading his wife into seducing another man, he would retire to the next room where his children slept.

For all his worship of women in his imagination, Sacher-Masoch treated them poorly in real life. He maneuvered his mistress, Anna von Kottowitz, into a liaison with an alleged exiled Polish count. When the count turned out to be a Russian petty thief who gave Kottowitz syphilis, Sacher-Masoch dismissed her immediately. He later told his first wife:

> Women have no character—only *caprices*. A woman could torture me to death and it would only make me happy . . . but I do not allow myself to be bored. I simply dumped her.[23]

He saw women as bearing great symbolic power, but not as his intellectual or spiritual equal.

> I know that I am spiritually superior to any woman. But I require the woman I love to be superior to me by being in complete control of her own sensuality and subduing me through mine. Consequently, my cruel ideal woman is for me simply the instrument by which I terrorise myself.[24]

This realization, unfortunately for him and his family, didn't help him change his ways.

Class transgression was a theme of his relationships. Just as Munby and Cullwick traveled on the Continent with her in the role of a lady, Sacher-Masoch and his mistresses traveled as servant and lady. As Hannah Cullwick was sometimes addressed with the common female servant name, "Mary," Sacher-Masoch took the generic male servant name of "Gregor," when he traveled with Pistor to Italy.

It was unsurprising that Sacher-Masoch's marriage to Aurora Rümelin was full of power struggles and abuse, though it was the wife who got the worst of it, as told in Rümelin's memoirs, *The Confessions of Wanda von Sacher-Masoch* (1907). It was a relationship founded on bad faith. Rümelin, a poor glovemaker, participated in a complicated prank on Sacher-Masoch and first met him while disguised with a veil and pretending to be the author of letters from "Wanda von Dunajew."

After the early death of their first child, Sacher-Masoch became more compulsive in his fantasies. "Brigands" was his favorite game. He would recruit Rümelin and other women to play bandits, fur-clad of course, who would rob and beat him. When Rümelin tried to assert control over their finances, he took a page right out of *Venus in Furs*.

> [H]e found it truly charming to be dependent entirely on me. He wanted to have a signed contract giving me the right to dispose of all his income. I could not keep from laughing; but he took the matter seriously and begged me to immediately draw up the contract. I recognized the advantages accruing from such an arrangement, and declared myself ready to do what he wanted. I sat at the desk and he brought me a beautiful sheet of parchment.
>
> "But," he added, "it is necessary that you put on a fur to write, so that I may have the sensation of being dominated by you!"
>
> I put on the fur and drew up the contract while he stood close by, apprehensive, yet satisfied. When the agreement was written he signed it, saying, "Guard it well. Now you are my mistress, and I your slave. Henceforth I shall address you only as 'Mistress.' *Command and I will always obey.*"[25]

Later, he told her that, if his fantasies were not enacted in real life, they would permeate his writing, which was their only source of income. He always looked for "the Greek," a man with whom his "Wanda" would have an affair.

Sacher-Masoch couldn't keep to boundaries; in front of their children he would call his wife cruel and heartless, and urge her to beat him. Eventually, he reached his wife's limit when she discovered his affair with his "old maid" translator. Rümelin beat her in front of the "frozen" Leopold before throwing her out. She then had his bed and all the furs and whips moved to another room. "*Free!* Delivered from the torment of ten years! Finally to belong to myself again! Never again to don a fur, never again to hold a whip, and never again to hear a word spoken about the Greek!"[26] As the saying goes, the cruelest thing to say to a masochist is "No."

Rümelin was financially dependent on Sacher-Masoch, and divorce law meant that leaving him would deprive her of everything, even her children. She only left her husband when pushed beyond the brink and, significantly, when she had another man in her life. Though nominally submissive, Sacher-Masoch was more controlling than Munby ever was.

By comparison, Munby and Cullwick had compatible fantasies and fetishes, and neither of them ever reached the point of their desires interfering with their ability to take care of themselves or form relationships. Though she defined herself as a slave, Cullwick had no class aspirations and made sure she had the financial means to support herself if she ever had to leave. She also had no children tying her to Munby. She could, and did, leave him. These cases show why Cullwick was right to be wary of marriage, that a supposedly higher status could instead deprive a woman of freedom and security.

Sacher-Masoch's novels and historical works made him well known in literary circles, but his recurring fantasies made him famous in a different world. People from across Europe sent him fan mail about how his ideas resonated with them, and wanted to share their own or even become part of his. The post and the newspaper personal columns led Sacher-Masoch into a shadowy world of false identities and anonymous encounters. One correspondent signed his letters "Anatole," a character from one of Sacher-Masoch's stories, in which a homosexual man meets a correspondent named Anatole, who turns out to be a woman. Sacher-Masoch convinced himself that this Anatole was really a woman, too. He, while blindfolded, met "Anatole" in a hotel room, who turned out to be a tall, beautifully voiced man. Undaunted, Sacher-Masoch immediately recast this stranger into the role of the Greek from his fantasy, and arranged a meeting between his wife and this Anatole. Rümelin, instead, met with a small, pale, hunchbacked man. Years later, Sacher-Masoch and Rümelin learned that the first of the "two Anatoles" had probably been the eccentric King Ludwig II of Bavaria, and the second Prince Alexander of Orange.[27]

Sacher-Masoch would probably not have been happy to learn that, a century after his death, he is primarily known for his sexuality, and his historical and literary achievements are largely forgotten. For that, he could thank Dr. Richard von Krafft-Ebing.

KRAFFT-EBING AND THE MAN FROM BERLIN

While the Marquis de Sade had been dead for decades before the word "sadism" was created, Leopold von Sacher-Masoch was alive when psychiatrist Richard von Krafft-Ebing coined "masochism." The writer wasn't pleased with this dubious honor. Both men taught at the University of Graz, though there is no evidence they ever met.[28]

Krafft-Ebing was a forensic psychiatrist by training, at a time when the discipline was struggling for respect. He was a popularizer of psychiatry, who gave public lectures and demonstrations of the power of hypnosis on women, which his critics slighted as sensationalist events.[29]

Krafft-Ebing coined "Masochism" for the sixth edition of his best known work, *Psychopathia Sexualis*, first published in 1886. Like many other books on sex, *Psychopathia Sexualis* occupied an ambiguous position between the academic and the pornographic. It was intended as a forensic reference for doctors and judges, to help them distinguish the criminal from the pathological, and many of the more explicit passages were written in Latin or French to discourage lay readers. The American publishers of the 12th edition wrote in the book's preface that it was not for sale to the general public, and should restricted to medical and legal professionals.

Despite this, *Psychopathia Sexualis* was immensely popular with lay readers. Between 1892 and 1978, there were at least thirty-four authorized English translations. Even when academic institutions wouldn't touch it, popular publishers would sell it as pornography, sometimes translating the Latin parts into modern languages. Apart from the case histories themselves, there were descriptions of the sexual rites of aboriginal peoples and of the nightlife and brothels of modern Europe. No other book did so much to satisfy the sexual curiosity of its readers.

"Masochism" as a term was a product of the symbiotic relationship between literature and psychiatry in the nineteenth century. Realist and decadent writers like Octave Mirbeau, Émile Zola, and Guy de Maupassant drew on medical texts for extremes of human behavior, while Krafft-Ebing and his colleague Alfred Binet looked to the writings of Rousseau, Sade, Sacher-Masoch, and Réstif de la Bretonne (whose name was the basis for *restifism*, an archaic term for foot fetishism).[30]

In *Psychopathia Sexualis*, Krafft-Ebing defined four basic categories of sexual deviance: *paradoxia* (sexual desire in childhood or old age, the wrong time), *anesthesia* (insufficient desire), *hyperesthesia* (excessive desire), and *paresthesia* (desire for the wrong act, anything other than coitus, or the wrong object, human or non-human).[31] Paresthesia included all sexual perversions, that is, any desire that diverted someone from the natural purpose of sex, procreation. This included what today would be called homosexuality, fetishism, sadism, and masochism, as well as necrophilia, zoophilia, "lustmurder," and exhibitionism. Krafft-Ebing viewed homosexuality, or "contrary sexual desire," as a problem of female traits in men, and vice versa. Masochism was a similar condition: submissiveness was normal in women but a perversion in men. Sadism, however, was an exaggerated, atavistic form of natural male sexual aggression. Fetishes were malfunctions of natural desire, caused by hereditary "taint."[32]

In the early years of his studies of sexuality, Krafft-Ebing worked mainly with lower-class inmates of prisons and asylums, whose desires were so uncontrollable that they interfered with their ability to lead a normal life or even drove them to criminal acts. In his private practice, he increasingly worked with middle-class patients who suffered from vague nineteenth-century ailments like neurasthenia. Hannah Cullwick and Arthur Munby, who quietly practiced their kinks in private and had no desire to disclose themselves to others, would not have become subjects for Krafft-Ebing's studies. A gentleman like Sacher-Masoch would never have considered the possibility that anything was wrong with him. Thus, Krafft-Ebing's experience with kinky people was with those who wanted to talk about their desires, or were forced to talk about them.

Krafft-Ebing's case studies ranged from the harmless (a man who wished to lather a woman's face and shave her with a razor) to the horrifying (examples of "lust murder" and necrophilia), with fantasies of bondage, flagellation, and humiliation in between. Many of them were short autobiographical sketches, whose authors described their responses to the mass media of the day. Harriet Beecher Stowe's *Uncle Tom's Cabin* figured in one of the case histories: (Case 57).

> Even in my early childhood I loved to revel in ideas about the absolute mastery of one man over others. The thought of slavery had something exciting in it for me, alike whether from the standpoint of master or servant. That one man could possess, sell or whip another, caused me intense excitement; and in reading *Uncle Tom's Cabin* (which I read at about the beginning of puberty) I had erections. Particularly exciting for me was the thought of a man being hitched to a waggon in which another man sat with a whip, driving and whipping him.[33]

The erotics of Atlantic slavery appear in the case study of Miss X (Case 84).

> Often I have dreamed that I was his slave—but, mind you, not his female slave! For instance, I have imagined that he was Robinson [Crusoe], and I the savage that served him. I often look at the pictures in which Robinson puts his foot on the neck of the savage. I now find an explanation of these strange fantasies: I look upon woman in general as low, far below man; but I am otherwise extremely proud and quite indomitable, whence it arises that I think as a man (who is by nature proud and superior). This renders my humiliation before the man I love the more intense. I have also fantasized myself to be his female slave; but this does not suffice, for after all every woman can be the slave of her husband.[34]

Freud[35] and other researchers of the time also reported flagellant patients who were aroused by *Uncle Tom's Cabin* and other abolitionist texts and images.

An anonymous correspondent from Berlin brought the works of Sacher-Masoch to Krafft-Ebing's attention. This "well-educated man," as Krafft-Ebing described him, also sent his detailed life history and an analysis of his fantasies, which he didn't consider pathological. He recognized himself in Rousseau's *Confessions* and in the writings of Sacher-Masoch and saw his desires as a form of medieval courtly love.[36] He also tried to compile a Sade-like list of "all maltreatments and humiliations which a woman can inflict on a man, and to classify them in clearly delimited categories and subcategories, which I indicated with Roman and Arabic numbers."[37]

The Berlin man told Krafft-Ebing of the "comedies" of pain and submission played out by prostitutes and their clients in Paris, Berlin, and Vienna: kicks, orders, schoolroom or nursery lectures, verbal abuse, flagellation and beatings, iron chains and handcuffs, or dried peas for the client to kneel upon. Masochistic men were said to be widespread, and there were many prostitutes who catered to such desires. Contact advertisements in German newspapers explicitly referenced the writings of Sacher-Masoch.[38] Instead of a few isolated deviants, the sexologist learned of an entire demimonde of "perverts" and those who catered to them.

The Berlin man was just one of the hundreds of correspondents who mailed their fantasies and life stories to Krafft-Ebing. Some sent him pictures as well, including a postcard from Paris's Moulin Rouge cabaret, showing a man in a tuxedo on all fours, with a woman astride his back and holding the reins of a bit in his mouth.

Some of the people who contacted Krafft-Ebing were deeply troubled by their sexual desires, describing themselves as an "error of nature," a "moral monster, devoid of human feelings," or an "unnatural human being, beyond the laws of nature of society."[39] They reached out in the hope of a cure. Krafft-Ebing employed electrotherapy, hydrotherapy, and particularly hypnosis to treat perversions, though he admitted the results were mixed at best. Others he told they had to accept their desires as unchangeable, and even suggested that one man, only attracted to crippled woman, should marry a woman with a limp and have a happy life.[40]

For the Berlin man and other correspondents, however, Krafft-Ebing was primarily a sympathetic ear. These people felt that their desires were inborn and accepted or even embraced them. In later editions, subjects said they weren't seeking a cure, since it was social condemnation that was the source of their problems. These homosexuals and fetishists didn't view their desires as morally or medically wrong, and they eloquently wrote of their wish for social acceptance. After years of people revealing their secrets to him, Krafft-Ebing became more supportive. There were perverts who were miserable, a danger to others or themselves, or both, but others just led lives of quiet desperation, and some were otherwise mentally healthy and socially integrated.[41]

More than half of Krafft-Ebing's patients and correspondents had bourgeois or aristocratic backgrounds. They were part of the literate culture of diaries and memoirs, of confession and storytelling. People told of their childhood experiences as their first inkling of their homosexuality or masochism; their efforts to repress these desires; their self-recognition through books like *Uncle Tom's Cabin, Robinson Crusoe*, Rousseau's *Confessions*,[42] and even earlier editions of *Psychopathia Sexualis*; compromises such as patronizing prostitutes; and finally a degree of self-acceptance and peace of mind.

In the wake of Rousseau's tell-all autobiography, in which he explored himself as a complex, authentic individual, many people felt the need to construct an identity. The traditional institutions that assigned identity—the church, the extended family, and the agricultural community—had waned in influence. In the new urban, industrial society, literate people had the opportunity to craft their own identities, borrowing terms from medical science and artistic fantasy. The inner self of desires and fantasies became more important than the outer self of roles and titles. Everybody wanted to tell the stories of their own lives. The result might be the published memoirs of a great man, an anonymous sexual fantasy sent to a magazine, or a self-written case history sent to Krafft-Ebing or another medical authority.

Instead of the traditional view of perverse *acts* being transient aberrations due to environmental influences (such as drunkenness, seduction, hereditary "taint," or an immoral society), Krafft-Ebing came to view perverse *desires* as fundamental aspect of individual character, granted by nature. To deny or repress them was to lead a false, inauthentic life. The same conditions that nurtured the ideal of romantic love also made the idea of the homosexual or sadomasochistic person possible.[43]

Krafft-Ebing retained the common belief that women were naturally sexually passive, and this belief informed his categorizing of case studies. He recorded no female sadists, fetishists, pedophiles, zoophiles, or exhibitionists. Out of 50 cases of masochism, only 3 were female, and out of 168 homosexual cases, only 25 were female.[44]

Krafft-Ebing wrote that exhibitionist, masochistic, and fetishistic behavior in women was normal, part of the natural drive to procreate. Women were supposed to show off their bodies, submit to men and fetishize masculine traits in them. Only excessive, one-sided emotional dependency on a man by a woman was an aberration, classified as "sexual bondage," and even that wasn't a perversion, in that it didn't interfere with intercourse and procreation. Masochism was a problem of men, related to homosexuality by the presence of feminine traits.[45] Given the submission expected of women in the nineteenth century, female masochism would not have been a problem, and therefore was invisible. Hannah Cullwick, for instance, would be regarded as merely an unusually devoted servant. As Miss X observed in one of Krafft-Ebing's case histories (Case 84), "every woman can be the slave of her husband." Likewise, fetishism as a perversion was supposed to be exclusive to men.[46]

Just as the French brothel system was intended to control sex and instead made it diversify, the psychiatric project to regulate and control sexuality instead fostered the beginnings of homosexual and sadomasochistic cultures. People across Europe gravitated to the writings of Krafft-Ebing and Sacher-Masoch, as reflections of their own desires. Mutual recognition laid the groundwork for their quest for legitimation, that their desires not be treated as crimes or pathologies.

The conditions that had nurtured the early form of the BDSM subculture were changing at the turn of the century.

In the first decades of the new century, fewer women were domestic servants, and those who were, were more like employees than slaves, demanding higher wages and respect. The class/gender gulf narrowed. Mass education projects, such as the charity school where Hannah Cullwick learned to read and write, had raised people's social expectations. Women entered white-collar work outside the home, gaining a measure of financial independence and breaking down the rigid gender division of labor.

Also, the position of all women had improved with legislation like the 1882 and 1893 Married Women's Property Acts, which gave married women the same rights over their property as unmarried women. Divorce law reform gave women the right to divorce and access to their children and property.[47] Not every woman was quite the slave of her husband anymore.

The trial of Oscar Wilde proved that gentlemen like Ashbee and Milnes could not rely on their social standing to place them above legal and social sanctions. There were now names for things like homosexuality and fetishism, as psychiatric ideas seeped into the mainstream. A man like Arthur Munby could no longer maintain (even to himself) that there was nothing sexual in his lifelong fascination for working women. There wouldn't be letters on flagellation or tightlacing in the same magazines as household hints anymore either. Even public schools would eventually admit that there was a sexual component to student beatings, though the practice continued sporadically into the late twentieth century.

Even if Krafft-Ebing had chosen another field of study, had not written *Psychopathia Sexualis* and created the psychiatric map of sexuality for the coming century, the sadomasochistic subculture would still have developed much as it did, though perhaps at a slightly slower pace or with different terminology. The man from Berlin was just one of many with similar fantasies and desires, and their loose network kept growing. They wrote letters, poems, and novels and privately commissioned and collected books and photographs. They patronized the sub-sector of the brothel industry that catered to their needs or they played out their fantasies in private, like Munby and Cullwick or Sacher-Masoch and Rümelin. The common language of the modern BDSM culture had begun.

Chapter Eight

Every Woman Adores a Fascist

It's uniform night at the fetish club. The multilevel, black-walled nightclub is full of camouflage-patterned pants and tank tops, watch caps and sailor hats. Sexy cops, nurses, surgeons, firefighters, and soldiers, all dance to industrial music. Uniforms are also a kind of costume, obscuring the individual wearer's identity.

A few are more invested in the image, and wear full-dress uniforms, salvaged from thrift shops and online stores. The image these particular garments present is of power and ability, a person who stands apart from everyday society. The uniforms themselves are slightly taboo, being worn by people who technically should not have them. The signifier is detached from the signified.

One of the partygoers, a young white man, stands slightly apart. His uniform is meticulously detailed and fits perfectly. The black jacket, breeches, knee-boots, gloves, and peaked cap make him look like a single, solid object. What really sets him apart is the armband, with the elemental colors of red, white, and black, and the jagged, four-pointed symbol burned into history as the sign of tyranny and genocide. This was the Nazi SS dress uniform, designed for an elite group of men, the culmination of centuries of evolution in masculine dress, a new uniform for a new kind of man.

In cloaking himself in the trappings of a despised and feared elite organization, he has put on a taboo. In all likelihood, he is not a fascist or white supremacist, any more than the women dancing in sexy nurse outfits are qualified medical professionals. But in a subculture that plays with power and taboo, he's gone further than anyone else present, just by wearing a certain outfit. That makes power radiate from him, not so much the power from capability, but the power from the breaking of taboo. In a room full of uniforms, he stood out.

The series of bloody wars and genocides that gripped the world in the first half of the twentieth century tested the new hope that human nature could be understood and controlled through reason. Fascism, as it rose to power in certain countries and formed popular movements in others, challenged the ideals of rationality, freedom, and democracy. Adolf Hitler's first speech as Reichskanzler on January 30, 1933, concluded, "[U]nquestionably, you are not to act, you are to obey and to conform; you have to submit to the primordial need to obey."[1] Why some people seemed to prefer slavish obedience to charismatic, uniformed dictators over liberty and self-determination required an explanation. One rationale was that the political dynamic of fascism was a symptom of a perverse psychological, or even specifically sexual, dynamic.

Centuries before, Shakespeare's *Measure for Measure* (discussed in chapter 2) linked the sexual repression of the Duke of Vienna and the judge Angelo to their stated need for strict law and order and their sexual cruelty, expressed through allusion and metaphor. Angelo's harsh rule is merely an excuse to indulge his sadism, while Isabella seeks out restriction and pain from his authority, indulging her masochism.

THE FASCISM QUESTION

The glib bit of folk anthropology that "Nazis were all repressed queers and perverts" grossly oversimplifies a complex relationship between sexuality and politics. The exact relationship between authoritarianism and sadomasochism is elusive. Certainly, there were anecdotal accounts of fascist leaders with fetishistic or sadomasochistic behaviors, but that doesn't necessarily mean that the rank-and-file Nazis had such proclivities, or that that was the basis of fascism. Another school of thought suggested that fascism and sadomasochism are the results of the libido being repressed by pleasure-hating, conformist society.

What is clear is that fascism has been associated with deviant sexuality. Just as earlier generations expressed their anxieties about Catholicism, the Orient, or slavery through anti-Catholic, Orientalist, or Southern fantasies, people of the twentieth century expressed their anxiety about fascism through a new genre of sexualized scenarios.[2]

French historian and philosopher Michel Foucault, himself a practicing sadomasochist, found the association of fascism with deviant and decadent sexuality puzzling. In 1974, he asked:

> How could Nazism, which was represented by lamentable, shabby, puritan young men, by a species of Victorian spinsters, have become everywhere today—in France, in Germany, in the United States—in all the pornographic literature of the whole world, the absolute reference of eroticism? All the shoddiest aspects of the erotic imagination are now put under the sign of Nazism.[3]

Elsewhere, Foucault denied the connection between fascism and the libido:

> Nazism wasn't invented by the great erotic madmen of the twentieth century but by the most sinister, boring, disgusting petite bourgeoisie you can imagine. . . . It's the infected *petit bourgeois* dream of racial propriety that underlies the Nazi dream.[4]

Foucault hedged his claim a bit, acknowledging there might be "localized" and "incidental" elements of eroticism in fascism. On the other hand, Leo Bersani in *Homos* says that "the polarized structure of master and slave, of dominance and submission, is the same in Nazism and S&M, and that structure—not the dream of racial 'purity' or the strictly formal dimension of the game—is what gives pleasure."[5]

DESTROY THIS MAD BRUTE

Well before the rise of fascism, propagandists juxtaposed deviant politics with deviant sexuality. A classic trope in propaganda is to impute to the enemy excessive and deviant sexuality, particularly if the intended audience prides itself on its sexual continence. The same artistic approach that informed Powers's *The Greek Slave* and Palmer's *White Slave* in the nineteenth century was applied to new conflicts.

French and English propaganda had deployed the image of the cruel, hypermasculine, oversexed, and mindlessly obedient German soldier since the Franco-Prussian War of 1870, if not earlier. In World War I, French and British propaganda about the German invasions of Belgium and France explicitly used rape imagery; both literally, in that actual rapes would occur, and metaphorically, figuring the entire conflict in sexual terms of masculine aggressors attacking feminine victims. One American propaganda poster showed a dark, gorilla-like creature with wide, staring eyes, an open, fanged mouth, and a Prussian spiked helmet labeled "Militarism," carrying a club in one hand and a swooning blonde woman in the other. The caption read, "Destroy this mad brute. Enlist."[6] Another shows, in silhouette, a soldier with a spiked helmet and a rifle pulling a young woman by the wrist.

Propaganda is not a genre of subtlety or ambiguity. It presents a Manichean view of unmistakable good versus evil, and a call to action. And yet, a curious thing happens when sex is used as a metaphor for war; both become seductive.

> These fantasies in which Britain, France and the United States cast themselves as the feminine victim of a virile Germany are often given romantic or erotic overtones. A French World War I poster called "Les Monstres" depicts a German soldier leaving a woman on the floor beside a tousled bed; the caption exclaims, "He might at least have courted her!!" It is odd to see courtship invoked in this picture of sexual violence. A British World War I cartoon by Louis Raemaekers titled *Seduction* shows a dark-skinned German slumped in an easy chair, legs crossed, with a pistol pointed toward a kneeling woman, whose dress is pulled down to expose one breast, as in depictions of Liberty. The caption: "Germany to Belgium: 'Aren't I a lovable fellow?'" These images, and many others like them, broadly imply sexual violence, but they also have what Ruth Harris calls an "almost pornographic" tone, since the terms of seduction, courtship, and romance hint at eroticism in Germany's imagined relationship to France and Britain.
>
> This Manicheanism and absolute prohibition are essential generators of eroticized images of fascism, which foreground the propagandistic construction of the enemy, questioning and sometimes parodying such representations and, above all, showing political prohibition—especially when based on sexual voraciousness—to be sexually exciting.[7]

Anne Desclos, alias Pauline Reage, author of *Story of O*, suggested that, as a young French girl during World War I, the threat of German military aggression influenced her sexual fantasies.

As a little girl, during that period [of World War I], I had a strange dream that kept recurring until 1942 or thereabouts, at which point I suddenly realized I wasn't dreaming it anymore. I was in my grandmother's room, where I slept, and the drapes by the door began to stir. We could hear footsteps coming up the stairs. I knew it was the German soldiers coming to arrest us. I grabbed a rifle and ran out onto the landing and began to fire at them, until I was killed by their gunfire. At which point I woke up.[8]

Susan Brownmiller, in her feminist analysis of rape *Against Our Will* (1975), also wrote about how her sexual fantasies were influenced at a young age by an image of WWI propaganda, a German "Hun" juxtaposed with a beautiful woman lying beneath him:

This was the middle of World War II, the German Army had marched through Belgium a second time, and I was a Jewish girl growing up in Brooklyn. I could not help but conclude that the Hun and the Nazi were the same and, therefore, I had to be Belgium. In the next year I fantasized myself to sleep at night with a strange tableau. A tall and handsome Nazi concentration camp guard stood near a barbed-wire fence. He did not menace me directly—after all, I had no idea what the actual menace involved. For my part, I lay there motionless, at a safe distance. I was terribly beautiful. . . .

[It] struck me as peculiar and dangerous even as I conjured it up, and soon rooted it out of my fantasy life.[9]

WORLD WAR II

In the interwar period, fascism's enemies attempted to impugn the masculinity and sexuality of the movement. As early as 1931, anti-fascists criticized the Nazis for appointing known homosexual Ernst Roehm as Party Chief of Staff, accusing them of both sexual deviance and sexual hypocrisy.[10]

Accusations of homosexuality were . . . particularly widespread in anti-fascist discourse; despite the Nazis' persecution of homosexuals, anti-fascists often co-opted the Nazis' own language to argue that Nazi leadership was a clique of homosexuals, not "real men" of the sort who had fought the fascists in Spain.[11]

Freudians tried to explain fascism as a manifestation of sexual dysfunction, such as Rodney Colin's 1934 essay claiming that Germans had turned to Hitler because of mass sexual frustration.[12] Fascism was the collective id unleashed, which had to be restrained by democracy as the collective superego. Fascism was also equated with primitivism, which parallels the nineteenth-century linking of deviant sexuality with "primitive" religions (giving us words like "fetish" and "taboo"). Germans were explicitly likened to Neanderthals and Cro-Magnons, via the pseudoscience of physiognomy. Freud's disciple Wilhelm Reich wrote that, "The formation of the authoritarian structure takes place through the anchoring of sexual inhibition and sexual anxiety."[13]

Although Nazisploitation is generally thought of as a post-WWII phenomenon, its roots were apparent during the war. The propaganda film *Hitler's Children* (1943)[14] illustrated the evils of fascism through sexualized attacks on a woman's body, including the threat of sterilization and a public whipping scene. *So Ends Our Night* (1941)[15] showed German women being sterilized for anything from color blindness to political defiance. Magazine headlines shouted "How Nazis Debauch Paris Womanhood" and "Sex Outrages by Jap Soldiers," and showed blonde women menaced by weapon-wielding men, the swastika or the imperial sun in clear view.[16]

Though some would say that World War II ended with a cathartic victory of good over evil, the Nazi returned again and again, particularly as a sexualized threat. Nazis came to have a symbolic function as a floating signifier for the abject in simplistic narratives of good and evil. Even feminists had their own rhetorical uses for Nazis, from Betty Friedan comparing American suburban female life to a "comfortable concentration camp" in *The Feminine Mystique* (1963) to Germaine Greer referring to "Nazi anthropologists" in *The Female Eunuch* (1970).

Beginning in the early 1960s, American men's adventure magazines spawned an even less reputable subgenre of "leg shackler" magazines that played out sadomasochistic scenes on their lurid covers, with women in peril while handsome Anglo men fought Nazis and Japanese. Over time, the scenarios became more extreme, and the male heroes dropped out, leaving only fascist men and women menacing captive women (and occasionally men) with a wide variety of tortures and mutilation. These magazines sometimes had the same illustrators and scenarios as the "weird menace" pulps of the 1930s, with the aggressor figure, once vaguely Oriental, now wearing a swastika. Later in the Cold War era, the magazines shifted to Communism as the deviant Other, exchanging the swastika for the hammer and sickle, but the scenes were basically the same. Russian or Chinese Communists were also depicted as sexually deviant and even physically monstrous, drawing in elements of Orientalism.

As the Vietnam War escalated and second-wave feminism emerged, heroism was no longer about saving distressed women:

> The new, unspoken heroes were not saviors, but the hardest and most degenerate torturers who wear Satanic hoods and are assisted by hunchbacked horror film outcasts. Even the long-despised swastika is seen as symbolizing a suppressed manhood that rids itself of women who humiliate and degrade by virtue of the superiority of their looks.[17]

On the other hand, the illustrators and writers were often known for their satire and black humor, and "the tongues were packed in cheek, and sometimes they spilled out. As long as buyers were roped in, publishers overlooked the dark 'in' humor."[18] Over the 1960s, leg shacklers shifted their attention to domestic enemies, such as juvenile delinquents, bikers, and hippies, before being superseded by soft-core and hard-core pornography magazines.

The American Nazisploitation magazines produced a strange offshoot in the Stalag novels published in Israel in the early 1960s. Stalag novels were pulpy tales of sex and violence, presented as Hebrew translations of English-language true-war stories, with macho, Gentile bylines like "Victor Boulder" and "Ralph Butcher." Their covers bore art pirated from American "leg shacklers." Typically a British or American male soldier or airman ("Stalags almost never featured Jewish characters."[19]) is captured, and held in a prison run by female guards, described with fetishized detail:

> There was nothing peculiar about the soldiers.... Nothing exceptional, but the physical fact that the soldiers *were women*. Two platoons of female SS storm troopers, wearing tight pants, shining boots, and vests from clothe that stretched across tall and upright breasts. Beneath the caps sprouted short army haircuts, but the hair was fine and the necks feminine and slim.[20]

Stalag novels differed from their American counterparts in emphasizing the domination of men by women, and by the seductive power of female guards. "Even as they plot rebellion, the soldiers are compelled to obey their sex-crazed dominators with a mixture of pleasure and revulsion."[21]

"The narrative structure common across the genre consists of three main phases: initial downfall; captivity and transgression; breakout and revenge."[22] This is the familiar ritual cycle of separation-transgression-integration, as seen in tales of Barbary Coast slavery, American captivity narratives, and antebellum slave narratives.

The fantastic prison camps of the Stalag novels were isolated realms of transgression, a world turned upside down. The Aryans were decadents, capable of anything, driven by irrational impulses. Gender roles were inverted: male Nazi officers were effeminate, while female Nazis were brutish.[23] "[W]hat makes this captivity special is the constant potential of transgression within it."[24] Nazis were depicted as "inherently bipolar," a civilized exterior failing to contain a beast within.

The transgression of the norms of the reader's Israeli society can only be atoned for by the destruction of the outside force. The novels end with escape and/or bloody revenge, setting the world to rights again. The Stalags coincided with the trial of Adolf Eichmann and the breaking of the taboo about discussing the Jewish experience of the Holocaust, and they were immensely popular with the postwar generation of Israeli youth dealing with specific anxieties of sexuality and national and ethnic identity.

Though the first true Nazisploitation movie was *Love Camp Seven* (1969), the genre flourished in the mid- and late-1970s, a time of increasing liberalization of film production, and a greater interest in making explicit the sex and violence that earlier filmmakers had to imply. The genre included both sophisticated films that explored the legacy of fascism and the Holocaust, and pulpy exploitation that dealt in shock and thrills, though the dividing line could be razor fine.

If there's an image that epitomizes 1970s kink, it's Charlotte Rampling in Liliana Cavini's *The Night Porter* (1974): singing a Marlene Dietrich song to SS officer Max and the German guards, topless, wearing an SS officer's cap, trousers, boots, and suspenders, as if she has adopted the appearance of her captors as protective coloration.[25] The scene ends with Max giving Lucia a gift: the head of the inmate who was brutalizing the others. By pretending to give her power, he has cast her in his fantasy as Salome, a frequent topic of nineteenth-century art about the seductive power of women.

Chronologically, the movie starts with Lucia as a young girl of ambiguous age in the prewar era, before she and her family are captured. Max, an SS officer, picks her out of a lineup of nude concentration camp prisoners, for his favorite. It's implied that Lucia went through her sexual awakening and maturation from girl to woman in a concentration camp, under Max's tutelage. Her ideals were men who had the power of life and death over her, and her only agency came through pleasing and even mimicking them, becoming a kind of mascot figure.

Other flashbacks in the concentration camp have the atmosphere of dreams or nightmares, or recollections by Max or Lucia of events so bizarre that they seem to be another world, with an extra layer of gauze added by the years. In this world, anything was possible.

Years after the war, Max lives quietly as a night porter in a luxury hotel, serving as servant, pimp, drug pusher, audience, and more for the people who live and work there. Lucia, now an adult, arrives at Max's hotel and threatens to reveal his secret but also to destabilize his detachment. Max's retired Nazi comrades may kill her to conceal his secrets, or he may have to do it himself. Lucia herself is torn between hate and love, revenge and mercy.

In *The Night Porter*, all relationships are ambiguous and reversible. Max is both servant and master of his guests. Lucia both threatens to reveal Max's criminal past and awakens feelings of love. When Max and Lucia finally meet face-to-face postwar, they go through a cascade of different emotions in a single shot: fear, hate, rage, guilt, shame, lust, and even love.

Max and Lucia barricade themselves in Max's apartment, until they begin starving, knowing they will be killed by one party or another if they go outside. They fall into their old patterns from the concentration camp: Max as protector/jailer, Lucia as prisoner/object of desire. At last, they go outside and are gunned down together. They are the ambiguity of desire in a world that wants only black and white.

The other best-known example of the Nazisploitation genre is *Ilsa: She Wolf of the SS*,[26] starring Dyanne Thorne in the title role. While *The Night Porter* aspired to art-house respectability, *Ilsa* headed straight to the grindhouse (see Figure 8.1).

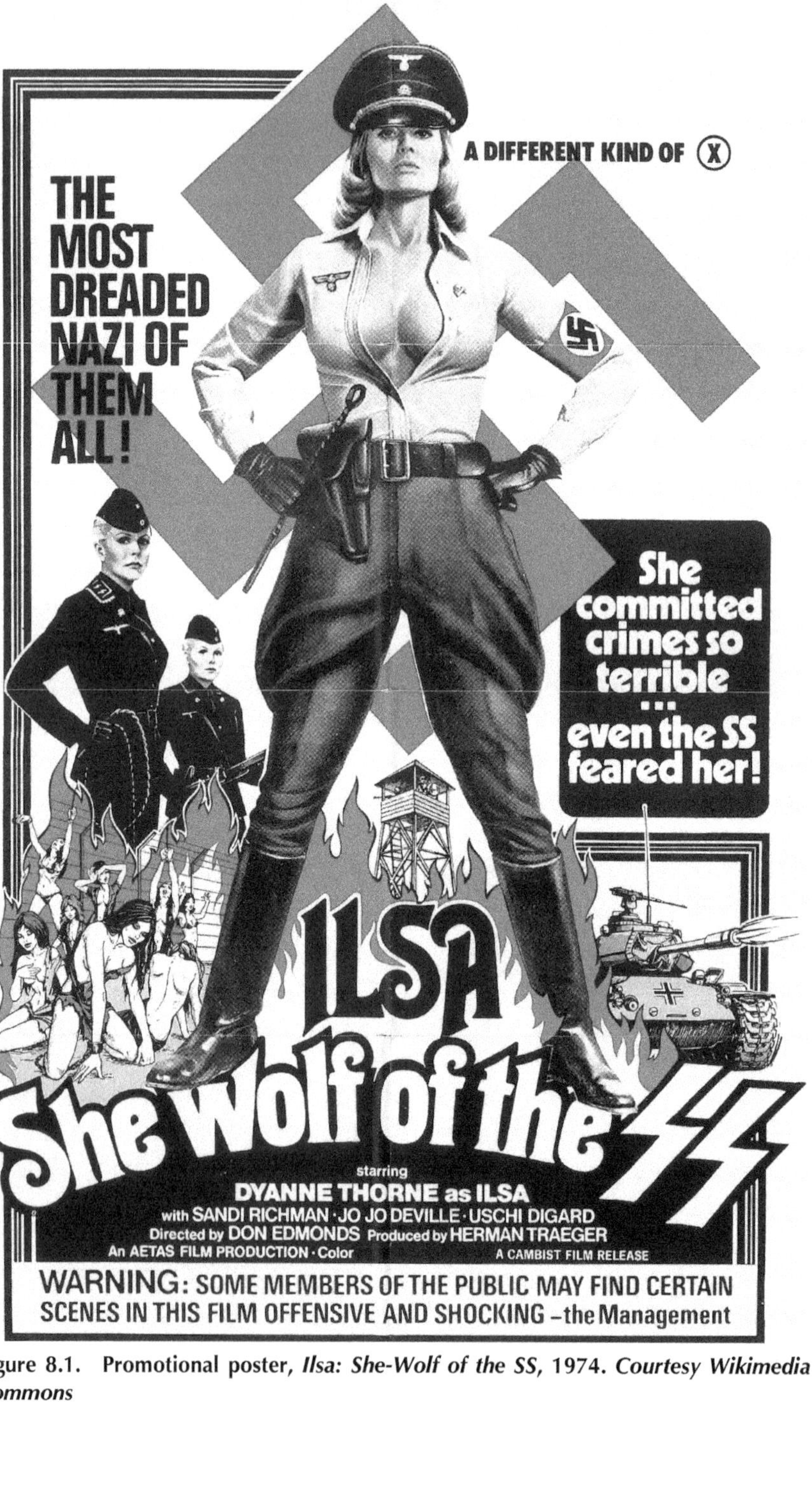

Figure 8.1. Promotional poster, *Ilsa: She-Wolf of the SS*, 1974. *Courtesy Wikimedia Commons*

David F. Friedman, *Ilsa*'s producer, was in the US Army Signal Corps in the mid-1940s, and worked on films about the newly liberated concentration camps, using the shocking images of emaciated survivors and stacked corpses. Later, Friedman worked on the anti-Communist film *Halfway to Hell* (1953), which used similar shock imagery, then produced and played a bit part in *Love Camp Seven* (1969), then produced the first *Ilsa* movie in 1974.[27] This is the familiar blurring of lines between propaganda and exploitation we've seen in treatments of Mediterranean and Atlantic slavery. *Ilsa* even begins with a title card and a voice-over claiming the film's historical accuracy, making it a bizarre parody of the real atrocities of Nazi concentration camps.

Don Edmonds, the director, described his conversation with Friedman:

> The things that are in *Ilsa*, I told him at the time, "You wanna see this stuff? Because I can put it on the screen for you. You want to pull back and cut away?" And he said, "No." And I said, "Then I'm going to give it to you, brother". . . And I did.[28]

In the film, the women sent to Ilsa's camp are divided into two groups. Some are sent for "work detail" of sexually serving the men in the guardhouse. The others are beaten, electrocuted, boiled, suffocated, and more in "experiments" overseen by the uniformed Ilsa and her female assistants. Ilsa's ostensible reason for this is to demonstrate that women can endure as much pain as men and prove that women can serve the Reich by fighting on the front line. Thus, Ilsa and her female subordinates are a feminist insurgency within Nazism, usurping male prerogatives like authority, violence, and sexual service.

Male prisoners get one night with Ilsa, after which she has them castrated. This changes with the arrival of the prisoner Wolfe, a German-American soldier with the ability to withhold ejaculation indefinitely. Ilsa is so taken with Wolfe's indefatigable penis that he alone survives a night with her intact.

Whereas Wolfe represents ideal masculinity, the general who oversees Ilsa's camp is a masochistic freak. He tops Ilsa from the bottom by demanding that she strip down to just her uniform tunic and stockings, then urinate on him. The camera focuses on Ilsa's face, grimacing in disgust and humiliation as she complies with his command.

At the climax of the film, Wolfe seduces Ilsa into letting him tie her to her bed, then leads the prisoners in revolt. One of Ilsa's bloody female victims tries to stab Ilsa to death, but she passes out or dies before she can finish the job. After the prisoners escape, German forces arrive, and an officer kills Ilsa, on orders from the general, and then burns the camp down so there is no evidence.

The last shot is of Wolfe and one of the female prisoners standing together, watching the fire; proper sexual and gender roles are restored by the death of Ilsa. The struggle of democracy versus fascism is displaced onto the struggle of patriarchal society against insurgent femininity. It's as if one deviant woman is somehow more evil than the entire Nazi hierarchy.

The Ilsa character was extremely loosely based on the notorious Ilse Koch, wife of Karl-Otto Koch, the camp commandant of Buchenwald and Majdanek. Koch and her husband were tried and imprisoned by the SS for embezzlement and murdering prisoners. After she was released for lack of evidence, during the Allied occupation of Germany she was captured and tried again for war crimes. Witnesses testified she had numerous affairs with camp guards and inmates, and exposed herself to inmates. Like her fictional counterpart, Koch was seen as a monster by both sides of the conflict.

Compare Koch to Delphine LaLaurie of antebellum New Orleans. A fire in her home in 1834 revealed dead, mutilated, and bound slaves in her attic. This set off a riot that forced LaLaurie and her family to flee to France. Long after her death in 1842, LaLaurie became a figure of folklore, legendary for her supposed lasciviousness and sadism toward her slaves. In the Italian exploitation/historical film *Addio Zio Tom (Goodbye Uncle Tom)* (1971),[29] LaLaurie was depicted as a beautiful woman who slinked around her mansion in a see-through gown while torturing male slaves. Whether the real LaLaurie's treatment of her slaves was worse than typical for her time and place is beside the point. This is the realm of myth, in which the deviant woman becomes the scapegoat for a deviant society.

Despite her character's death at the end of *Ilsa: She Wolf of the SS*, Dyanne Thorne reprised her role in three sequels, each of which associated Ilsa with a different tyrannical regime: Middle Eastern petro-states in *Ilsa, Harem Keeper of the Oil Sheiks* (1976),[30] Latin American dictatorships in *Ilsa, the Wicked Warden* (1977),[31] and Stalinist gulags in *Ilsa, the Tigress of Siberia* (1977).[32] At the end of each film, Ilsa is defeated if not killed, but she comes back, apparently not aging and immortal. The films serve as a repetitive ritual, with the Ilsa figure as a sacrificial scapegoat, embodying all seductive, deviant politics and sexuality, who is destroyed, only to rise again. The image of the monstrous, sexually deviant woman can be attached to any deviant political system.

Ilsa's symbolic sisters were *les femmes tondues*, women of post-WWII France who allegedly committed "horizontal collaboration" with German occupiers, and during the Liberation were publicly shaved bald, stripped naked, and paraded through the streets as punishment. The *Ilsa* films and the ritualized abuse of *les femmes tondues* both provide female scapegoats who embody unacceptable politics (violence and collaboration, respectively), express them through deviant sexuality (female sadism and female promiscuity, respectively) and are publicly punished, restoring moral/sexual order to the universe. However, that conflict is never permanently resolved, and the ritual must be repeated; thus, there's always a sequel.

Pier Paolo Pasolini's *Salò* (1975)[33] furthered the association of fascism with deviant sexuality. The film is loosely based on Sade's *120 Days of Sodom*, with the story transplanted to an isolated Italian villa at the end of World War II. The Italian fascists assume that it is only a matter of time until the Allied forces arrive and execute them, so they take the opportunity to use the last of their absolute power. Like Sade's libertine aristocrats, they create a miniature world in mockery of the real world, parodying government and religion.

While *Ilsa* displaced the evil of fascism onto one aberrant woman, Tinto Brass's *Salon Kitty* (1976)[34] viewed fascism as a more universal relationship dynamic of abject obedience, sadist and masochist, pimp and whore. To blackmail his way into power in the Third Reich, SS officer Wallenberg coerces brothel keeper Madame Kitty into dismissing her troupe of bodily and ethnically diverse prostitutes and replacing them with his handpicked cohort of Aryan whores. These women are introduced in scenes that emphasize their abnormal cruelty: women and brownshirt men tease each other in a pig slaughterhouse, a woman is more devoted to the image of Hitler than her own family, and a Hitler Youth girl crushes a Jewish boy's wind-up toy beneath her shoe.

Wallenberg orchestrates a military-like exercise in which the women couple with an equal number of strapping Aryan men in a gymnasium. Next, the women are placed in cells with a veritable zoo of people deemed degenerate by Nazi ideology (e.g., a lesbian, a Jew, a Romany, a man missing his legs) and told to have intercourse with them. Wallenberg watches with clinical detachment. In his view, the ideal Nazi woman will fuck anyone and anything on demand. Fascism's professed ideals of maternity, domesticity, and racial purity are subordinate to the requirement of obedience, the desire to exalt himself and see others willingly debased.

Kitty's brothel allows the possibility of love (even lesbian love), while Wallenberg's fascism is decadent, sterile, narcissistic, and fetishistic, fixated on the trappings of power. Out of uniform, he still wears Nazi-themed clothing, such as the silver lamé suit with SS insignia he sports while snorting cocaine. Even naked in the steam bath, where he is killed, Wallenberg wears Nazi forearm bands.

The success and controversy of films like *The Night Porter*, *Salò*, and *Salon Kitty* led to a boom of Nazi-exploitation films in the late 1970s, though they were more about the grindhouse thrills of *Ilsa* than meditations on totalitarianism. These furthered the association of fascism, or rather the iconography of fascism, with deviant and decadent sexuality, as well as a sense of imminent doom that resonated with the alienation and nihilism of the times.

YOU DON'T THINK I'M A NAZI, DO YOU?

Within the kinky subculture, fascism-based scenarios or attire have always been a controversial and minority interest. However, the practice attracts attention and criticism out of proportion to its actual popularity. Anti-s/m critics frequently used fascist imagery and role play as a synecdoche for the BDSM subculture as a whole.

It would be an overstatement to say that all gay men were attracted to the Nazi image. To be certain, there is a resemblance between the SS officer in dress uniform and the classic Tom of Finland leatherman, beautiful male figures in militaristic, black uniforms. (Tom of Finland's men are tough, but they are tender, not cruel.) Yet the SS uniform and the leatherman are both the products of centuries of evolution in male clothing and shifting ideas about the image of the ideal man. Had the Third Reich never happened, black, red, and white would still be an effective color combination, and black clothing on men would still be a symbol of an ascendant elite.

Nonetheless, military uniforms, symbolizing the perfected man, exerted a powerful hold over the gay male imagination, and the SS dress uniform represented an extreme of that, with the additional element of a powerful taboo, a sacred mystery in the ritual.

Arnie Kantrowitz, a founding member of GLAAD, described his brush with Nazi imagery in the early 1970s, when a friend urged him to wear his leatherman cap:

> [A]s I accepted the hat, I noticed a small pin that I hadn't seen before, attached to the band. It was a swastika, held in the talons of an eagle. "Never mind," I said. "I don't want to wear this." . . .
> "Oh, that doesn't mean anything. It's just part of the look. It's nothing to make a big deal about. [. . .] It's only part of the game," he answered, "only an image of power. You don't think I'm a Nazi, do you?"[35]

Kantrowitz saw the swastika appropriated as a symbol of the Hell's Angels, a gesture of defiance to mainstream society, and later picked up by gays. "Many gays . . . see the Angels and other cyclists as Romantic antiheroes, rebellious individualists whose toughness bears imitating. . . . [I]t is only a short step from eroticizing the swastika bearer to eroticizing the genuine fascist."[36] Regardless of history, Nazi imagery was potent precisely because of its transgression of the postwar taboo (a taste shared with BDSM's cousins, punk and heavy metal music culture). It became a favorite target of anti-SM and anti-butch critiques, both inside and outside the gay culture.

Gay male leather magazine *Drummer* launched in 1975, at the height of Nazisploitation. The first three issues included ads for the gay National Socialist League, with the Nazi insignia, that parodied the song "Tomorrow Belongs to Me" from anti-Nazi film *Cabaret* (1972) with the slogan "Tomorrow Belongs to You." Dropping the ads under pressure from both inside and outside the magazine's staff resulted in a lawsuit from the gay Nazis, which *Drummer* lost. Despite criticism, *Drummer* continued to run Nazi-themed pictorials and fiction intermittently through the 1980s and 1990s, often with an element of parody, such as an ad showing an SS officer dominating a *Drummer* reader, with the caption, "You Vill Read *Drummer*." Personal ads also referenced the fascist type. Jack Fritscher, *Drummer*'s founding editor in chief, argued that the gay male appreciation of the Nazi aesthetic was filtered through a healthy layer of parody and camp, like laughing at comedies like *The Great Dictator* (1940) and *The Producers* (1967), or enjoying the stylized dramas of *Seven Beauties* (1975) and *The Night Porter*.[37]

Outsiders were troubled by the fetishization of fascism in sadomasochism. In 1975, *The Village Voice* published Richard Goldstein's "S&M: The Dark Side of Gay Liberation."[38] The article provides a snapshot of the New York gay leather scene in the mid-1970s, when it was already bemoaning its visibility and the consequent presence of "fluff" tourists and poseurs. The author started with "the association between SM and authoritarianism, even genocide" though he acknowledges that over the last twenty years a more tolerant attitude has emerged. His article ended with an interview with gay leather artist "Rex," described as a "Naziphile," who said:

[T]he greatest SM trip in history was the Nazis. It's so rousing, so Teutonic. It touches, I think, a chord in man. The Nazis were a brilliant test-tube example of modern man. And it will come about again, through the chaos and mediocrity of capitalism. As we enter this great financial crisis, the scruples will fall left and right. [. . .] It's coming—the spying and the concentration camps, a world run by gangsters—but without the style and the imagination of the Nazis.

"Rex" saw Americans as the new people destined to battle Asia. He played a scratchy recording of the music from Nazi propaganda film *Triumph of the Will* (1935), and talked about how "many people in those camps received some sexual gratification from what happened to them." ("I'm starting to feel nauseated," writes the author.)

Born the year World War II ended, "Rex's" view of Nazism was purely aesthetic. It had nothing to do with German history or politics, or anti-Semitism. This was the postwar generation, who did not experience World War II or the Holocaust directly but mediated through the Adolf Eichmann trial, fiction, and nonfiction books and films, and other secondhand phenomena.[39]

The emergence of Nazi chic, associated with deviant sexuality, gay and straight, was met with consternation from liberal intellectuals.

In 1975, the *New York Review of Books* published Susan Sontag's essay "Fascinating Fascism" in which she reviewed two seemingly unrelated publications. The first was the photo book *The Last of the Nuba*, by Leni Riefenstahl, a German actress and filmmaker best known as the director of the Nazi propaganda film *Triumph of the Will*. Sontag considered the photo essay on the African Nuba people an example of the "mystic warrior on the brink of annihilation" kind of thinking that fostered Nazism.

> Fascist aesthetics include but go far beyond the rather special celebration of the primitive to be found in *The Nuba*. They also flow from (and justify) a preoccupation with situations of control, submissive behavior, extravagant effort, and the endurance of pain; they endorse two seemingly opposite states, egomania and servitude. . . . Fascist art glorifies surrender, it exalts mindlessness, it glamorizes death.[40]

That the world considered Riefenstahl's new art worthy suggested to Sontag that we had not completely purged ourselves of fascistic impulses, and sadomasochism was another indication of that.

The second book Sontag considered was *SS Regalia*, a catalog of uniforms, equipment, and other historical artifacts, which led her to the same question asked by Foucault.

> In the sex shops, the baths, the leather bars, the brothels, people are dragging out their gear. But why? Why has Nazi Germany, which was a sexually repressive society, become erotic? How could a regime which persecuted homosexuals become a gay turn-on?[41]

Sontag's answer was that BDSM is the result of too much freedom, too much choice, which naturally tends toward depersonalization, without intimacy or connection.

> Sadomasochism is to sex what war is to civil life; the magnificent experience. . . . As the social contract seems tame in comparison to war, so fucking and sucking come to seem merely nice, and therefore unexciting. The end to which all sexual experience tends, as Bataille insisted in a lifetime of writing, is defilement, blasphemy. To be "nice," as to be civilized, means being alienated from this savage experience—which is entirely staged.[42]

The fad for Nazi regalia indicates . . . a response to an oppressive freedom of choice in sex (and in other matters), to an unbearable degree of individuality; the rehearsal of enslavement rather than its reenactment.[43]

Sontag had little good to say about BDSM: "The color is black, the material is leather, the seduction is beauty, the justification is honesty, the aim is ecstasy, the fantasy is death."[44] Like Goldstein, she viewed fascist symbols within BDSM as the ultimate form, rather than just one branch within many.

In the late 1970s and 1980s, lesbian-feminists adopted Sontag's thesis and frequently invoked fascism, or other forms of violent authoritarianism, in their critiques of lesbian sadomasochism. In this discourse, the minority of lesbian sadomasochists who wore fascist symbols or enacted fascist-derived scenarios stood in for the whole.

The anthology *Against Sadomasochism: A Radical Feminist Analysis* (1982)[45] included several works that drew connections between kink and fascism. Editor Robin Ruth Linden cited the infamous 1971 Stanford Prison experiment that suggested that ordinary people will act sadistically given the slightest excuse.[46] "By generalizing from the prison simulation to sadomasochism, we can infer that enacting dominant and submissive roles would be habituating rather than cathartic."[47]

Sarah Lucia Hoagland's "Sadism, Masochism and Lesbian-Feminism" also claimed, without support, that fascism corresponded with deviant sexuality.

> Have we forgotten or failed to inform ourselves that some nazi men found the torture of Jews highly erotic? Have we forgotten or failed to inform ourselves that some nazi men experienced orgasm while watching Jews being beaten, tortured, mutilated, gassed, destroyed? It is just not true that all areas of eroticism should be explored by Lesbian-feminists or anyone else.[48]

In her essay "Swastikas: The Street and the University," Susan Leigh Star described walking in the Castro district of San Francisco, and seeing people wearing leather and chains, and magazines with Nazi Germany uniforms.

> In particular, the swastikas trigger my troubled street sense, although by now I think I've generalized the response. Somebody in black leather is a

bit like the man in the proverbial alley. Simple fellow (or sister) passer-by in the alley, I'm not going to stick around to find out [if they are dangerous]. A similar analysis could be made of whips and chains but the swastika example best illustrates my feelings about symbols of sadomasochism.[49]

Star wrote that a psychological experience cannot be separated from historical context. Wearing a swastika, or employing whips and chains, for whatever reason, cannot be separated from their effect on other people: the Jews or homosexuals or women who see them as signs of danger, the fascists who see them as signs of acceptance of their ideologies. She said that she would reevaluate those symbols if and when she is certain the real-world oppression they reference is extinct.[50]

Sheila Jeffreys's essay "Sadomasochism: The Erotic Cult of Fascism,"[51] written in 1984 when she was part of Lesbians against Sadomasochism, cited various fictional movies and plays published in the postwar era to suggest a link between sadomasochism and fascism. Jeffreys argued that fascist symbols, even in jest, should not be tolerated, because fascism was still a threat, and especially to queer people.

> Fascists get exactly the same "fun" out of wearing swastikas that S/M proponents do, power from other women's fear and distress. One serious danger that will result from tolerance of nazi insignia in the gay scene, under the guise of "fun," sexual practice, or fashion, is the paralysis of our will or ability to act in the face of actual fascist violence. It is as important now to challenge and reject the sporting of nazi emblems as it was in Germany in the twenties and thirties as fascism took hold.[52]

Jeffreys added, "I would say that most [S/M proponents] are not fascists, even though experiencing pleasure from the terrorising of other lesbians by wearing fascist regalia comes pretty close, but promoters of fascist values."[53] She also saw normative heterosexuality as inherently sadomasochistic, and masochism as the powerless, especially women, eroticizing their oppression.[54]

> The construction of S/M sexuality is a mighty clever ploy for the oppressor. Our resistance is undermined in our very guts if our response to the torture of others or to the trappings of militarism is erotic rather than politically indignant. It is very hard to fight what turns you on. This is a problem

which feminists fighting porn have already recognised and understood. It feels humiliating and paralysing to be turned on by the very degradation of women that you wish to challenge. The only way to fight is to turn that pain into anger.[55]

There's an element of Judeo-Christian thought in this, in which the body and its pleasures are necessarily opposed to the mind and its political/ spiritual development.

The collection *Unleashing Feminism* (1993)[56] took a slightly different view. Jamie Lee Evans's essay opened with:

> I believe the not-guilty verdict against the batterers of Rodney King was a decision based on racism as well as a product of analysis brought forth via a culture indoctrinated with violence and sadomasochistic beliefs.[57]

Her theory was based on a statement from jurors in the King case, who said they thought that King was partly in control of the situation in which he was beaten.

> The only way anyone could think that someone on the bottom of a beating was in control, is by way of sm thinking. The common belief and propaganda in sm is that the bottom is "in control." We are told that they are in power of "determining" *how long, how much and how severe* their violent violation will be. Sound familiar? . . .
>
> There was no "safe word" in the Rodney King beating because the truth of the matter is *there is no safe word when you are being beaten!*[58]

Irene Reti drew connections between sadomasochism and authoritarianism, again without evidence.

> [S]adomasochism was an integral part of the Holocaust; there were many "real Nazis" involved in "kinky sexual scenes." One of the purposes of this essay is to demonstrate that fact. Whips, chains, racks, shackles, and other instruments and methods are our inheritance—passed down through history.[59]

Irene Reti wrote that SM doesn't just resemble or take inspiration from fascism; historical violence *is* SM. "Sadomasochism has been around for a long time, but the Holocaust was a particularly recent and virulent occurrence of SM." She does backpedal somewhat on the next page: "Obviously the people in the camps were not enjoying themselves, nor were they there out of any kind of choice. But I think we must ask ourselves—*why is this enjoyable*? What are these rituals doing in our sexuality?"[60]

Likewise, D. A. Clarke said that sadomasochism sugarcoats fascism.

> It was Dr. Einstein who said that you cannot simultaneously prevent and prepare for war; I firmly believe that you cannot simultaneously oppose and worship violence. People who find whips exciting and bruises alluring, Nazi regalia attractive and slavery titillating, will have a hard time suspending their love affair with evil for long enough to oppose it.[61]

In these essays, the connection between sadomasochistic sexuality and fascist politics was seen as a given, without much in the way of support. Sadomasochism was said to be both the beginning of the slippery slope to fascism and its driving psychology.

As World War II and the Holocaust faded further into the past and became more mythology than history, the SS officer became the perfect prefab villain, divorced from any historical specificity. In the hard-core BDSM videos produced by Hungarian porn company Mood Pictures, women in Nazi uniforms are just another set of stock characters, and the explicit references to the July 20 *putsch* are just a premise for the flagellation action.

> [I]n our day and age, the myth of Nazi Germany that is perpetuated by the mass media has usurped the actual events that occurred more than half a century ago in such a way that the historical referent has been lost, not "even though" but "precisely because" it is repeatedly resurrected in popular culture. These fictional reincarnations do not even attempt any "real" connections to the past, but are rather exclusively driven by concerns of the solipsistic present.[62]

They don't reference actual atrocities, but other cinematic depictions of atrocities. Compare this to Anna Freud's theory of fantasy as repeatedly reworked scenarios. We've already reached the point at which Barbary Coast slavery is acceptable fodder for fantasy, regardless of the suffering of actual captives centuries ago. It is only a matter of time until Nazi and

Holocaust imagery sheds its moral weight and become just another set of images.

The same patterns played out in the US-Iraq war, though not necessarily in the way expected. When US Army private Jessica Lynch was lost in Iraq, the initial story followed the standard captivity narrative of American history: separation, peril from foreign men, rescue. In reality, far from slavering beasts eager to defile white womanhood, the Iraqis who found Lynch rescued her, desperately struggled to keep her alive, and were prevented from returning her because no Iraqi could get near a US outpost without being shot at.

The neo-colonialist narrative of America as a civilizing force in Iraq took another hit with the appearance of reports and pictures of the abuses of Iraqi prisoners in Abu Ghraib. American soldier Lynndie England became an icon, photographed pointing at naked prisoners' genitals while grinning, or holding a leash wrapped around the throat of a naked prisoner lying on the floor. These pictures catalyzed discussions about the morality and efficacy of torture in time of war, and added terms like "stress position" and "waterboarding" to the cultural lexicon.

A few years later, the Mexican adult comic *Relatos de Presidio* ("Stockade Tales") printed a cover with illustrations based on the iconic Abu Ghraib pictures, though England was depicted as more shapely and enticing. It took only a few years for Abu Ghraib to become a topic for satire and erotica.

To answer Foucault and Sontag's question, Nazisploitation is a by-product of the ongoing process of history transforming into myth. By associating a threatening Other with the transgression of taboos, symbols are created that may be manipulated in rituals. Earlier generations adopted the symbols of the threatening, and often defeated, Other: the fez and cummerbund of the Turk, the nun's habit and black hassock of Catholicism, the mohawk and buckskin of the "Indian" warrior. Repeating this with the symbols of the great transgressors of the twentieth century is unsurprising. When we restage the battle of good and evil, purity and impurity, sacred and profane, somebody has to play the bad guy.

The difference between fascism and sadomasochism lies not in the scene, but in the interpretation of it. A sadomasochistic narrative is about both of the parties involved, with the constantly shifting point of view identified by Freud. A truly fascist narrative is only about the fascist. What we see in works ranging from D. H. Lawrence's authoritarian novels to Jean Genet's plays to Sylvia Plath's poem "Daddy" ("Every woman adores a fascist . . .") are relationships that may not be consensual, but are reciprocal.

As Laura Frost wrote:

> In sadomasochistic fantasy, the characters are engaged with one another's desires and move, however circuitously, toward pleasure. In scenes of fascist violence, consent, recognition, and exchange among the characters are missing, as is erotic pleasure. These distinctions are lost when we read purely for thematic content, that is, when we note merely the fascist images in sexual scenarios. These texts must be read with an attention to erotic investment and inticement, for shifts in agency, and for the differences between historically faithful representations of fascism and a clearly distorted fantasy of fascism.[63]

Other writers have distinguished between the fascist mentality and the sadomasochistic mentality, despite superficial appearances.

> Georges Bataille . . . distinguishes fascist "sadism" from sadomasochistic eroticism as a form of sexuality that does not literally destroy. In *At the Mind's Limits*, Jean Amery, writing on his survival of Nazi imprisonment and torture, directly addresses the question of whether the Nazis were "sadomasochists" in the conventional sense. He asserts that Bataille's explanation of sadism/cruelty is resonant with his own experience with the SS. "[The Gestapo] were bureaucrats of torture. And yet, they were also much more. I saw it in their serious, tense faces, which were not swelling, let us say, with sexual-sadistic delight, but concentrated in murderous self-realization."[64]

An actual Nazi brought forward in time to view *Ilsa: She-Wolf of the SS* or one of the *Drummer* pictorials would be appalled by these parodies. The swastika was now associated with everything the Nazis thought they were saving Germany from: homosexuality, decadence, effeminate men, masculinized women, deviant sexuality.

Even so, the unironic, sincere use of fascist imagery continued in various forms in Europe and America. In the mid-2010s, and especially during the 2016 US presidential election season, the so-called alt-right came into public view. Savvy in the use of modern media, this loose conglomeration of groups re-re-appropriated fascist symbols and imagery. The "Unite the Right" protesters who gathered in Charlottesville, Virginia on the weekend of August 11, 2017, deployed torch-lit night marches, slogans like "Blood and soil," and symbols like the *Schwarze Sonne* (Black Sun) or an eagle carrying a fasces, or bundle of rods. They are drawn to those symbols precisely because they are transgressive, because they frighten and enrage their perceived enemies.

The alt-right is driven by the fragile paranoia and alienation of a certain strain of heterosexual white male, and they project their chosen persona of masculine power. In the sexual realm, this includes a contempt for feminism and a preference for reactionary gender roles. Proud Boys, a self-described "pro-Western fraternal organization" founded by *Vice* magazine co-founder Gavin McInnes, urges members to refrain from masturbation and pornography. Jack Donovan, an out gay writer and skinhead icon, expresses his contempt for consensual BDSM while lauding all-male gangs as the ideal society.

The movement's fascist iconography, sincere or not, is definitely attached to the fascist politics of white supremacy, anti-Semitism, misogyny, and anti-democracy. They're not kidding around.

Chapter Nine

The Velvet Underground

There is an informal uniform to sadomasochistic gatherings, visible at any play party or fetish night. Even people who aren't fetishists per se will adopt elements of this style to indicate their belongingness to this subculture. The overwhelming color is, of course, black, a color with complex associations. Style gestures toward extremes of masculine ruggedness, derived from military uniforms or working clothes, or feminine display, with cleavage, wasp waists, visible garters, and stockings. Female attire walks a fine line between the "spikiness and hardness" of high heels and corsets, and the vulnerability of exposed legs and breasts. The style is immediately recognizable, but it wasn't designed. Instead, it was cobbled together out of a century of accumulated associations.

In the three decades following World War II, America developed several different sadomasochistic subcultures that evolved in near-complete isolation, with only occasional direct contact. The men who built the gay leather subculture knew almost nothing about the artists and distributors who built heterosexual SM culture, and vice versa.

GAY LEATHER

After the war, a generation of men returned home to peacetime. Whether due to awakened homosexuality in the all-male society of the military, or just a distaste for the new American dream of job and family, many of these men created an alternative culture that continued the outdoor homosociality and initiatory experience of military life. This was eventually refined into the leatherman culture, which does not completely overlap with gay SM culture.

It should be noted that, long before the postwar leatherman style evolved in the mid-1950s, there was a gay sadomasochistic culture in America, going back at least to the 1930s. Not well organized, it relied on coded language like "Sadie Mazie" for SM.[1] Samuel M Steward describes his early life in S/M before there was a Scene:

> There was no crowd as there is today. There were isolated individuals who might tie you up and beat the hell out of you. Ah . . . but it was dangerous. And you didn't know . . . in the early days, even as late as the forties, you didn't . . . ah . . . there was no codification of it. No ritualization of SM as there is today. It was catch as catch can. But . . . ah . . . Sadie Mazzies were looked down on by all of us ordinary, normal homosexuals in the twenties and the thirties. We thought that was too extravagant. And that didn't . . . that happened only in Berlin![2]

Even finding equipment was difficult.

> [I]n the 1930s, I had become interested in S/M. . . . In those days there were no leather shops, no specialty stores; and leather jackets were unheard of and unavailable except in police equipment outlets that would generally not sell to civilians. I finally found my first one in Sears-Roebuck's basement in Chicago. And I had unearthed—literally, for his saddlery shop was in a cellar on North Avenue—a little man who braided a few whips for me, and even found a "weveling" Danish cat-o'-nine-tails crocheted from heavy white twine, and located also a handsome crop of twisted willow wood.
>
> My introduction to S/M had begun with my answering a personal ad in the columns of the *Saturday Review of Literature*, a weekly publication out of New York City. In those days some of the wordings and contents of the ads were mildly outrageous for the times, growing wilder until the publishing of them was entirely stopped by the guardians of our American purity. The one that caught my attention [in August 1947] ran something like:
>
> > *Should flogging be allowed? Ex-sailor welcomes opinions and replies. Box . . .*[3]

Answering that ad put Steward in touch with Hal Baron, a former sailor dedicated to connecting every S (sadist) with an M (masochist) that he could. He introduced Steward to other men who had answered the ad.[4]

Steward, then a college teacher, was interviewed by the controversial Dr. Alfred Kinsey, and became an unofficial collaborator on Kinsey's sexual research. The two men shared interests in sexuality and record keeping; Steward kept a comprehensive list of his many sexual encounters in his "Stud File" of index cards, often noted as "sadie-maisie" or "sad-mashy."[5] Kinsey invented the term "S/M" (pronounced "ess-em") as part of his group's elaborate alphanumeric code for discussing sexual topics discretely. In 1952, Kinsey arranged a meeting between Steward and Mike Miksche, a freelance illustrator and erotic artist under the alias "Steve Masters," as M (masochist) and S (sadist) respectively. Kinsey filmed this two-day encounter, the first homosexual encounter so recorded for the archives, as if documenting the mating habits of a rare species of lemur.[6] (The film was financed by money earmarked for "mammalian studies."[7]) Miksche was connected to Bob Milne, the hub of New York's circle of gay sadomasochists.[8]

Later in his life, Steward pursued many other men whom he hoped would be the "S" of his fantasies, often to great disappointment. Chuck Renslow, the Chicago-based publisher of beefcake and leather magazines and owner of the Gold Coast leather bar, sent Steward young hustlers, and each had to read a numbered "handout" before the session on how Steward was to be (mis)treated. Titled "What This Particular M Likes," it included instructions like "Please remember: he is your absolute slave" and "Piss in his mouth (a little, not too much . . .)" and "Give him a few whacks on the ass with your belt. Or use whip if one present."[9] Like Sacher-Masoch, Steward wanted nothing left to chance.

When leatherman culture began formalizing in the late 1950s, the aging Steward couldn't adapt. His ambivalence about other homosexuals made him solitary and antisocial, and he believed that his desire for sex with rough, working-class or criminal-class, heterosexual men that was always on the brink of real violence, could not be domesticated. He wrote an essay called "Pussies in Boots":

> An artificial hierarchy, a ritual, and a practice have been superimposed over a very real need of the human spirit [to locate that which is authentically masculine] . . . [but] the entire affair has become a ritual, a Fun and Games sort of thing, and in essence there is no difference today between a female impersonator or drag-queen and a leather-boy in full leather-drag. Both are dressing up to represent something they are not. . . .

It is difficult to say at what point in such a "movement" the degeneration sets in, and the elements of parody and caricature make their first appearance. Perhaps the decay began when the first M decided that he, too, could wear leather as well as the big butch S he so much admired. And so he bought himself a leather jacket.[10]

Thom Magister described the early days of the leatherman culture built by men like Steward, Renslow, and Baron:

In the early 1950s the leather scene in California was a strictly serious business. The men involved in S/M action lived by a code. There was no tolerance, as there is today, for phonies and onlookers, although there were always plenty of them. Since there were no popular leather magazines, porn videos, or even books to inform the novice, everything was passed on by legend and word-of-mouth tradition—just like any other nomad tribe. The worlds of S/M, leathermen, and leather-bikermen were intertwined. Gay bikers and straight bikers commingled with little conflict. Their commonality was leather, Harley-Davidson bikes, and painful memories of a war that had disfigured them physically, emotionally, and spiritually. This was not carefree youth on a spree. These men were angry. Hell, they were pissed off! And they could never, ever, go home again. Among outcasts there is little distinction or discrimination. Certainly a kinky sexual preference seemed of little consequence. Just your everyday oddity in a world light-years from reality.

There were gay bars and leather bars and biker bars and tea rooms and truck stops and all the other gathering places of men hungry for sex with other men. But there was, under the surface, another group—hidden—on the prowl among the general population of leathermen. These were the true sadists and masochists who were both serious and devoted. There were no markings—no signals—no keys, no bright, multicolored hankies of identification, no displayed handcuffs and cock rings—just burning eyes and attitude.[11]

Too young for the war, Magister was mentored by veterans through a protracted initiation into "the work" (not "play"). This was a world of apprenticeship, extended courtship, dominants outnumbering submissives, and subtle identification signals like wearing your belt buckle to the right or left of center, to indicate masochist or sadist. The terms and titles used were quite different from those used by later generations.

The terms "S" and "M" were interpreted solely as "sadist" and "masochist" in Magister's circle in L.A. in this period, and "master" (not capitalized) was used only to describe a man who had learned ("mastered") a particular field of kinky technique so thoroughly that he could be creative with it and teach it to others. Someone might be referred to as, say, "a bondage master" or "a master of knives," but never as "Master So-and-So." If a title was needed, "Sir" was used. And no one was called "slave" at all, either during a session or in terms of a relationship dynamic.[12]

Another leatherman of the postwar era, Len G., joined a group of former military men in the Tidewater area of Virginia who met covertly. He described the group's own jargon, which used "Master" and "slave" to distinguish between the masculine men/boys and the others.

The [Tidewater] area was/is considered "Southern," and the lingo was common to the South. Thus "Master-slave" was an almost automatic reference to a more or less enduring Dominant/submissive relationship. "Top," "bottom," "boy," "Man," "Master," "slave," "Sir," "you" were the terms . . . used in the circles that I was involved in.[13]

In this time, the archetypal leatherman look, the signifiers of normative masculinity exaggerated to the brink of absurdity, emerged from the complicated history of gay male fashion, which is always imperfectly mimetic, a tangled mix of "passing, minstrelization and capitulation," to quote sociologist Martin P. Levine.[14]

Even before the trial of Oscar Wilde, there was the trial and acquittal of Ernest Boulton (aka "Fanny") and Frederick Payne (aka "Stella") in 1871, two homosexual men who were also cross-dressers *and* sex workers.[15] Ever since, those three categories have been conflated in the public mind (sometimes with justification). Gay men have overlapped with and been in fashion dialectic with other marginal groups (sex workers, soldiers, sailors, aristocrats, police, punks, bikers, artists, etc.) for a variety of reasons: camouflage, recognition both covert and overt, political statements, defensive intimidation, generational differentiation, heightening male beauty, conspicuous consumption, personal fetishes or parody.

Black leather, and black clothing in general, brought a complicated, even contradictory, set of associations to the process. John Harvey's *Men in Black* (1996) suggested two related themes of black clothing.

The first is that black is the preferred wear of ascendant elites, before they achieve their goals and slide into decadence. Not only was the British Empire at its peak run by men in black (except in the tropics, where colonial officers wore gleaming white), so were the Spanish and French empires. Black clothing signifies a rejection of the existing social classes, and creation of a new class of power and destiny, one that means business. This fits BDSM culture's sense of itself as avant-garde, providing the wearer a sense of initiation into a new society that is self-disciplined, exciting, and daring. It is the attire of a person undergoing regeneration, in a liminal state. The newsletter of Oswald Mosley's British Union of Fascists wrote, "[W]hen you have put on the Black Shirt, you will become a Knight of Fascism, of a political and spiritual Order. You will be born anew."[16]

The second theme is that black suggests violence, which may be outwardly directed, as when worn by the soldier or the outlaw (i.e., the sadist), or inwardly, as when worn by the ascetic or the mourner (i.e., the masochist), or delivered from above (i.e., the judge or priest). The near-universal black of Charles Dickens's England indicated a society built through and permeated with violence, justified by Calvinist-capitalist ideology.

> The black of mourning may originate in a violence of grieving, and a violence against the self is part of the whole story of asceticism; but it is violence not only against the self, but against others, including the innocent.[17]
>
> It has become a folk intuition, that in putting on black leather you are putting on power: it may be the power that defies the law, it may be the power that enforces it. . . .
>
> Given the complicated relations of Eros and Thanatos in human sexuality in any case, it is not hard to understand how black, with its acquired associations with discipline, sex and power, can be an efficient trigger and excitant, the more so when the practitioner, rapt in sexual mechanism, binds with black leather, or its deader-still surrogates black plastic or black rubber, the tender human body.[18]

Leather coats were already associated with dashing race drivers and aviators, particularly the mythologized pilots of the Great War, the International Brigade in the Spanish Civil War, and other adventurers. In the interwar period, leather jackets became common wear for American working men, giving them a bit of flair that matched a pair of Levis for dressed-down simplicity. The archetypal black leather motorcycle jacket was the Schott Perfecto, designed by Irving Schott in 1928 in New York City as the first jacket to include a zipper.[19]

World War II took it to a new level, with millions of leather jackets and coats produced for soldiers, particularly the motorcycle troops in Africa, and officers. It became part of the calculated images of leaders like Patton, Rommel, and MacArthur. After the war, in America the black leather jacket was worn by opposing cultural forces: police, the front line of law and order, and hipsters, who rejected peacetime society. One of the most prominent factions of the latter were bikers, who wore leather jackets in part for protection.

The 1947 Hollister, California, motorcycle race and hill-climb and subsequent riot was a flashpoint for this culture clash, creating a new archetypal "monster" of American society: the biker. The incident was fictionalized into *The Wild One* (1953), starring Marlon Brando as the brooding, sexually magnetic, leather-clad Johnny.[20] Schott provided the jackets for the film, including the "'W-style' One Star" worn by Brando.[21] Actual Hell's Angels did wear leather jackets and sewed their colors on them, but abandoned them in the mid-1950s to avoid police attention and to flaunt their disregard for the law and safety, preferring the denim vest with colors. For them, leather jackets became the mark of the poser.[22]

British rockers also adopted the full black leather look, starting with transplanted American singer Gene Vincent (styled by BBC producer Jack Good after Sir Laurence Olivier's costume in *Richard III* [1955]), and followed by Bob Dylan, Elvis Presley, Jim Morrison, and others.[23]

For gay men, the biker look, which evolved into the leatherman look, was one part aspirational (gesturing toward Brando in *The Wild One* and other icons of outlaw masculinity, to reject the effeminate stereotypes of the past), one part protection (you looked tough to deter enemies), one part camouflage (if you didn't own a bike, you could always claim it had broken down; some even carried a helmet), one part fetish (nothing quite like leather), and one part seduction (becoming what Quentin Crisp called "the great dark man" gay men dreamed of). The gay male object of desire was no longer the straight man who had to be coaxed or bribed into sex with another man, but the confident, masculine man who subtly announced his sexuality to the world. The look straddled at least three groups: bikers, gay men into leather who didn't do S/M, and gay men who did do S/M.

> While the associations of sadomasochism (S/M) were definitely there for some men, for others it was just an extension of the strict codification of gay dress. It projected an air of dark, brooding masculinity, with associations of the rebel, of Marlon Brando in *The Wild One* (1954), of the dominator.[24]

Leathermen developed subtle codes for the display of keys on the body to indicate dominance or submission, which expanded into the handkerchief color and placement code to indicate specific sexual roles and interests. These codes usually varied between regions, doubtless sowing confusion.[25]

More than any other artist, the leatherman look was made into an icon by artist Tom of Finland, real name Touko Laaksonen. Even in childhood, Laaksonen was attracted to men in uniform and drew simple comic strips of police officers. As a young man in Helsinki during the war, he was drafted and enjoyed fleeting encounters with the uniformed men of Finland, Russia, and Germany. After the war, he worked as a freelance artist in the bohemian scene, but avoided the homosexual bars for their atmosphere of flamboyant effeminacy. His ideal was the capable, virile man, which he continued to draw in secret, until 1956, when he mailed a drawing of a young, bare-chested logroller to an American physique magazine. The drawing, attributed to "Tom of Finland," was a hit. Over his career, the artist produced about thirty-five hundred pieces that revolutionized gay male visual identity, perfecting the icon of masculinity. Brando's iconic role in *The Wild One* was one of Laaksonen's greatest inspirations.[26] Laaksonen's men in their black leather caps, jackets, pants, and boots were masterful and muscular, but he drew them with a rounded quality that took the hard edge off. These men were tough but tender, not cruel, often with a sly smile on their lips that was an open invitation to the viewer.[27]

John Rechy's 1963 novel *City of Night* suggested just how strong this icon was in a scene of a sex worker dressed up by a client:

> There's a black leather jacket with stars like a general, eagled motorcycle cap, engineer boots with gleaming polished buckles. He left the closet door open, and I could see, hanging neatly, other similar clothes—different sizes.

It was not enough to have the clothes to wear. The john had the clothes already and then got other men to wear them. The flesh-and-blood person merely animated the outfit.

In John Preston's highly popular novel *Mr. Benson* (serialized in *Drummer* magazine between 1979 and 1980), the leatherman outfit of "heavy black boots, button-fly jeans, a washed-out Levi's shirt and an old, greasy, leather jacket" signified Aristotle Benson's authentic masculinity, and indicated protagonist Jamie's shedding of his "disco doll" persona and his initiation into the ways of true male homosexuality.[28]

In the years to come, a certain amount of misinformation, mythologizing, and outright lies grew up around the so-called "Old Guard" of gay men in S/M. There's no mention of the term in Larry Townsend's *Leatherman's Handbook* (1972). The term itself first appeared in print in Rover's column in the December 1973 issue of *California Scene Magazine*, referring to gay bikers in general, not necessarily S/M practitioners. It wasn't used specifically for kinky gay men of the early days until the late 1980s, when it was a derogatory term for conservative elements within the scene, contrasted with the New Guard. Ironically, it later became associated with a combination of high protocol and uniforms, sought by some kinky people of all sexualities as authentic.[29]

The early generations of leathermen were not a monoculture of practice or custom. There were internal dialectics between those who had actually served and seen combat and those who hadn't, or those who were actual outlaw criminal bikers and those who had steady jobs and paid their taxes, or those who pushed the boundaries and those who defined the rules of safety. Joseph W. Bean described this tension between what he called "greasers" and "club-men":

> The circle I was in worked (meaning we did SM scenes) in planned parties with rules and with a host who was playing what eventually became the role of the dungeon master. We dressed carefully, groomed ourselves neatly, and tried with all our might to follow Social Rule One: Don't frighten the villagers. This meant not behaving in ways that would attract attention from outsiders, more than anything else. . . .
>
> We were aware—me last of all it seems—of others who worked differently. Their lives are pretty much described in the famous [William] Carney book, *The Real Thing*. There don't seem to be rules and there definitely are no dungeon masters. Same world, same time, different approach. In the real world as I knew it, the Real-Thing men could be seen as . . . too rebellious to

bear the rules of the world in such a way that they could hold and succeed in jobs or have careers. If we were neat to a pre-Beatles fault, they were studies in slovenliness. I have to admit that they were very sexy to me, but their sexual appeal was mostly in the fact that I was scared to death whenever I saw them. The important thing is that I knew they were not us.[30]

The formalized style considered Old Guard by later generations was actually the New Guard in Bean's early career. A generation later, Bean witnessed the new New Guard appear, men who wore rubber and body piercings and led their submissives on a leash in the street.

From its earliest days, the BDSM culture has suffered from a permanent crisis of authenticity, the split between the originals and the posers, endemic to all subcultures. In part, this is simply generational, with every member believing that at some point after they joined, the newcomers were all inauthentic wannabes. Conversely, a member's doubts about his own authenticity created the belief that somewhere and in some other time, "real S/M" existed, producing myths like the Old Guard or the fabled, centuries-old European slave-training houses.

In the new, media-saturated age, no subculture could stay truly underground forever. No less than *Life* magazine ran a story and pictorial in the June 25, 1964, issue, "Homosexuality in America." The article opened with a page-and-a-half photo of leather-clad men in the shadowy interior of the Tool Box leather bar in San Francisco, a mural of leathermen by Chuck Arnett in the background. Gay leathermen were portrayed as a deviant group within a deviant group.

> On another far-out fringe of the "gay" world are the so-called S&M bars ("S" for sadism and "M" for masochism). One of the most dramatic examples is in the warehouse district of San Francisco. Outside the entrance stand a few brightly polished motorcycles, including an occasional lavender model. Inside the bar, the accent is on leather and sadistic symbolism. The walls are covered with murals of masculine-looking men in black leather jackets. A metal collage of motorcycle parts hangs on one wall. A cluster of tennis shoes—favorite footwear for many homosexuals with feminine traits—dangles from the ceiling, Behind it a derisive sign reads: "Down with sneakers!"[31]

Like it or not, when many Americans imagined "a homosexual," what they envisioned was a short-haired man in jeans, leather jacket, and a leather cap. For pre-Stonewall homosexuals who advocated discretion, leathermen were sartorially and sexually problematic. For others, it provided an alternative homosexual identity to the nelly stereotype. Regardless, *Life* magazine had opened the gay closet and revealed to the world the black leather chaps, jacket, and hat hanging there.

David Stein described the effects of exposure on the early leatherman scene:

> Pre-Stonewall gay S/M was a *very* small community: perhaps a couple of hundred serious tops and bottoms around the country and a few hundred more hangers-on. Nearly everyone knew everybody else, or at least everyone who mattered. It was not an easy group to join. The primary entry points were maybe a dozen "real" leather bars. . . .
>
> By the time I was coming out into S/M, it had ceased to exist. It was swept away by the sexual revolution of the 1960s. Once the lure of S/M was discovered by those outside the ranks of aficionados, the trappings of the scene, stripped of its essence, became fashion. Leather bars, at least for men, proliferated, and publications featuring fetishes and kink were sold on newsstands. Thousands, then tens of thousands of gay men adopted a carefully studied Tom of Finland look, but the sexual flavor of choice for the vast majority, once out of their clothes, was still plain vanilla.[32]

Leathermen could not last as a small, underground tribe. Mass media exposed it, and the apprenticeship model of initiation and education would not scale to larger numbers of people. The scene had to evolve.

STRAIGHT KINK

Though not as well documented as the gay male leather culture, the heterosexual sadomasochistic underground existed during this period, in a more diffuse form. The formation of a subculture was hampered by the sparse population and official censors attacking the major communications channels like the postal service and magazine publishing and distribution.

The look of fetish and bondage in this period was defined by a small number of artists working in and around New York City. Operating on the border of legality and legitimacy between the mob-connected pornography publishers and the mainstream, these men largely worked under pseudonyms, and their biographical details are sketchy, while their publishers frequently changed their company names and places of business. In the days before the wide availability of hardcore imagery, publishers used fetishes like catfighting, spanking, bondage, and high heels as a way of separating their products from typical "bathing beauty" erotic photography, while (hopefully) keeping the law at bay by not showing nudity or sexuality.

The main media for kink stories and imagery were digest-sized magazines with a general interest in the "bizarre" or "exotic," sold by mail-order or on the top shelves of magazine stores; photo sets sold by mail order from small advertisements in magazines; short silent film loops, usually of women spanking, wrestling, or just dressing and undressing, and sold to the underground stag film network; and soft-core paperback novels in which euphemisms like "throbbing manhood" and "moment of union" were the limits of explicitness. Publishers lent their writers copies of *Psychopathia Sexualis* and other sexology works for inspiration. These stories were published in cheaply produced, typewritten books, with high markups. Contributors were paid in cash or in checks from dummy corporations, and quite well for the time, which is how the publishers got skilled artists to do the all-important book and magazine covers, and moonlighting mainstream writers for the formulaic contents.[33]

The early kink scene was formed in the tension between those who saw kink as a market niche to exploit for profit and those who saw kink as a kind of personal art form. As with the gay male kink culture, there were forerunners of the heterosexual kink culture in the prewar period. The best known was costumer and entrepreneur Charles Guyette. He contributed to and advertised in *London Life* in the early 1930s and became the center of an underground network of fetishists and artists/artisans. Though not a photographer or artist himself, he networked fetish talent together, including bringing art from France to the USA. He was arrested in 1935 and served time in a federal penitentiary, then returned to his business under a variety of aliases and fronts. He moved his business into g-strings, theatrical footwear, and other exotic costumes for burlesque performer and fetishists at a time when, such garments were only custom made.

In the early 1940s, Guyette made contacts in the girlie magazine publishing world and connected or otherwise influenced the next generation of fetish artists, such as John Coutts and Eric Stanton, and entrepreneurs such as Irving Klaw and Leonard Burtman.[34]

Born in Singapore, educated in England, and residing in Australia, John A. S. Coutts adopted the pen name of "John Willie" for his bondage and fetish photography and illustration. He published his own digest-sized magazine, *Bizarre*, a highly idiosyncratic publication (volume 2 came out in 1946, and volume 1 came out in 1954, just after volume 13), which refined the format of prewar proto-fetish magazines like *London Life* and *Photo Bits*, making only the faintest pretense of being a general-interest magazine. Coutts was both a fan of *London Life* and frustrated by what he saw as its conservatism; he wanted to outdo it.[35]

Each issue featured photos of models in bondage or fetishwear, pictures clipped from mainstream newspapers and magazines, short stories, and fetish letters, covering bondage, corsetry, high-heeled shoes and boots, gagging, cross-dressing, amputees, masks, spanking, and humiliation. As with all fetish correspondence, there is the question of how many, if any, of these letters were mailed in from readers and not written in house. Some were more plausible than others. One man wrote in with tips on how to smuggle cameras into movie theaters to take pictures of the film, and he included a list of movies with bondage scenes in them. This is a distant ancestor of the video captures traded on the internet today.

At least one letter was for real. "Ibitoe," later known as Fakir Musafar, one of the founders of the body modification and modern primitive culture, wrote in volume 21 about his self-driven body modification efforts, with photos. Ibitoe's story didn't quite fit in with stories of domestic discipline, but it seemed to have been included out of a general interest in the bizarre.

Some of the stories referred to Victorian-era clothing and social relations, with "Memoirs of Paula Sanchez" purporting to be a nineteenth-century account. Other features waxed Orientalist. Volume 19 had "Saudi Arabian Nights," supposedly based on "Flesh for Sale," an article published in the *New York Post* in 1956, which claims that the slave trade continues in modern-day Saudi Arabia. Accurate or not, the author of the article instead switched to "the report of a British agent who was through the area in the early 30's," privileging this anonymous "agent's" account over the more recent news article. The "agent's" account goes into pornographic detail about the alleged slave markets, describing the slaves and how they were dressed and bound and speculating about Russian female aristocrats ending up as slaves. A letter in volume 26, "Eastern Diplomacy," is another classic Orientalist fantasy set in Turkey circa 1917, full of harems and flagellation. Another letter by "Darlene" (vol. 24) had a white man forced, by blackmail, to dress as a black woman and to pick cotton.

Most of the illustrations and photography were by Coutts himself, featuring long-limbed women bound and gagged, or in elaborate fancy dress costumes that combined bondage with whimsy. He also continued his *Sweet Gwendoline* comic strip, originally published in *Wink* magazine, using the "virtue in distress" storyline as a vehicle for more bondage. Writing in a wry, jocular tone, Coutts was more of a naughty uncle than a sadistic torturer, and his illustrations and comics were more English pantomime than Sade. Even in his essays about keeping wives bound and gagged, there was nothing nasty about it.[36]

Coutts never found a distributor. He did the work himself, selling to stores on consignment. This gave him complete artistic freedom and kept him under the radar of authorities.[37]

Coutts epitomized the auteur side of the kink subculture, while others were more commercial. Since 1939, brother and sister Irving and Paula Klaw ran a bookstore in New York City that branched into selling pictures of movie stars and models. Shortly after the war, their customers came to them for something a little more specialized. Paula Klaw recollects:

> Customers brought us that particular interest—bondage, girlie stuff, garter belts and high heels. They were mostly wealthy lawyers and doctors. A couple of them offered to put up the money for the project—models, photography and all, providing we kept their names anonymous . . . and that's why and how we did it. We really did it as a service to them. We hired the models and the studios and these guys showed us exactly what they wanted done. They taught us. [. . .] We ran ads in all the girlie magazines. [. . . We recruited models] through agencies and photographers. We recruited photographers at first and they had a list of girls in their little black books who were ready. One model told another. Some volunteered and came down because they wanted to work. These men taught me how to tie the knots, but they were really afraid to touch the women . . . so they instructed me how to do it. I learned quickly how to tie knots and I then went on to become a photographer as well.[38]

The Klaws expanded their semi-underground operation into books, magazines, and film loops. One of their models for fetish and bondage shoots was Bettie Page, who quickly became famous with her brilliant smile, hourglass figure, and trademark black bangs. With the body of a goddess and the face of an angel, Page always seemed to be smiling in her photo shoots and film loops, and was photographed by pinup artist Bunny Yeager and crime photographer Weegee. Perhaps more than anybody else, Page made S/M look fun. After Page disappeared from public view in the late 1950s, she became an icon for future generations of kinksters.

Coutts intensely disliked Klaw, seeing him as an exploiter of both amateur and professional artists. The two men epitomized the two intersecting subcultures that produced the American postwar heterosexual SM style: Coutts was a "producer-practitioner," who came to bondage and fetish with an artist's eye, while Klaw focused on creating as much niche product as possible, as quickly as possible.[39] Coutts described Klaw's photo shoots as being full of men solely there for the voyeurism, something he never allowed in his own studio.[40]

Irving Klaw carefully stayed outside the boundaries of obscenity. He made sure that models wore two pairs of panties in the photo shoots, to ensure no pubic hair showed, and didn't deal in pictures that showed men and women together.[41] Nonetheless, the Klaws had frequent legal troubles through the 1950s and early 1960s, forcing them to destroy some of their stock, and they eventually moved back to celebrity photography. Before then, they developed the artists who defined a genre of erotica, such as Eric Stanton and Gene Bilbrew, both students at the School for the Visual Arts in New York City.[42]

Arguably the second-best-known fetish artist after John Willie, Eric Stanton (born Ernest Stanzoni or Ernest Stanten, depending on the story) was a Brooklyn-born fan who turned pro at the end of the 1940s. He wrote to Irving Klaw and claimed he could do better than the female wrestling pictures he purchased. Klaw took the young Stanton up on his offer and hired him.[43]

Stanton started out drawing catfights, then mimicked Willie's style, drawing delicate women in elaborate bondage costumes. He studied at the Cartoonists and Illustrators School, and shared office space with classmate Steve Ditko, a future Marvel Comics artist. Stanton later developed his own painting and illustration style and preferred subject matter: powerful, buxom Amazons, often dressed in masculine clothes, with a penchant for wrestling. A private client gave Stanton the idea for what he dubbed "Princkazons," giant women with massive breasts and penises. They reflected the anxiety men felt about the idea of the liberated woman, simultaneously drawn to them and fearful of them. Most of his work was on commission, doing high-heeled shoe fetish and forced-feminization stories.[44] He also self-published by mimeograph, and later by photocopier, a series of *Stantoons* comics, with over one hundred issues published into the 1990s until his death.[45]

Born in Los Angeles and a former doo-wop singer, Gene Bilbrew, who often signed his work "Eneg," was one of the few African Americans working in this field. He was formally trained and developed a cartoon-influenced style of illustration that became a mainstay of Leonard Burtman's fetish digest magazine *Exotique*, plus the covers of many pulp gay and drug paperbacks. Unfortunately, Bilbrew struggled with drug addiction, and as publishers began using photographs for book covers in the late 1960s, his opportunities dried up as his work deteriorated. He eventually died in 1974 of a drug overdose in the back of Eddie Mishkin's adult store, where he had been living.[46] Bilbrew's death marked the end of an era, as hard-core film and photography was increasingly in demand and there was little place for illustrated erotica.

Leonard "Lennie" Burtman took the Klaws' business model to the next level, going beyond mail order to national distribution of fetish media, though he still struggled with persecution from local law enforcement, postal authorities, the FBI, and even the Catholic Church. A California transplant to New York City, and by some accounts a failed scientist or engineer, Burtman was also a practitioner as well as a producer. He became the nexus of a circle of kinksters who gathered at his Manhattan apartment for parties.

He started working as a pinup and fetish photographer, and by the mid-1950s was distributing his own fetish photosets and films. He published the digest-format *Exotique* magazine from 1955 to 1959, modeled after Willie's *Bizarre*, though with an emphasis on fetish fashion instead of bondage. Most of the covers and artwork were by Bilbrew and Stanton. It also featured one of Burtman's wives, the burlesque dancer and fetish model Tana Louise, as model and columnist. He produced a 35 mm feature narrative film, *Satan in High Heels* (1962), starring Meg Myles in a leather suit, spurs, and riding crop, singing "The Female of the Species." This was the first mass-distributed film made with intentional fetishistic content.[47] Burtman also developed *Bizarre Life* magazine, the first specialty SM magazine published in 8.5×11 format.[48]

Burtman sold his wares via post (with a mailing list of tens of thousands of names) and via professional distributors to adult retail shops nationally, but not by direct retail. Over the 1960s, changes in distribution and production systems affected the content produced by Burtman. In the 1950s and early 1960s, he had a high degree of creative control over his work, informed by his contacts in the practitioner networks. In the mid-1960s, Burtman had financial problems, and he was bailed out by America's top porn distributor, Reuben Sturman. Under Sturman's influence, Burtman had less creative control, and magazines like *Bizarre Life* were less idiosyncratic and more homogeneous, as well as more explicit in nudity, with men and women featured together. Some pictures were just recycled content, lacking Burtman's innovations. The bizarre style was no longer an eccentric niche market; it had been assimilated as just another category of mainstream porn.[49]

Burtman was eventually convicted of bribery, not obscenity, and served a federal prison term. In 1972, he returned to California with his second wife, Jutka Goz (alias Jennifer Jordan and Mistress Jeanette), and resumed publishing, though keeping a lower profile.[50]

As one generation of BDSM producers declined, another rose. Yogi Klein, Leonard Burtman's cousin, and a woman known only as "Ms. B" founded the House of Milan in Chicago in the fall of 1964. The business was partially modeled after Burtman's empire, and Klein bought some of the pieces in Burtman's *Bizarre Costume Catalog* (many of which were exorbitantly priced to discourage sales, because they were unique pieces). It became the first public retail outlet for fetish clothing in the United States. In the 1970s, Ms. B took over the business, brought in outside investors, moved to California, and renamed the company HOM. It became one of largest producers of SM and fetish erotica in the United States, dealing in contact magazines like *Latent Image*, glossy SM and fetish magazines, adult videos, sex toys, and clothing.[51]

MISS SM APPEAL

Taking advantage of increasingly relaxed censorship, mainstream culture continued to provide glimpses of sadomasochistic imagery, creating a kind of jigsaw puzzle for those with the right frame of mind to assemble into a picture. Fetishistic and sadomasochistic scenarios were used to dance on the border of censorship.

As it had since the silent era, mainstream Hollywood continued to sprinkle its films with harem slave girls, captive princesses, bare-chested gladiator slaves, and floggings. We have no way of knowing how many people had their first moment of kinky recognition watching something like the off-camera whipping scene in *Tarzan and the Slave Girl* (1950) or the spankings in *Kiss Me Kate* (1953) or *McLintock!* (1963), or the humans captured and caged by beasts in *Planet of the Apes* (1968).

When the film market for "nudies" was oversaturated by the early 1960s, producers started making "roughies" or "kinkies," which provided violence, bordering on horror, in place of explicit sexuality, to escape the censors. Some drew on established women-in-peril scenarios, such as *White Slaves of Chinatown* (1964) and *Invitation to Ruin* (1968). Others depicted secret societies of vengeful, castrating lesbians, like *The Daughters of Lesbos* (1968). One of the best known examples was Russ Meyer's *Faster Pussycat! Kill! Kill!* (1965), about female race car drivers fighting over money in the desert, which became a cult classic.[52] This genre also influenced the Nazisploitation subgenre discussed in chapter 8.

Even television played its part, with sexuality sublimated into fantastic scenes of bondage and mind control in order to slip by the censors. The 1966 *Batman* TV series turned the bondage and costumes of the old adventure serials into high camp pop art, full of absurd death traps. The spy TV fad of the 1960s provided numerous opportunities for confinement, mind control, torture, and other kinkiness. The UK mod-spy TV series *The Avengers* provided Mrs. Emma Peel, memorably played by Diana Rigg. One theory claimed the name was a play on "Miss S-M Appeal," and given that she was beautiful, capable of defeating men hand-to-hand, and given to tight-fitting jumpsuits and boots, she definitely had that. Fans particularly remember the episodes "A Touch of Brimstone," in which she appeared in stockings, a corset, and a spiked collar as the Queen of Sin, and "Death at Bargain Prices," in which she wore a leather catsuit with straps and zippers. The series' other female leads also had a penchant for leather and kinky boots. They were the femme fatales of an earlier generation turned into heroines.

Mainstream fashion had its own flirtation with the biker image, continuing the tradition of women adopting pieces of male attire. Motorcycle magazines advertised ladies' companion leather jackets in the 1950s, but they remained a subcultural style. That changed when Yves St. Laurent designed for Dior a black leather women's jacket for winter 1960, based on Paris street fashion. The outrage over this contributed to St. Laurent being fired from Dior and eventually launching his own house.

As early as September 1960, *Elle* had female models in leather jackets on Harley-Davidsons, and by 1968, Marianne Faithfull wore black leather pants and fur as the *Girl on a Motorcycle*. Versace's fall 1992 line was full of tight-fitting black with straps and metallic buckles.

Leather also has the perhaps unique quality of suggesting both the primitive and the futuristic. Designers Pierre Cardin, Christian Dior, and Mac Douglas made use of this quality, along with other fetishized materials like rubber and vinyl, to create the smooth, basic forms of fashion and design in the "Space Age."[53]

John Sutcliffe turned his fetish for leather into a business in 1957, after various attempts to treat what was then seen as a mental illness. While working as a photographer, he took a lady friend for a ride on his motorcycle, who enjoyed it until the weather turned. They tried to find a leather riding suit for women, but could only find suits cut for small men. Sutcliffe bought some skins of red leather, borrowed a sewing machine, and his friend loved what he made. So did other women, even for street wear, and Sutcliffe found his calling as a self-taught designer and dressmaker. He founded Atomage, providing leather, and later rubber, wear. In 1967, a company called Granville Chemicals commissioned Sutcliffe to make a skin-tight, full-length leather suit, including hood, boots, gloves, and goggles, for a mystery model. On the eve of an auto trade show, the leather woman stalked through the streets of London as a publicity stunt. Contrary to some stories, Sutcliffe did not provide the leather garments for *The Avengers*, though he did supply the costumes for the stage version of the show. His designs did appear in films and on stage, crossing the boundaries of fetish and fashion.[54]

Producers like Klaw and Burtman drew upon loose, clandestine networks of fetishists for models, photographers, and creativity. Little is known definitively about these networks in the 1950s and 1960s. One of the few books about this particular subculture was Michael Leigh's *The Velvet Underground* (1963), which described how magazines and newspapers ran personal ads with code phrases like "exotic," "bizarre," "adventurous," "broad-minded," or "uninhibited." This was the new incarnation of a tradition that goes back at least to the Victorian era.

> Superficially, the magazines themselves are harmless enough. They show nudes and lingerie models, and run articles and short stories dealing with sexy, innocuous, situations. They never go too far. They may discuss spanking but never discipline as such, and they never mention what is known as bondage.[55]

The main channel of communication was mail contact services. Fill in a form, mail in the fee, and you would receive regular bulletins with descriptions of advertisers and box numbers for replies. Some of these contact networks were adjuncts to pornography (magazines or photosets) or adult toy businesses, selling bondage and discipline gear, leather fashions, and so on. Some of the people were amateurs, some were sex workers.

There were risks in getting involved in this hidden world. Sending "obscene" material through the mail was a crime at the time, punishable by a fine up to $5,000, up to five years imprisonment, or both; the legacy of Anthony Comstock.[56] Furthermore, some of the people used or ran these services to obtain nude pictures for publication without having to pay models or photographers.[57]

There was no particular distinction between what we would now call swinging/swapping and BDSM. People were surprisingly willing to offer explicit letters and pictures (including their faces), sometimes for trade, sometimes on loan. A Minnesota man offered himself and his wife for sexual shows, including bondage (with a disturbing reference to "numbed limbs and muscles"), torture, and sexual humiliation. An Ohio man described what sounds suspiciously like a fantasy of being taken to a house by a man and two women to be dominated by them. There are other anecdotes of sadomasochistic acts. These people didn't have a good grasp of their own limits, and there was no shared body of knowledge about physical safety, much less emotional safety. Decades before "safe, sane and consensual," these people worked without a net.

The Velvet Underground provided the name for the proto-punk/Goth band the Velvet Underground, and their debut album *Velvet Underground and Nico* (1967) featured the track "Venus in Furs," based on Leopold von Sacher-Masoch's novel. Both Leigh and the members of the Velvet Underground saw the world described in this book as something revolutionary or at least transgressive, the resurgence of the primitive into the modern world (though one condemned and the other approved). The people described in the book didn't see themselves as particularly transgressive or avant-garde. Leigh wrote, "They are not the so-called dead beats, the alleged beatniks or what used to be called Bohemians. . . . To the casual observer, they are respected and respectable members of their communities."[58] They were the heirs of Munby and Cullwick, who quietly lived their kinks in private and were not political in the way that was borrowed from gay liberation.

The artists and performers of this era, who worked on the fringe of legality, with little reward or respect, are now remembered through a soft haze of nostalgia. Coutts's *Bizarre* and Burtman's *Exotique* were collected into coffee table books by art publisher Taschen. Tom of Finland was commemorated by a series of Finnish postage stamps in 2014. Bettie Page abruptly quit modeling in 1957, but her image grew from an underground pinup queen to a style icon and female role model. What was once kept under the counter would adorn the fridge magnets of later generations.

By 1970, the pieces were there, but they had yet to come together. The heterosexual sadomasochistic culture was still scattered individuals or couples, linked by loose networks. The sexual revolution and the growth in subcultures would change that.

Chapter Ten

Unknown Pleasures

In the early days of the internet in the 1990s, just getting in touch with kinky people was difficult. I managed my crude online calendar of local events, made with hand-coded HTML, but the main emphasis was print media. I designed and printed posters and flyers for local events, which I distributed by hand to fetish/punk clothing shops, adult stores, LGBT bookstores, and piercing parlors. A few local alternative free weeklies carried announcements of workshops and play parties. It was still likely that there were many people who might want to be part of our subculture but didn't have the awareness or the courage to make contact. Imagine how it was a generation before that.

The early 1970s were a time of significant and far-reaching change in the sadomasochistic subculture(s). In the wake of the sexual revolution and the Stonewall riots, American and European society grew increasingly liberal sexually. Kink was more visible and more organized than ever before, though still widely misunderstood and scorned. The sadomasochistic subculture's evolution roughly paralleled gay culture: a shift from a loose network of those in the know, to aboveground, formal organizations for education and support.

However, there were important differences. Gay culture came to view coming out of the closet as a profound act, both politically and personally. Kink culture retained a strong emphasis on privacy and keeping a low profile. For kinky people, "coming out" meant attending the semi-public educational, social, and play events instead of playing in private with partners, while still keeping one's sexuality secret from one's family, friends, coworkers, and other public spaces. In that respect, the heterosexual BDSM culture lagged a decade or more behind the gay culture.

The swinger networks and contact magazines of the earlier decades connected people, but didn't provide education or psychological support. Beginning in the early 1970s, kinky people founded the first formal, open organizations for heterosexual sadomasochists, whose primary functions were education and socializing. The new kink organizations were open invitation, instead of the secretive and insular clubs of the previous decades.

The early heterosexual BDSM scene had strong links with the gay leather scene and the professional domination scene by necessity. Leathermen and pro-dominatrices were the primary sources of information on technique and safety for straights, and they had access to venues open to kinky educational, social, and play events. The master-apprentice model practiced by leathermen couldn't scale to larger numbers of people, and education shifted to a teacher-classroom model.[1]

HETEROSEXUAL KINK

The first modern, aboveground BDSM organization was the Till Eulenspiegel Society, founded in 1971 in New York City. Pat Bond, a heterosexual male submissive, started out seeking dominant women.

> I started checking the ad sections of the underground press, planning ads that would appeal to dominant women. The idea then occurred to me to run an ad for "M's" to get their heads together, since I knew that there must be many others like myself with similar problems. Getting together to devise a positive program for ourselves seemed far preferable to me than remaining as we were—isolated, repressed & frustrated.[2]

In 1970, Bond placed ads in *Screw* and the *East Village Other*, which read:

> Masochist? Happy? Is it curable? Does psychiatry help? Is a satisfactory life-style possible? There's Women's Lib., Gay Lib., etc. Isn't it time we put something together? Write P O box 2783, Grand Central station.[3]

Bond received five answers, and three of them agreed to come to a meeting at his apartments. Two actually arrived. One was a female M (masochist) named Terry Kolb, who joined with Bond in founding the organization. Later, Kolb chose the new organization's name, the Till Eulenspiegel Society (TES), after a character from German folklore. Theodore Reik's *Masochism in Modern Man* (1941) described him as a trickster who was happy while he was carrying a heavy load up a hill because he imagined how easy it would be going down the hill not carrying anything. But he was sad when he descended because he thought of the next time he would have to carry a load up the hill.

They placed more ads in *Screw* and *Evo*, though the *Village Voice* rejected their ad, which Kolb took as a civil liberties issue. This got the attention of more people in the NYC area, gay and straight, in their twenties and thirties, who attended meetings. Kolb's campaign to make the *Voice* run the group's ad also won some publicity by being covered in Howard Smith's Scenes column. TES was an activist and social group that held its first public forums and meetings in 1971 and marched in the Gay Parade in 1972.

In its first few years, TES's membership was fairly evenly divided between gays and straights, and "S"s and "M"s, with many "switchables." Women were always underrepresented, but some of the most active members were female, such as Terry Kolb.[4]

On the other side of North America, the Society of Janus (SOJ) was founded in San Francisco in 1975. Cynthia Slater, the group's cofounder and a pro-domme, said that education came first, meeting partners second, and emotional validation and support third. Slater joined San Francisco Sex Information in 1972 and got the organization to become SM positive.[5]

> The groups they [Slater and her male lover] discovered by reading *Berkeley Barb* ads were mostly swing-swap-n-clap clubs. Commercial. Heterosexist. Very much "I'll kiss-off my wife for yours." The women were traded around like fuckable commodities on the New York Stock Exchange.
>
> At the same time, Slater grew tired of her non-S&M friends whose "heavy vicarious curiosity" became a judgmental mindfuck. "They never really shared themselves other than saying, 'I'm not into that.' At the same time they'd be squirming on the edge of their seat and clenching their wet thighs. I felt ripped off. Even psycho-sexually molested." . . .

> Finally, she and her lover decided that in order to meet other S&M people, without the bullshit of the existing clubs, they'd have to start their own organization. It was August, 1975. Their first move was a newsletter, advertised in the *Barb*, listing the monthly meetings at Cynthia's house. In those early days—before gay men started joining—a lot of heterosexual men persisted in "dogging the women," Slater says. "That was the only reason they came."[6]

Much like TES, Janus was founded to correct the bias of the existing scene, in this case, to favor straight and bisexual women. Instead of the tribal initiation atmosphere of the early gay leather scene, these gatherings were more human potential movement, with rapport and consciousness-raising sessions. Jack Fritscher described Slater: "She sprinkles her talk with pop-psych vocab. 'Validating' comes up a lot. The 'OK-ness' of being a Top or a Bottom. Slater stops well this side of [cult-like human potential seminar] est." Jay Wiseman recalled:

> When I started going to Janus events [1977 or 1978] (which at the time consisted of one event a month), it was about 85% gay men, about 13% lesbians, with literally a sprinkling of hetfolk like me. Among other things, it meant that "we" had to be careful about what we did and said. While "on paper" Janus was a pansexual organization (I don't think that the word pansexual was in widespread use at the time), in reality it had a very strong gay male leatherman atmosphere. Thus, being low-profile, relatively quiet, and courteous was a distinctly good idea if you were het.[7]

Teaching safety proved to be difficult. Patrick Califia recalls:

> It was hard going because so many of the people in the SM community then were rather damaged and fringey. Just pushing the notion of safe play was an uphill battle sometimes. Getting people to have enough self-esteem that they could separate consensual from nonconsensual activity. A lot of members were program vampires who came to the educational events but never incorporated any of that information into their personal lives; they wanted Janus to put on a series of sex shows that they could jack off to.[8]

Janus borrowed venues for educational and social meetings, including the gay male fisting club the Catacombs, the Shotwell Meeting House, and a disused brewery, with flogging demonstrations held inside an empty beer vat. Orientation discussion meetings were held at Xanadu Pleasure Gardens, a house with live peacocks and reportedly the largest hot tub in San Francisco. Noni Howard ran her orientations like a scavenger hunt, and sent orientees searching through the house to find improvised toys, instilling the idea that you didn't need special toys for play.

This is also where Slater met Dossie Easton, future coauthor of *The Ethical Slut* (1997), and Patrick (then known as Pat) Califia, future author of the lesbian sex guide *Sapphistry* (1980) and the lesbian kink story collection *Macho Sluts* (1988). Other kink notables like the Reverend Jim Kane, Guy Baldwin, and Jay Wiseman were involved. Like most communities, Janus had its fractious politics and personality conflicts, but also moments of solidarity, like helping Jay Wiseman when he was injured and unable to work, or supporting Slater in the final years of her struggle with HIV-related illnesses.

Janus had an intimate yet awkward relationship with gay culture. Slater, Easton, and Califia hung out at gay leather bars, where they weren't always welcome, and Slater had a habit of crushing on gay men. Califia pushed hard for Janus to march for the first time in the 1978 Gay Freedom Day Parade. Even though floats built by leather bars were commonplace, Janus's contingent met with harassment from parade organizers and anti-violence and anti-pornography groups.[9]

Women also drew upon the gay male leather culture for education, venues, and support, once they got over the cultural barrier. Califia recalls:

> The women who were doing SM community leadership in the 70s did more than just go to the leather bars and talk to people. We played there. A lot of the bars had back rooms then. It was one of the few public places where you could strut your stuff. And it was one of the ways we made contact with leathermen. They could SEE that we were into the same thing that they were into. Some of them were pissed off about this but a few of them thought we were interesting and a good time, and became allies.[10]

In the early 1980s, while Janus struggled to launch a Los Angeles chapter, it began to shift from a predominantly gay male membership to heterosexual, for a variety of reasons. As heterosexual kink culture grew, it developed its own, more diverse practices that didn't mesh with established gay male kink. Fakir Musafar (once known as Ibitoe in John Coutts's

Bizarre) recalls that, during a program on Spirituality and Piercing, one man in leather got up, shouted, "This isn't SM!" and stormed out.[11]

Cynthia Slater wanted Janus to be a pansexual organization, open to all, but the influx of straights, and particularly what Guy Baldwin called "some really arrogant and predatory het men," pushed gay men out. "We [i.e., gay men] had a place to go back to, the women, both lesbian and het did not. It is no accident that it was about this time that the women's groups began."[12] This was the chronic problem of heterosexual kink organizations: too many straight men, particularly submissives, who often lacked social skills. The group had to implement a "no cruising" policy at orientations.

The larger problems were the gentrification of San Francisco's "south of Market" or SOMA district, which once held a strip of leather bars and related businesses; and the arrival of AIDS, which sickened and killed gay men. Janus's membership and leaders were devastated by the loss of too many advisers, friends, and lovers, including Cynthia Slater in 1989. Fearing a poorly understood disease, straights stopped playing alongside gays.

Within the gay community, folk theories of AIDS scapegoated leathermen for the disease by linking it to promiscuity, sadomasochism, anal fisting, the use of amyl nitrate, or the "absence of love."[13] Randy Shilts's book *And the Band Played On* (1987) constructed a moralistic narrative that implied that AIDS resulted from the alleged dehumanization of gay male sexuality.

> Slowly, the relational aspects of the sexual interaction dropped away. Intimacy disappeared and, before long, people were wearing outward signs of sexual tasks, hankies and keys, to make their cruising more efficient. . . . Stripped of humanity, sex sought ever-rising levels of physical stimulation in increasingly esoteric practices.[14]

During the moral panic that led to the closure of bathhouses, a key gay community institution, leather sex clubs like the Cauldron and the Catacombs posted information as it became available, and safer sex knowledge spread from person to person through public sex venues. Nonetheless, the belief that closures would control the problem shut down most of the specialized leather, SM, and fisting clubs, even without direct city action, and few leather businesses could afford to fight the city legally. The damage was done to South of Market's social and economic capital, and commercial development finished it off.[15]

The devastation of an entire generation of leathermen left the next generation of SM culture without mentors. The broad gap between generations created the perceived split between "old leather" and "new leather." Gayle Rubin wrote:

> Formerly the transmission of cultural norms and expectations was largely accomplished through interpersonal contact such as mentoring, friendship, and sexual liaisons. Now many of the experienced men who would have welcomed and educated newcomers are gone. Consequently, men currently coming into leather often get much of their education from books and classes rather than from personal contact.[16]

The leather community did socially evolve to meet the crisis. The modern title system, which began in 1979 with the first International Mr. Leather (IML) contest in Chicago, served as an important AIDS fundraiser, and in the 1980s, IML winners became spokespeople for AIDS-related issues. Small-scale Ms. Leather title contests started in the San Francisco area in 1981, and in 1987 the first International Ms. Leather contest specifically said the titleholder should be a "spokesperson." The Folsom Street Fair and Up Your Alley, which started in 1984 and 1987 respectively, showed that the South of Market neighborhood was still vital and kinky. By the end of the decade, the leather community in San Francisco was smaller, but tighter and more socially integrated, with alliances between gay men, lesbians, and straights. Play parties open to all genders and orientations began, and the 1986 Gay Freedom Day Parade had a SM Community contingent.[17]

Other organizations based on the TES and Janus model of social plus education for heterosexuals sprang up around North America. Starting in 1986, Nancy Ava Miller drove her van across America creating chapters of PEP, People Exchanging Power, an educational support network, often struggling to get meeting spaces or put ads in newspapers.[18] She wrote, "S&M groups are important because folks will practice S&M whether or not they have a group, pornography, literature, or videos. Therefore, support groups are good so people know what they're doing when engaging in this form of erotica so they don't risk injuring someone."[19] On HIV, she added,

> People will not stop relating to one another erotically just because of disease or because some moralistic, self-proclaimed pundit insists that the only way to prevent AIDS is through abstinence. . . . And S&M offers many avenues for erotic pleasure and exploration that will not transmit the AIDS virus: bondage, nipple play, spanking, foot worship, cross-dressing, and fetish attire, to name just a few.[20]

PEP also had a vital role in support for kinky people who may have been isolated and fearful of their own desires.

> People skulk in that first night. They feel bad about themselves, worried, guilty, frustrated, lonely; they feel abnormal because of their longings, their obsessions. . . . I do PEP because I don't want anyone to go through what *I* went through, not knowing there are other people out there.[21]

While some PEP groups folded almost immediately, others lasted decades. PEP-DC, which she founded in 1987, became Black Rose in 1989.[22]

The ascent of the heterosexual BDSM community unfortunately coincided with the alienation and devastation of its forebearers—gay leathermen. The dream of a pansexual kinky utopia died as it was conceived, and straight, gay, and lesbian kink cultures separated to evolve in parallel, though with a certain amount of crossover. HIV also forced kinky people to consider the safety of their play. In the mid-1980s, safety techniques became more systematized, and organizers started hosting clean and sober parties.[23]

LESBIAN BDSM

The culture of lesbian sadomasochism followed its own distinct trajectory through the 1970s and 1980s, largely in isolation from gay and heterosexual kink. Lesbian sadomasochism as it is known today is largely defined by the political struggle between pro- and anti-SM lesbian-feminists; the actual practices of lesbian sadomasochists in the 1970s and early 1980s are not well documented, and there is little or no known record of lesbian BDSM in earlier decades.

American second-wave feminism in the 1960s saw lesbians as "the lavender menace," as Betty Friedan put it in 1969. They had to guard against any taint by association with any form of deviant sexuality or gender expression. In 1970, lesbians crashed the second Congress to Unite Women, wearing "lavender menace" T-shirts, and read their manifesto.[24]

Then, in a remarkably short period of time, lesbians went from the barbarians at the gates of feminism to the standard-bearers. Ti Grace Atkinson is said to have proclaimed, in the early 1970s, "Feminism is the theory, lesbianism is practice." (That she may have never said this, or was misquoted, is beside the point.)[25]

However, this acceptance only applied to certain types of lesbians: femme but not too femme, monogamous, bourgeois and domestic (and white), and vanilla. No women of color, no bisexuals, no sex toys, no strap-ons, no "roles" (i.e., butch-femme), no fisting, no cruising, no porn, and definitely no S/M. The newly conceived identity of the lesbian-feminist asserted a new model of "real" female sexuality. The irony was that it was perfectly compatible with mainstream (i.e., patriarchal) society's stereotype of female sexuality, as had been dominant since at least the mid-nineteenth century. Furthermore, some proposed that "lesbian" was a political identity, not a sexual identity, and not at all analogous to male homosexuality. Lesbian sexuality was not sexuality at all.

Lesbian sadomasochists, as an identity group, emerged in roughly the same period, and they starkly defied the new prescription of authentic female sexuality.[26] From the beginning, lesbian sadomasochism had a complex and difficult relationship with lesbian-feminism.

Perhaps recorded lesbian sadomasochism began in October 1974,[27] when *Lesbian Tide* published "The Spirit Is Feminist but the Flesh Is?," by Karla Jay. In the opening paragraph, Jay claimed, "I've seen countless sisters rant against any sort of sexual inequality in a lesbian relationship only to hear later that their favorite sexual 'sport' is sado-masochism."[28] Jay's offhand mention and the apparent lack of response from readers suggests that lesbian SM was a known practice, if not common or widely accepted. However, she added, "[S]ocial pressure has also forced some sado-masochists and lesbians living as prostitutes to live in this second closet."[29]

Jay explored the controversy among lesbians over sadomasochism along with other practices, such as dildo use and prostitution, and asked whether one could or should control one's sexual fantasies. She favored individuals following their own consciousness, but acknowledged she had no resolution.[30]

The next year, Barbara Lipschutz (aka Barbara Ruth, aka Drivenwoman) published "Cathexis (on the nature of S&M)" in *Hera*, reprinted in 1977 in *Lesbian Tide*.[31] Lipschutz idealized lesbian sadomasochism, proclaiming it was not only feminist but superior to heterosexual vanilla sex in providing women pleasure, because of women's supposedly greater relational abilities.[32] In her follow up article, "Coming Out on S&M," in 1976, Lipschutz linked SM and lesbianism as personal truths that were difficult to admit in public.[33]

In 1976, *Lesbian Tide* printed a transcript of a consciousness-raising session in which women discussed sadomasochism in a variety of ways: as body work for expressing emotions ("being restrained has helped me with releasing energy in my pelvic area that has been blocked"), as intense expressions of devotion ("Taking or having complete control, or having another woman give me that much control, total control, to me is one of the most beautiful experiences I've ever had"), as uncertain territory ("Sometimes I wonder how far I would really go, either as a sadist or masochist"), or part of a continuum of all sexuality ("Sexuality, any kind of sex, then bondage and dominance, and then sado-masochism is all on a continuum of control. Most sex in this society is based on control, on giving and taking. I think this can be real unhealthy or real wonderful and beautiful").[34]

Later came Patrick Califia's article "A Secret Side of Lesbian Sexuality," published in the *Advocate* in 1979. The essay positioned sadomasochists as caught between two enemies.

> It's obvious that conservative forces like organized religion, the police, and other agents of the tyrannical majority don't want sadomasochism to flourish anywhere, and sexually active women have always been a threat the system won't tolerate. But conservative gay liberationists and orthodox feminists are also embarrassed by kinky sexual subcultures (even if that's where they do their tricking).[35]

Califia recalled later:

> I was terrified when I wrote it. I kept getting up in the middle of typing to lie down until my nausea subsided and my hands stopped shaking. When

that issue of *The Advocate* hit the newsstands, it was days before I could actually look at my words in print.[36]

Califia described the lack of organizational infrastructure for S/M lesbians, even in the post-Stonewall years.

> Lesbian S/M isn't terribly well-organized yet. . . . We don't have bars. We don't even have newspapers or magazines with sex ads. I sometimes think the gay subculture must have looked like this when gay life first became urbanized. Since our community depends on word-of-mouth and social networks, we have to work very hard to keep it going. It's a survival issue.[37]

Activist and academic Gayle Rubin described it thus:

> When I came out as a lesbian sadomasochist, there was no place to go. A notice I put up in my local feminist bookstore was torn down. It took months of painstaking detective work to track down other women who were into S/M. There was no public lesbian S/M community to find, so I had to help build one.[38]

S/M lesbians had to find allies in gay men and pro-dommes for education and venues such as the Catacombs fisting club and other gay leather bars that allowed women.

Society of Janus, which had strong support from bisexual and lesbian women, launched Cardea, a women's outreach group, in 1976. Initially a discussion group, Cardea began giving demonstrations. Cynthia Slater spoke at the Bacchanal lesbian bar in Albany in 1976, and according to Patrick Califia, "It was the most explicit information about S/M eroticism the community had heard so far, and more than a few women who would later join Samois began 'coming out' that night."[39]

The volunteers eventually burned out, but the core group of lesbian women founded the Samois Collective in 1978, named after the estate of a lesbian dominatrix in *Story of O*.[40] This followed the tradition of coded names for homosexual groups like the Mattachine Society and the Daughters of Bilitis. Gayle Rubin described their membership as "lots of refugees from Lesbian Nation, a good number of bar dykes, and many women who work in the sex industry."[41] Lacking their own bars or baths to cruise in, they held play parties in peoples' homes, creating tension over whether

Samois was a political or a social group. The group organized educational presentations and worked to be included in the 1979 Gay Freedom Day Parade, along with potlucks, workshops, fashion shows, playroom tours, and other events.

Even more than its predecessor organization, Samois had to fight for recognition and resources, often against other women. Their publications, like the forty-five-page booklet called *What Color Is Your Handkerchief?* (1979)[42] and *Hanky Code for Women* (1979), were initially refused by feminist bookstores or hidden in back shelves. Samois published an anthology of fiction and nonfiction, *Coming to Power* (1981), which proved highly popular and broke lesbian sexuality out of the box pushed by orthodox lesbian feminists. Samois's 1981 meeting at the Women's Building (after warnings from the management not to do anything "offensive"[43]) brought together S/M lesbians from all over North America, interested in starting their own organizations. The organizational strains caused Samois to fragment, and the group folded in 1983. Successor groups included the Outcasts and the Exiles, which was still active in the 2010s.[44]

On the US east coast, the vanguard of lesbian sadomasochism was the Lesbian Sex Mafia (LSM), founded in 1981 for "politically incorrect women." One of the organizers, Dorothy Allison, described it:

> The Lesbian Sex Mafia was to be an old-fashion consciousness-raising group whose whole concern would be the subject of sex. To be sure that we would remain focused on our own outrageousness, we chose our deliberately provocative name and concentrated on attracting members whose primary sexual orientation was s/m, butch/femme, fetish specific, or otherwise politically incorrect. We drew more women from the lesbian bars than the feminist movement, but we deliberately brought back the principles of CR (using xeroxes of guidelines from 1973 that I found in my files). We insisted that within the group we would make no assumptions, no judgment, and no conclusions. We began by asking each other what it would be like to organize for our sexual desire as strongly as we had tried to organize for our sexual defense.[45]

Much like Samois, LSM was founded to meet the needs for community and education, including play parties and workshops, and formed close ties with GMSMA (Gay Male S/M Activists). The two groups co-sponsored Leather Pride, a fundraiser for the Gay and Lesbian Pride Parade.[46]

S/M lesbians were in an awkward position, under attack from two different angles. From one side, cultural conservatives, such as the Save Our Children movement led by Anita Bryant, focused on the minority and fringe elements of the gay community. "This created a mean-spirited and frightened attitude in the mainstream gay movement. Pedophiles, transsexuals and transvestites, tearoom cruisers, hustlers, young gays and S/M people were disavowed and urged to keep quiet and become invisible."[47]

On the other side, lesbian-feminists shunned or outright demonized S/M lesbians, either as a defense against conservatives or as an attack on what they saw as patriarchal false consciousness.[48]

Only a few months after Karla Jay's essay was published in *Lesbian Tide*, Ti-Grace Atkinson addressed a meeting of the Till Eulenspiegel Society and took the opposite stance from Jay.

> Your "enemy" is not the Establishment *per se*. In *fact*, you claim *as your life force* the distillation of the *essence* of that Establishment. Your *enemy* is the *resistance* of the Establishment to *recognize* you as its *own*.
>
> I think that a proper analysis of the Establishment's resistance to openly embracing S/M would clue you in to the hostility of Women's Liberation to you. S/M is the cat the Establishment does not want out of the bag—*not* because it does not understand your blood kinship, but because it does not want women to understand in such overt and brutal terms the very nature of the power relationship. And, I must add, the nature and function of sex itself—at least as the Establishment would have it.[49]

Atkinson said that if forced to choose between freedom and sex, a true feminist would always choose freedom.[50] In her view, female masochism came from women's oppression, a symptom that would be shed in the process of liberation. "The fact that oppressed people, not only women, have masochistic sexual fantasies is a reflection of a passive political position."[51] Female sadism was not even mentioned.

Atkinson's talk was widely reprinted and cited in debates over SM, notably in the 1982 anthology *Against Sadomasochism* with the title "Why I'm Against S/M Liberation."[52]

Also in 1975, Susan Brownmiller published *Against Our Will*, her groundbreaking feminist treatise on rape. She briefly discussed the gay leather subculture and sadomasochism.

Hardly by accident, sadomasochism has always been defined by male and female terms. It has been codified by those who see in sadism a twisted understanding of their manhood, and it has been accepted by those who see in masochism the abuse and pain that is synonymous with Woman. For this reason alone sadomasochism shall always remain a reactionary antithesis to women's liberation.[53]

Atkinson and Brownmiller both located sadomasochism as part of heterosexuality, which meant male domination and female submission. Their beliefs echoed those of many other second-wave feminists, and in those terms, "S/M and feminism were not just strange bedfellows, but a theoretical impossibility."[54] These thoughts also contributed to mid-1970s feminist protests against sexualized violence in the media. At the time, popular culture flirted with S/M chic, often associated with fascism or nihilistic decadence, such as *The Night Porter* (1974), the film adaptation of *Story of O* (1975), the exploitation/hoax film *Snuff* (1976), and the billboard promoting the Rolling Stones's *Black and Blue* album (1976), which showed a bound woman with the caption "I'm Black and Blue from the Rolling Stones and I love it."[55]

Although Atkinson and Brownmiller did not directly speak on lesbian sadomasochism, kinky lesbians became the marginal population that lesbian-feminists targeted for exclusion. In the late 1970s and early 1980s, the categories of "lesbian" and "feminist" were highly unstable. In such circumstances, people shore up their boundaries by identifying marginal populations and trying to exclude them. At the same time as second-wave feminism began addressing issues of sexuality, lesbian S/M organizations like Samois and the Lesbian Sex Mafia were just beginning to make themselves known. Sadomasochism, even if practiced consensually by lesbians, was deemed the worst kind of patriarchal oppression. S/M was also used to stand in for pornography as a whole, for shock value, with no consideration that women could consent or take pleasure in S/M.[56] Lynda Hart called this a moral panic.[57] This conflict came to be known as the Lesbian Sex Wars.[58]

In San Francisco, WAVPM (Women Against Violence in Pornography and the Media) frequently attacked S/M, and particularly Samois, despite the women who were members of both groups. It used a slide show about pornography as a recruiting tool, which juxtaposed bondage photos with police pictures of battered women, and presented the images without context or discussion.[59] WAVPM shut Samois out of the national Feminist Perspectives on Pornography conference, refused to engage in debate or dialog with S/M lesbians, and even denied having a policy on S/M. In 1980, WAVPM announced a forum on sadomasochism in the lesbian community. Samois members were invited, but they decided that they were being set up and picketed the forum, passing out leaflets titled, "This Forum Is a Lie about S/M." Inside, the WAVPM named sadomasochism as a disease of a patriarchal society, and linked it to everything from violence in lesbian relationships to white slavery. At this point, even some of the audience questioned WAVPM's statements and how they had handled the forum, causing a loss of credibility.[60]

In the same year, the National Organization for Women passed a resolution condemning "pederasty, pornography, sadomasochism and public sex" as male-identified and violating feminist principles.[61]

A major clash of the Lesbian Sex Wars came in 1982 at the Scholar and the Feminist IX Conference at Barnard College in New York City (commonly known as "the Barnard Conference"). The planners decided to apply feminist analysis to SM rather than "setting off controversy in the ruts available to feminists now." However, they were also critical of the tactics and ideologies of anti-pornography feminists, and refused to allow Women Against Pornography to participate in the committee or present at the conference because they "would destroy the spirit of open inquiry."[62]

Prior to the conference, a small group of anti-pornography activists called the Barnard administration and the Women's Center and claimed that the conference's planning committee had been manipulated or controlled by sadomasochists. This pressure made the Barnard administration confiscate and destroy the conference's program less than twenty-four hours before the event started, and reprint it without any mention of the hosting institution, after the event was over.[63]

The conference itself saw more problems. Anti-SM feminists, united under "Coalition for a Feminist Sexuality Against Sadomasochism," smeared the conference with a protest outside, staffed by women wearing T-shirts that read "For Feminist Sexuality" on one side and "Against S/M" on the other. They distributed a leaflet[64] that named specific women as perverts and exploiters of women, and misrepresented the conference as solely concerned with and uncritical of pornography, S/M, and butch/

femme, when these were only a few of the topics related to women's health and sexuality discussed.[65] They successfully framed the terms of the debate in feminist media as pro- versus anti-SM.[66]

At the speak-out organized by the LSM the next day at the Lesbian Herstory Archives, SM lesbians wore their leathers publicly and spoke on the topics the Barnard Conference was accused of promoting.[67] They described their personal experiences, and especially their feelings of being excluded from the feminist movement.[68] Dorothy Allison declared her lesbian feminist bona fides, then explained:

> I had a slight problem. "We love softer" was what lesbian feminists said, and I liked big, tough, pushy women. I lived in a feminist closet for 6 years; I was celibate for two years and wrote lots of bad short stories. But I became less good at hiding eventually. Also, if you're hiding, you're not connecting, you're not getting any.[69]

For years afterwards, Allison received awkward phone calls from lesbian colleagues who wanted advice about their sexual practices, which they could barely put into words because of their shame and ignorance, proof of the need for kink education. She was also harassed with anonymous phone calls at her place of work.

The arguments and counterarguments over the Barnard Conference and the coalition's actions continued in the feminist media for years afterward, which reinforced the misperception that the conference was primarily about lesbian sadomasochism.[70]

The debate through the 1980s over feminism and S/M was largely academic, and heavy on theory instead of practical knowledge.[71] In the anthology *Against Sadomasochism* (1982),[72] sadomasochism was described as, at worst, patriarchal false consciousness and, at best, an immature holdover from less enlightened times. Instead of being a primitive form of psychological development, it was a primitive form of political consciousness.[73] The anthology was based on a WAVPM forum about lesbian sadomasochism (to which Samois was not invited).[74] It included contributions from notable feminist academics and writers like Ti-Grace Atkinson,[75] Judith Butler, Audre Lorde, and Alice Walker.

Some of the essays were satires that portrayed sadomasochism as childish or self-destructive.[76] Others linked SM with fascism and other historical forms of oppression, as an insult to the real sufferers of the oppression of the Holocaust or slavery, as a way of normalizing authoritarianism in the present, or as a reactionary backlash against feminism that even gay men and lesbians were caught up in.[77]

Some of the essays took a social-constructivist position to criticize the idea of "consent" and of inherent desires. A certain strain of lesbian-feminist argued that "lesbian" was not a psychosexual type but a chosen social and political identity, a conscientious objector to heteronormativity. Likewise, the sadist or masochist was not "born that way," but just playing out their predetermined part in the social order. If the goal was removal of power from all human relations, fantasy or reality, then sadomasochism was unacceptable.[78]

Some of the writers followed a kind of Christian sin-and-repent narrative, with the author recounting personal experience with the seductions and pleasures of sadomasochism, a crisis, a new consciousness, and the promise of salvation through non-sadomasochistic sex. Marissa Jonel's "Letter from a Former Masochist" ended with a tepid endorsement of non-kinky sex:

> It is my hope that by sharing my experiences other lesbians in similar situations can find hope and know that it's possible to leave—that it is possible to go from the drama and high energy/emotion of sm back to "vanilla" sex. "Vanilla" sex is *not* unexciting.[79]

A few of the authors were surprisingly ambivalent about SM. They admitted their sadomasochistic desires and fantasies, which conflicted with their political principles. The solution appears to be varying degrees of personal repression.[80] Maryel Norris, in her essay "An Opinionated Piece on Sadomasochism," wrestled with this question.

> Isn't the thought as sick as the act would be? Or, as I believe, do fantasies serve a useful purpose in venting frustrations? No one is harmed. Punching a pillow is better than punching one's lover. And I allow myself my fantasies.[81]

Some lesbian-feminists tried to reclaim lost territory by positioning certain sexual acts as politically acceptable, instead of leaving them under the umbrella of SM. In one lesbian erotica anthology, five out of twelve stories contained acts that could be seen as SM, though neither the anthology nor the stories were specifically billed as SM. "This is, in part, a defusion of sm's claim to centre stage by redefining as neutral acts that have become discursively constructed as sm, for example, anal penetration and fisting."[82] SM-based terminology, like "top" and "bottom," permeated the discussion among vanilla lesbians.[83]

Pro-sex and pro-BDSM lesbians created their own discourse in anthologies like *Coming to Power*, journals like *Cathexis* (launched 1983) and *Outrageous Women* (launched 1984), and magazines like *Bad Attitude* and *On Our Backs* (both launched 1984). They positioned themselves as rebels against both mainstream society and the orthodoxy of radical lesbian-feminists.

Bad Attitude and *On Our Backs* could be hyperbolic and reactionary,[84] but they were crucial in forming the identity category of the SM lesbian, and they couldn't be separated from the lesbian-feminist criticism. The letter columns showed a wide variety of attitudes toward lesbian sexual expression and SM, but the discussion was what mattered.[85]

The follow-up to *Against Sadomasochism*, published a decade later, was *Unleashing Feminism* (1993).[86] The authors' argued that lesbians and other queers had lost their revolutionary principles and were being assimilated into mainstream consumer culture. Some of the essays portrayed the "lesbian sex wars" as a microcosm of a larger, almost apocalyptic conflict.

Kathy Miriam's "From Rage to All the Rage: Lesbian-Feminism, Sadomasochism, and the Politics of Memory" saw lesbian BDSM as the same old sexual values seductively repackaged as hip for queers, part of a retreat from more political views of identity.[87] Jamie Lee Evans bluntly declared, "I believe the not-guilty verdict against the batterers of Rodney King was a decision based on racism as well as a product of analysis brought forth via a culture indoctrinated with violence and sadomasochistic beliefs."[88] Her theory was based on a statement from jurors in the King case, who said they thought that King was partly in control of his beating. "In sadomasochism . . . the backgrounds of masochists are usually of those who have been victimized and those who are sadists are usually people who hold power positions in their family, workplace, etc."[89] (Note that she offered no evidence for this claim.)

A key point of this debate was: What exactly was the nature of female sexuality without male domination? Would it be purely loving and egalitarian? Could the aggressive aspects of sexuality under patriarchy be expunged? For lesbian-feminists, that was the goal, though this kind of ideal sexual experience appeared to be a somewhat uncommon event. Kathy Miriam quoted Sheila Jeffreys, discussing egalitarian sexuality as if it were some kind of elusive cryptofauna, more theory than practice.[90]

When *Unleashing Feminism* was published, lesbian-feminism as a political philosophy and practice was only about twenty years old. People tried to make two separate concepts, lesbianism and feminism, not just compatible but synonymous, and exclude people who didn't fit. Radical lesbian-feminists defined themselves in opposition to lesbian sadomasochists, and reciprocally, lesbian feminists defined themselves against the prescriptions of radical lesbian-feminists. "The sadomasochist's attack on lesbian-feminism (egalitarianism is a mask for good girl patriarchal morality) is a symmetrical rebuttal of the feminist critique of sadomasochism as a product of conditioning."

Both sides took pleasure in their roles in the drama.[91] The first issue of *On Our Backs* included a satirical article by "Andrix Workin" (i.e., radical feminist Andrea Dworkin) titled "A Cup of Tea Is Preferable to Any Sexual Encounter."[92] Likewise, anti-SM feminists wrote their own satires, such as Vivienne Walker-Crawford's "The Saga of Sadie O. Massey," or "Smokers Protest Healthism" by "Paula Tiklicorrect" in *Against Sadomasochism*.[93]

Despite the vehemence of the conflict in the early 1980s, the lesbian sex wars for the most part faded out. Lesbian BDSM organizations, events, and publications expanded across North America into the 1990s and beyond. Publications like *Cathexis* and *Outrageous Women* included advertisements for BDSM toys, guest houses, and other publications, indicating a growing BDSM economy.[94] The International Ms. Leather contest launched in 1987.[95] The narrow sexual orthodoxy prescribed by radical lesbian-feminists was superseded by women-owned sex-toy shops, strip clubs, and bathhouses. Pro-sex lesbians apparently won, if only by default.[96]

POLITICAL GAY LEATHER

While the established culture of leather bars and clubs continued into the 1970s and 1980s, Gay Male S/M Activists (GMSMA) was a radically new organization.

As with TES and Janus, GMSMA started with a single individual using the communications media available to reach out to the like-minded. In this case, it was Brian O'Dell, who came out as a gay activist before he got involved in S/M. In the summer of 1980, O'Dell "tried a gambit that would have never have occurred to anyone who kept his sexuality and his politics separate"; he posted a letter to the *Gay Community News* looking for gay men in New York City to talk about kink, and included his real name and phone number. Over the next six months, what began as a handful of men nervously meeting in a living room grew into something much larger, and the first publicized meeting was in January 1981.[97]

GMSMA, like LSM, differed from existing S/M organizations like the Chicago Hellfire Club and San Francisco's 15 Association. Instead of operating like a private club in which a new member or attendee had to be sponsored by an existing member, GMSMA had an open roster, with no sponsorship or qualification required.[98] Whereas earlier gay leather groups kept under the radar, and even TES and Janus had discrete names, GMSMA was high profile and included both "gay" and "S/M" in its name, chosen to echo the old Gay Activists Alliance. This was enough for the group to be banned from using the new Gay and Lesbian Community Center. Then-president Richard Hocutt attended an open forum and publicly confronted the center's board. The crowd agreed with Hocutt and GMSMA was allowed to use the center.

GMSMA had three pillars: educational, social, and political. By far, education was the first priority, and the group taught both technique and understanding through workshops, seminars, and special interest groups to those new to the scene. Play parties were never a big part of GMSMA, but it organized many other social functions, often at the Mineshaft leather bar. The group, modeled after the National Gay Task Force, also did activist work, such as convincing a psychiatrist to stop advertising that he could "cure" sadomasochism, sending letters to the editors of the *Advocate*, the *Native*, *Drummer*, and other publications about their depiction of leatherpeople, and opening communication with police forces through the Gay Officers Action League.

In 1986, GMSMA won recognition from a coalition of gay and lesbian organizations planning a march on Washington the next year, and a seat on the steering committee. The group put together a national network to organize their contingent in the march, and in so doing had to come up with policies on who belonged in their contingent, and what their demands were.

The 1987 conference and march on Washington put the GMSMA and the general kink scene in contact with the larger network of queer activist organizations, and GMSMA was involved in many other queer and leather political actions in the 1980s and 1990s.[99]

GMSMA settled on two important concepts that proved to be far-reaching. The first was that any person who thought they belonged to the kink community, did, regardless of gender, sexuality, ethnicity, physical ability, age, level of experience, or degree of involvement in the scene. The second was GMSMA's sole demand: that all adults have the right in private to express affection in any manner that is "safe, sane and consensual," a phrase that became a guide to an entire generation of kinksters.

The earliest known use of the phrase "safe, sane and consensual" (SSC) appears in the August 1983 report from a committee to draft a new statement of identity and purpose for GMSMA. David Stein, one of the group's founders, says, "it seems very likely that i was its author" though he linked the phrase to a 1981 essay by Tony DeBlase in the run book for the Chicago Hellfire Club's Inferno 10 event, which mentioned "safe and sane enjoyment of men by men." Stein also linked it to the common reminder to "Have a safe and sane Fourth of July" that he often saw as a child. The phrase was accepted by the board and became part of GMSMA's media, particularly after the 1987 March on Washington, appearing on the SM contingent's correspondence, press releases, newsletters, and T-shirts. In the 1993 march, the slogan was even more prominently displayed across the contingent's banner.[100]

Adopted by the heterosexual and lesbian communities as well, SSC became something more than originally intended, an overall philosophy of S/M instead of the beginning of the discussion on how to do S/M.

In the wake of the first generation of BDSM organizations, groups with similar philosophies and practices appeared across North America, including Gay Men's S/M Cooperative (GMSMC) in Philadelphia; Avatar, Leather & Lace, and Threshold in Los Angeles; Vancouver Activists in S/M (VASM); Sigma in Washington, D.C.; and Bound & Determined in western Massachusetts; and local chapters of the Seattle-based National Leather Association.[101] In less than twenty years, S/M changed from something that belonged to small fraternities of men or sex workers to a continent-wide subculture that was vastly more visible and welcoming.

———•◉•———

The heterosexual BDSM community did not have, and probably never could have had, a city district to call its own, the way leathermen could claim SOMA in San Francisco before 1980. While there were active communities in major North American cities providing support and education in the late 1980s, their reach did not extend into smaller communities. Despite various books, magazines, and other forms of media exposure, there wasn't a way for a critical mass of kinky people to communicate with one another, the way gay men did in their own districts.

That was soon to change. The next stage in the evolution of BDSM culture was coming.

Chapter Eleven

alt.sex

My first contact with the kinky community was on the internet, via 14.4k acoustic modems and their characteristic screech, specifically the USENET forums of the early 1990s. One such contact was with a woman who lived on the other side of the continent. We began an e-mail-only Master-slave relationship that lasted for more than a year, with a signed contract, exchanged gifts, and daily reports. We are still friends more than twenty years later.

I only learned about local BDSM organizations through her, as she had access to a guidebook for LGBT and related organizations. Her encouragement helped me make that first step and meet other kinksters face-to-face.

When the internet rose to prominence as a new communications medium in the 1990s, sadomasochistic pornography was one of the many erotic genres that drove its expansion. The back pages of the *Computer Shopper* contained ads from erotic clubs and services.[1] The internet also had a more profound effect on the emerging sadomasochistic subculture, enabling it to expand and diversify to an unprecedented degree.

Since as far back as the late nineteenth century, people had used personal ads in newspapers and magazines to find and meet people for sexual interests. They combined anonymous expressions with connections based on interests instead of geography. If the Victorian flagellation ads and letters—anonymous, blurring fantasy and reality—were the seed of kink culture, the internet made it blossom. The internet, from the early days of local bulletin board systems to the USENET to the World Wide Web, raised this style of communication to an unprecedented degree. As a medium, it could be as niche and specific as the private newsletters published by BDSM organizations, yet be available to the general public if they chose to look. There was slang and jargon, but also the educational means to learn it.[2] Furthermore, the online space enabled kinky people to represent themselves to the world and each other.[3] It was a medium that fostered a strong, disinhibiting intimacy despite the narrow range of communication.[4]

The new social space of the internet also had gender and class implications. One woman wrote about her online experiences on the web and in BDSM chat rooms:

> From a primary, domestic network I found the wonders—and the wanderers—of surfing. Anything you had ever wondered about could be put in the search box and moments later a myriad of information arrived. I had entered virtual reality as a seeker of the real. Through my foray into surfing I found the decidedly unreal, and the out-of-this-world. My brain ran amuck. Here was a medium which would not judge me should I search for the less socially acceptable facts of life. . . . I felt, as many others have, that I was walking on the wild side. I started to write erotica as an outlet for my frustrated creativity. I found many women were doing the same thing. Most of us were expressing ourselves in ways that had never been acceptable to society or family in our roles as mothers, wives, daughters, co-workers, and so on. From the safety of my office chair, I had slipped over to the wrong side of town.[5]

Kink was no longer spatially located in the "wrong side of town," the marginalized, masculine world of adult stores, bars, brothels, porn studios, and swing clubs. Now, it was potentially everywhere there was a telephone connection, including female-gendered spaces like the home.

EDUCATION

This put vastly more people in reach of the sadomasochistic community's knowledge and support. When mainstream media such as book publishers or television news treated sadomasochism as sick or evil, the internet gave people access to information and support without such gatekeepers.

For private citizens, the earliest connections to the internet were bulletin board systems (BBSes) accessed via phone lines and acoustic modems.

Gloria Brame, future coauthor of *Different Loving* (1994), a groundbreaking collection of essays and interviews with kinksters, first ventured onto a BBS with kink material in late 1985.

> So, I logged onto the BBS and began reading messages which shocked me. I'm not sure now if part of that shock wasn't simply the shock of recognition. At the time, I was mildly horrified and fiercely embarrassed. All the things that, normally, are shamefully hidden were, in this forum, publicly and matter-of-factly flaunted. People talked about weird sex and extreme practices the way my parents talked about going to Dunkin' Donuts—with cheerful and eager anticipation.
>
> The candor among this band of perverts was captivating. Straightforward discussion of topics that most people considered taboo? Confessions of sexual quirks that most people (including myself) didn't have the balls to admit having, even to ourselves? There was something else: I had by then already made my commitment to art. The life of the artist, I knew from the first, was all about a commitment to living in truth. In their own way, these kinky adventurers were sexual artists. In short, I loved it![6]

Unlike the initiations of earlier generations of sadomasochists, such as David Stein's nervous first foray into a leather bar, Brame's moment of personal transformation came when she posted a message on the BBS introducing herself and describing her fantasies. "Writing that first message was the most difficult step I've ever taken. And it was at that moment, I think, that I truly became a sadomasochist. Because what drove me then was the knowledge that I was taking a step towards my sexual destiny."

Online services like Compuserve and America Online developed their own kink communities. On Compuserve, Gloria Brame founded the Human Sexuality Forum's Variations II group in 1987. On that forum, she met her future husband, Will Brame, and together with Jon Jacobs they coauthored *Different Loving* (1994).[7] Instead of kinky people having to view themselves refracted through sensationalist magazine pieces or psychology textbooks, this collection of interviews and essays were kinky people self-representing. In that regard, it was a descendant of *The Leatherman's Handbook* and *Coming to Power* but directed at a mass, primarily heterosexual audience. Another part of the internet was USENET, tens of thousands of newsgroups. Of the top-level hierarchies, the alt section was relatively unregulated, and the alt.sex subsection experienced an explosion of newsgroups devoted to alternative sexualities.

The newsgroup alt.sex.bondage ("asb" for short), founded in 1991, was a town square for kinky people all over the world.

> On any day in asb there will be around 30 new topics and responses. During one 24-hour period in early February, readers posted questions about a rumored Donahue show on "Private Parts Punishment," about the cast list for a movie based on an Anne Rice novel, and—from Austria—about the design of a "Leatherpride" symbol. A self-confessed "clueless" university student wanted more specific and basic information: "What is it that you enjoy about dominance and submission? How do you feel before/during/after a scene, and what is it that causes such an intense release? How did you get involved in B&D/S&M in the first place? Was it a gradual introduction, or a sudden submergence?"
> One new post contained a woman's reminiscence about the first time she was flogged by a man: "You gave me the sweet gift of wanting me and making me feel comfortable. The actual zero to sixty was, as I recall, just a few days over a week? And the wonder is, I thought if I ever did such a thing I would feel ambivalent afterwards. But all I really feel is blessed. Thank you." Others were requests for songs about dominance and submission, a eulogy for a dead friend, and an announcement for a new S/M 'zine. Such a broad range of postings has shaped asb into a kind of sexual town square with a real-time message board full of constantly shifting information and ideas.[8]

Amid the personal ads and pornography, asb's regulars worked out the ethics and philosophy of sadomasochism.

> One other subject that comes up again and again in asb is the power dynamics in S/M and bondage. How much power should one person have over another in a dominant/submissive relationship? . . . The nature of this lifestyle is constantly debated in asb. Even bondage supporters sometimes attack the idea of voluntary slavery. ("Submission does damage and weaken; it does so by definition! To state otherwise is a consummate hypocrisy!") Many slaves defend their lives as part of a spectrum of consensual behavior: ("I have examined my life as a slave, and found that for me it is a wonderful and empowering experience. Acceptance of yourself is what really counts.") This debate has been going on for almost as long as asb has existed, and the arguments seem no nearer to any kind of conclusion. As in the real world, debate of such a fundamental question will probably go on forever—in what's known online as a Holy War.[9]

Beginning in 1991, these questions were distilled into the alt.sex.bondage FAQ (Frequently Asked Questions) list by Rob Jellinghaus (also known as Johnson Grey), a Yale graduate and former Microsoft intern.[10] He addressed questions like, "What do B&D, S&M, D&S, 'top,' 'bottom' mean?" "What is a 'scene,' and what is 'negotiation'?" "When is pain not pain?" "Is SM degrading or abusive? Were most SM people abused?" or "My fantasies scare me. What if I get too into SM?"

Part technical manual, part self-help book, the ASB FAQ was the first information resource for many people exploring kink, in a time when there were few books or other resources available, and few channels that would carry them. It dealt with sadomasochism in a very practical, hands-on way, rather than a moralistic or medical position, and was written in a welcoming yet pragmatic style. Asb was later supplanted by soc.subculture.bondage-bdsm after the former was overrun by spam advertising, and the FAQ list migrated with it.

SOCIALIZATION

This accessibility also changed the nature of the community. The medium affected the content of the communication. In earlier decades, becoming a part of the sadomasochistic community involved, first, locating one of a small number of secretive groups located in major cities in the United States and Europe and, second, actually gaining admission. This involved a kind of "coming out" experience, or a second one in the case of non-heterosexual kinksters, at some social and physical risk. Learning kink etiquette and technique came from potential partners.[11]

Now, connection to the sadomasochistic community was as close as connecting to a chat room or newsgroup from the comfort of one's own home. No need to buy the outfit to pass a club or bar's dress code to connect to the culture, to cultivate the image before cultivating the knowledge.[12]

> The observer effect has held powerful sway in cyberspace, where large numbers of newcomers emulate the behavior of loquacious veterans and eagerly adopt the prevailing mores, etiquette, and slang. The net effect seems to be a growing emphasis on the technical elements of D&S and on its enormous potential as casual, safe-sex play. One of the more intriguing

phenomena has been the proliferation of "play parties" and "munches," regional social events organized by and for D&S cybernauts who meet for "3-D" interfacing.[13]

The sheer number of people entering the scene accelerated the cultural shift from the tribe-like structure of earlier generations of leathermen to the remote learning structure of the new scene. The primary mode of interaction shifted from "sight and then touch"[14] to text.

Internet communication was also important for changing the way in which kinky people formed their identities through shared interests instead of family, neighborhood, or work relationships.[15] Instead of medical texts or pornographic novels, kinky people could now form their identities through communication with each other and manage the stigma from the greater society. Virtual communities like asb provided validation and support from the like-minded, reassuring people that they weren't freaks or monsters. Users could post and read personal accounts that normalized sadomasochism in the face of condemnation, through articulating norms of consent and safety, and claims of benefit and self-fulfillment. They taught and learned the specialized vocabulary like "top," "bottom," and "switch," and reclaimed stigmatizing words like "pervert" and "deviant," much as homosexuals reclaimed words like "fag" and "dyke." They also denied deviance at all, claiming that kinky people were just another part of society, or even more enlightened than "vanilla" people who were not as concerned with consent or personal exploration.[16]

Beyond creating a semi-public space for learning and socializing, the internet also provided virtual worlds for fantasy and experimentation with roles in safe, anonymous, largely consequence-free spaces, variously known as netsex, cybersex, or TinySex. Kinky channels on IRC (Internet Relay Chat) developed a complicated and highly coded protocol for in-Scene communication, which some Scene veterans disdained. Polly Peachum, partner of Jon Jacobs, wrote of the difference between the "real" Scene, as she saw it, and the online Scene:

> So I had to assume that subs are being told regularly to do this lowercasing because most people in IRC chat rooms actually believe it is only right and proper for a submissive to lowercase her name. Am I the only one that finds this belief incredible, even preposterous?

Uppercasing and lowercasing one's nickname doesn't seem like such a big deal, and, in fact, it is a mighty convenient way to identify your place on the power continuum to attractive members of the opposite persuasion (maybe we should call this the "Hanky Panky Code"). Unfortunately, this practice suggests to people new to both D&S and IRC that all that submission consists of is a conglomeration of outward postures and attitudes, an idea amplified by many elements of the D&S subculture. Walk the walk, talk the talk, capitalize your name correctly and not only will everyone accept you as a genuine submissive but you will be a genuine submissive. If only it were actually that easy![17]

Other venues for BDSM interaction were the persistent text-based virtual environments known variously as MUDs, MUSHes, MUVEs, or MOOs, and their three-dimensional successors such as Second Life and The Sims Online.[18] A MOO called Strangebrew was one of the BDSM specialty communities, which offered educational essays as well as functionality like a specific command for submissives to lower their eyes or "cast" to others.[19]

In text-based virtual environments, people could program their MUD by writing prose descriptions of imaginary but persistent rooms, which could be specifically programmed for bondage, or programming a bullwhip with various "verbs" attached to it, or a character with scripted dialogue and behavior. Typing "@usage here" would reveal the instructions for a bondage room, such as "To fasten a player securely in the restraints on the four-poster bed, type the following: restrain <player> in wrist_straps, restrain <player> in ankle_straps." Doing so would restrict the player's range of actions in the MUD, though the room could also be programmed with a safe word: "If you need to get free, type @release, panic_button, or safe_word. This releases all the restraints in the room and sets all related properties to 0."[20] Much of the burden of creating the sexual experience was through writing descriptions, a collaborative, improvised fantasy. Even people who had never been spanked could be aroused by reading and writing descriptions of being whipped bloody.[21]

This experience emphasized the visual and intellectual instead of the tactile and the internal. Textual description filled in the gaps in the sensory experience by describing the sounds, touches, and smells. Even the visuals of Second Life, The Sims Online, and the like supplemented the previous generation of text-based worlds, but didn't replace them.[22]

This branched out into forms of sexuality and identity that were difficult or impossible in real life, such as furries (human-animal hybrids) or vore (being eaten).[23] It also created new forms of consent violation. In LambdaMOO, a user known as "Mr. Bungle" used a "voodoo doll" software tool to dictate the actions of other users's text avatars. The nascent community had to consider how to deal with this problem, and eventually banned the offender.[24]

Fans of John Norman's Gor series of sadomasochistic fantasy novels made particular use of this new technology. In effect, Gor already was a virtual world, described in great detail over more than twenty books at the time, and borrowing from the fantasies of the Orientalists of the previous centuries. Goreans replicated Gor in Second Life and similar virtual worlds, which allowed the extension of the BDSM aesthetic to a level impossible in reality, including gore and death.[25] The first Gorean public SIM, Port Kar, opened in 2005, with many private spaces before that. By 2006, there were over one hundred public Gorean spaces.[26] The online Gorean culture remains active in the 2010s, often using semi-obsolete chat programs like the Palace. Online Gor developed internal divisions between role players, who treated it more like a fantasy game, and lifestylers, who aimed to express their sexual roles and conservative ideas on gender, and adhered to the books closely, deriding other styles as "Disney Gor." A third subset were those who practiced BDSM in real life as well as in virtual life, and saw virtual worlds as a place to play at a higher level than was possible in real life.

There was considerable variety in how closely the virtual communities followed the books, how immersive the experience was, and how exclusionary the communities were to newcomers. Out of a list of fifty Gorean SIMs, only seven had explicit rules about consent, while in the others, nonconsensual enslavement was a possibility (provided the person didn't just exit the SIM).[27] Part of the appeal of Gor is that it is an extremely ordered world: "Everything in Gor is codified, and everyone knows their place and is proud of their identity."[28]

The spread of the Scene via the internet also meant that the Scene was "colonized" by people who had the means to connect to the internet—that is, access to a computer and modem, and the technical skills to use them. These were the already privileged: mostly male, white and middle-class, with a particular technocratic mind-set that often makes a person ill-suited to conventional heterosexual courtship.

Role-playing and group sex and scenes (whether of the consensual S-M, fetish, or other variants) can work very well with a technocosmology: They all call for explicit and simple rules. Map out and apply the algorithm. Don't rely on those vague subtle possibly apocryphal cues that nongeeks *say* they rely on. . . . This is not to say that all nerds lack social or courting skills, or go in for what are called in the personals columns "alternative lifestyles," or these days can't be into rollerblading. But a strong intersection exists between nerds and fringe sex.[29]

The Culture Shocked column in the *San Francisco Bay Guardian* called this particular combination of deviance and geekiness the "nervert":

> Nerds are well aware that they'll strike out every time in the Ken-and-Barbie land of Marina-style bar scenes. The sexual mainstream has already rejected them. So nerverts seek out situations in which the rules about what is and isn't desirable are simply different. One positive consequence of being a lifelong social outcast: it makes you more open to interesting alternatives.
>
> Yet the unwritten rules of human contact remain hopelessly obscure to the real nerd, who fails to grasp the kind of implicit social cues that most people take for granted. This is endlessly frustrating to the supremely logical nerd mind, which thrives in a RTFM ("read the fucking manual") environment in which there's a knowable system that can be examined and mastered. Human beings—they don't come with $*&%@ manuals!
>
> But consider this predicament as a lucky "freedom from social skills" and you'll see that it makes nerverts uniquely suited for highly structured sex games and all kinds of role-playing fantasies—from naughty nurse to D&D. They can at once escape the impossible task of just "acting normal" around others, and deliberately, systematically create their own worlds.
>
> While nerds don't do well with emotional nuances, they do respond well to the open communication, honesty, and well-defined rules inherent to S-M and safer-sex practices. All this pragmatic processing is like a Rosetta stone for the subtle cues nerverts can't read on their own. What a relief.[30]

Online, those who had any real-life experience in BDSM were outnumbered by those who had little or none (whether due to lack of opportunity or lack of courage), so the agenda was set in favor of the latter. Conventions that had begun online crept into other media and real life, like lowercase names for submissives and uppercase names and pronouns for dominants.

BDSM community lore has it that the very first munch, a casual gathering for kinky people at a public bar or restaurant, was organized by STella, a Stanford university student, and announced only on alt.sex.bondage. Thirteen people gathered at the Flames coffee shop in Santa Clara, California. STella later refined this idea into the weekly "BurgerMunch" at Kirk's Steakburger in Palo Alto, California, starting in April 1992. The event grew rapidly as more people learned about it online, and the group took over the patio area and even began to do some limited play. Due to friction with the management, the BurgerMunch was forced to relocate to Antonio's NutHouse in November 1992. Stella asked to keep the "BurgerMunch" name, and split it off into a private play event. The other group formalized the idea that the Munch should be a no-play event, nonthreatening and welcoming to newcomers.[31] This signified a transformation from the old San Francisco that had fostered the queer communities to the new San Francisco of tech business.[32] Munches were promoted through e-mail lists and online calendars and, later, FetLife postings; not mimeographed posters on leather bar walls or LGBTQ community center bulletin boards. The venues were distributed and networked, often suburban, not concentrated in a distinct area as San Francisco's SOMA before HIV and gentrification. The primary population of the Scene shifted from gay urban men to straight or bi men and women from San Francisco's suburbs, the kind of people who worried about "good schools." This was another iteration of the generational divides we've seen before in the evolution of the kink culture.

In the social network era of the late 2000s, FetLife rapidly became the premiere social network for kinky people. Founded by Montreal software engineer John Baku in 2008, it had an advantage that other competitors to Facebook didn't have, that many people wished to keep their kink lives separate from their vanilla lives. Baku claimed FetLife had a near-even split between men and women and an even split between straight and non-straight people. FetLife differed significantly from earlier kink-based social networks, such as Bondage.com, Alt.com and CollarMe.com. The search functions were deliberately limited, making it more difficult to search for, say, dominant females 18–35 and send harassing e-mails to all of them. FetLife was designed from the beginning as a community, not a hookup site. Kink wasn't just what some people did to get their rocks off, it was a part of their lives. It was recognized as a culture and a community, not just a marketing niche.[33] It was also free. "It is not another paid dating site where you can't do anything unless you are a paid member. FetLife is free as in Facebook and MySpace free. No scams, no tricks; we built the site for us and we are cheap bastards, so if we wouldn't pay how can we expect anyone else to :-)."[34] FetLife was definitely a product of the post-internet kink culture.

In the 1990s and 2000s, the online space fostered the visibility, growth, and diversification of sadomasochistic subculture. Unfortunately, the online medium also let it become a target.

Chapter Twelve

Sex and Power

Because sexuality in Western societies is so mystified, the wars over it are often fought at oblique angles, aimed at phony targets, conducted with misplaced passions, and are highly, intensely symbolic. Sexual activities often function as signifiers for personal and social apprehensions to which they have no intrinsic connection. During a moral panic, such fears attach to some unfortunate sexual activity or population. The media become ablaze with indignation, the public behaves like a rabid mob, the police are activated, and the state enacts new laws and regulations. . . . The system of sexual stratification provides easy victims who lack the power to defend themselves, and a preexisting apparatus for controlling their movements and curtailing their freedoms. The stigma against sexual dissidents renders them morally defenseless.[1]

Whom do I tell? That's a question that kept occurring to me as my career in the BDSM world progressed. Should I be political about kink, or is BDSM best kept as a delicious secret, reserved for the initiated? I've had a few Scene names, but I stopped bothering with them years ago. The Scene is full of people I only know by their first names or Scene names or Fetlife handles.

Some Scene people are meticulous about their privacy, fearing consequences in the professional or familial realms if discovered. Others are merely discreet. They don't go to great lengths to conceal their identities but aren't "out" in the way that gay people talk about it, as a social and political act. My own shift was a gradual process. As the internet grew, my name appeared in kink contexts with greater frequency, until anybody could type my name into a search engine and see my connection. The concepts of "privacy," and "public versus private," have changed significantly since I started in the early 1990s.

Of course, as a white, heterosexual, cisgender male, with no family to lose, who works in a field where people seldom care about such things, I can afford to say that. For other people the consequences of exposure are too great.

Even though kinky people gather at munches in family restaurants with kids eating nearby, and play parties advertise in local newspapers, the BDSM culture retains a strong ethos of privacy. In part, this is for the thrill of initiation into a secret, underground world. It is also a measure of the privilege of heterosexual kinksters that they can remain secret. This is a major gulf between straight and queer kinksters, and it prevents kinky people and groups from building alliances and becoming a politicized culture.[2]

Even in the 1990s, when Anne Rice's sadomasochistic erotica could be bought in any shopping mall bookstore, and the image of the dominatrix was used to sell breath mints, the BDSM community's position was far from secure. With BDSM's visibility in the 2000s came an unstable dialectic between acceptance and abhorrence.

In the history of external attacks on sadomasochism, kinky people are frequently the incidental targets in conflicts that do not directly concern them. By its nature, sadomasochism can be frightening and confusing to the uninitiated, yet attention-grabbing, almost guaranteed to spark moral panics. If the sight of two people of the same gender kissing in public was no longer enough to mobilize anti-gay sentiment, then perhaps graphic descriptions of fisting or bullwhipping would have the necessary impact. Homophobes seized upon the icon of the leatherman and activities like fisting and sadomasochism to paint all homosexual men as depraved perverts. Likewise, anti-pornography feminists and conservatives used the most graphic sadomasochistic images to represent and condemn the entire range of pornography. Even worse, potential allies in the queer community may scramble to distance themselves from the targeted kinksters in an effort to present themselves as no more threatening to the mainstream than heterosexuals.

Foucault wrote that sexuality functions as a "dense transfer point for relations of power."[3] Whether they want to be or not, kinky people are involved in political struggles.

LET'S GET ORGANIZED

One of the fronts in this conflict is the psychiatric, and the lingering pathologization of sadomasochism. In the United States, the authoritative guide to psychological illness is the *Diagnostic and Statistical Manual of Mental Disorders* (DSM), published by the American Psychiatric Association (APA). The APA voted to remove homosexuality from the DSM in 1974, though this was not completely implemented until 1986.

The diagnoses of sadism, masochism, and paraphilias had their own history in the DSM, as the reference slowly and haltingly moved into alignment with the consensus of the emerging BDSM culture.

The first edition of the DSM in 1952 had no diagnosis for sexual masochism.[4] Sexual sadism was part of the diagnosis of sexual deviation, "deviant sexuality . . . not symptomatic of more extensive syndromes," under the general heading of Sociopathic Personality Disturbance, though without any diagnostic criteria.[5]

In the second edition of the DSM in 1968, sexual sadism and sexual masochism were classified as sexual deviations and still lacked particular diagnostic criteria: "[S]exual interests are directed primarily towards objects other than people of the opposite sex, toward sexual acts not usually associated with coitus, or toward coitus performed under bizarre circumstances as in necrophilia, pedophilia, sexual sadism, and fetishism."[6]

In the DSM-III (1980), sexual sadism was reclassified as one of the paraphilias. While the criteria allowed for consenting partners, it was still pathologized: "[T]he repeatedly preferred or exclusive mode of achieving sexual excitement combines humiliation with simulated or mildly injurious bodily suffering." Or "[B]odily injury that is extensive, permanent, or possibly mortal is inflicted in order to achieve sexual excitement."[7] Questions of consent or harm were irrelevant; the desire itself was a sickness.

Sexual masochism was also classified as a paraphilia, and finally given distinct criteria: "A preferred or exclusive mode of producing sexual excitement is to be humiliated, bound, beaten, or otherwise made to suffer."

Or "The individual has intentionally participated in an activity in which he or she was physically harmed or his or her life was threatened, in order to produce sexual excitement."[8]

The revised DSM-III (1987)'s definition of sexual sadism still did not consider the consent of partners.

> A. Over a period of at least six months, recurrent intense sexual urges and sexually arousing fantasies involving acts (real, not simulated) in which the psychological or physical suffering (including humiliation) of the victim is sexually exciting to the person.
> B. The person has acted on these urges, or is markedly distressed by them.[9]

Sexual masochism now had a two-part diagnosis, including acting on fantasies: "A. Over a period of at least six months, recurrent, intense sexual urges and sexually arousing fantasies involving the act (real, not simulated) of being humiliated, beaten, bound, or otherwise made to suffer." And "B. The person has acted on these urges, or is markedly distressed by them."[10]

The DSM-IV (1994) was a turning point in the consideration of sadomasochism. The criteria for both sexual sadism and sexual masochism included a qualification: "The fantasies, sexual urges, or behaviors cause clinically significant distress or impairment in social, occupational, or other important areas of functioning." This "distress or impairment" could come about from imposing on an unwilling person. This definition, therefore, allowed for consensual, non-pathological relationships and experiences.[11]

One of the reasons for this change was the work of the DSM Project, a grassroots coalition of psychotherapeutic professionals dedicated to changing the categorization and diagnostic criteria of kink. Race Bannon, a writer and educator who had been involved in gay male leather since 1973, was the leader, and he was joined by Guy Baldwin, author, psychotherapist, and leather titleholder. Their advocacy helped change the DSM. Bannon and Baldwin also founded Kink Aware Professionals, a referral list of BDSM-friendly therapists.[12]

In the text revision edition published in 2000, the criteria for sexual masochism was unchanged, while the criteria for sexual sadism was one of the few changed from the previous edition. "The person has acted on these sexual urges with a non-consenting person, or the sexual urges or fantasies cause marked distress or interpersonal difficulty." It made clear that acting on sadistic urges was not in itself sufficient for diagnosis, and the person had to either violate consent or experience distress.[13]

The 2013 revision was the biggest change yet, distinguishing between a paraphilia or fetish and a paraphilic disorder, and between masochism and a masochistic disorder. The new diagnoses were "sexual sadism disorder," "sexual masochism disorder," and "fetishistic disorder," emphasizing that the condition must cause distress.

> A paraphilia is a necessary but not a sufficient condition for having a paraphilic disorder, and a paraphilia by itself does not necessarily justify or require clinical intervention.[14]

> In contrast, if they declare no distress, exemplified by anxiety, obsessions, guilt or shame, about these paraphilic impulses, and are not hampered by them in pursuing other personal goals, they could be ascertained as having masochistic sexual interest but should not be diagnosed with a sexual masochism disorder.[15]

> Many individuals who self-identify as fetishist practitioners do not necessarily report clinical impairment in association with their fetish-associated behaviors. Such individuals could be considered as having a fetish but not fetishistic disorder.[16]

> Clinical assessment of distress or impairment, like clinical assessment of transvestic sexual arousal, is usually dependent on the individual's self-report.[17]

In this revision, the National Coalition for Sexual Freedom participated in the revision of the DSM's criteria for sexual sadism, sexual masochism, and paraphilias.

The National Coalition for Sexual Freedom (NCSF)[18] was formed in 1997 as an alliance of five established American BDSM organizations:

- National Leather Association—International
- Gay Male S/M Activists
- The Eulenspiegel Society
- Black Rose
- Society of Janus

The driving force of this new coalition, and later its spokesperson, was Susan Wright, a science fiction, fantasy, romance/erotica, and nonfiction writer who had been active in the New York City leather community since 1991.[19] In 1997, she founded the SM Policy Reform Project to overturn the National Organization for Women's anti-SM stance, which succeeded in 1999. During this project, many kinky women told Wright about being discriminated against or losing custody of their children in divorces. This made her see the need of a national BDSM advocacy group, even though many activists told her it wouldn't work.[20]

The second version of the DSM Project was under the NCSF, and mainly run by Wright. She attempted to contact members of the APA's Sexual and Gender Identities Workgroup and the Paraphilias Subworkgroup with little result, until she met Dr. Richard Krueger in person after a panel and explained to him the problems with the current version of the DSM. "Legal complications" and "interference in social relationships" did happen in the lives of sadomasochists, Wright told Krueger, but that was because they were a persecuted minority, not because they were mentally ill. This was not unlike the way a homosexual person could suffer distress from having to live in social isolation or feel shame about their desires.[21]

Wright later sent Krueger the NCSF's accumulated research and arguments, including two surveys on violence and discrimination and the results from the Incident Reporting and Response program, and Krueger forwarded them to the rest of the workgroup. During this time, the NCSF also circulated its DSM Revision Petition to medical professionals. The final petition delivered to the APA had over three thousand signatures.[22]

The immediate impact to the revised DSM was in child custody cases involving kinky people, one of NCSF's main areas of interest. One-third of the roughly five hundred discrimination cases NCSF tracked each year involved divorce and custody issues. In one example, in 2010, St. Louis sex blogger Kendra Holliday lost her job at a local nonprofit because of a connection on social media to her blog. Six months later, she publicly came out, which resulted in her ten-year-old daughter being expelled from school and her ex-husband suing for custody.[23] Other examples include the 1996 Houghton case, in which a heterosexual couple's children were placed in a foster home at the urging of an overzealous police detective on the basis of photos and a videotape showing the couple in sadomasochistic acts, stolen from their house[24]; and a 2003 case in which a man demanded custody of his son from his ex-wife and her boyfriend and play partner, based on a doctor's claims about what the ex-wife and her lover *might* do in the future, informed by the wording in the DSM.[25] Reducing the stigma attached to alternative sexuality helped correct the imbalance in such cases.

CRIMINAL PROSECUTIONS

Another front between sadomasochism and mainstream culture is the police and courts, usually in terms of sex in public venues, sodomy, or assault. Consent is a key component of BDSM ethics, but it is not clearly recognized by British, Canadian, or American law as a defense.

Some jurists could not understand the concept of consent as a defense at all. In 1967,[26] Marvin Samuels, a California ophthalmologist with a sideline in making and performing in pornographic films, was arrested and charged with conspiracy to prepare and distribute obscene matter, two counts of assault by means of force likely to cause great bodily injury, and a final count of sodomy. These charges were because of two sadomasochistic films Samuels had made with other men.

Samuels was an associate of underground filmmaker Kenneth Anger, who had made homoerotic, sadomasochistic short films such as *Fireworks* (1947) and *Scorpio Rising* (1963).[27] Anger offered to develop some of Samuel's films and to connect Samuels with the Kinsey Institute, which collected such films. Anger sent one of Samuels's rolls of film to a developing company, which noted the content of the film and called the police. When Anger came to collect the film, he was arrested and questioned. Acting on information from Anger, police searched Samuels's house and questioned him. Samuels revealed he was a well-known "S" (sadist), and he made the film with a man he had met at a gay bar, who volunteered for the beating. Samuels also claimed the blows administered in the films were faked and the visible marks on the masochist's body were makeup.

The defense argued that the scenes depicted were consensual and therefore not assault. In some jurisdictions, consent is not a factor in assault charges, necessitated by domestic violence cases, but in this case the appellate court completely rejected the claim of consent.

It is a matter of common knowledge that a normal person in full possession of his mental faculties does not freely consent to the use, upon himself, of force likely to produce great bodily injury. Even if it be assumed that the victim in the "vertical" film did in fact suffer from some form of mental aberration which compelled him to submit to a beating which was so severe as to constitute an aggravated assault, defendant's conduct in inflicting that beating was no less violative of a penal statute obviously designed to prohibit one human being from severely or mortally injuring another. It follows that the trial court was correct in instructing the jury that consent was not a defense to the aggravated assault charge.

In this case, at least, the court saw it as self-evident that these could not be the acts of sane people. Samuels's "M" had to have been mentally incompetent to volunteer for such treatment, and therefore he could not have consented. There was no discourse the court would accept to make Samuels's bottom capable of consent.

In other cases, sadomasochists were deemed to be always already consenting. In a 1978 US case, two men were acquitted of rape and assault because of testimony that the alleged victim had masochistic fantasies and had sent one of the accused a birthday card jokingly calling him "a brute, an animal and a Sex Fiend!"[28] In a 1994 UK case, a jury found a man not guilty of rape with only two minutes of deliberation, and without hearing from the defense, after hearing that the alleged victim wore a rubber miniskirt, kept a riding crop near her bed, and had intimate parts of her body pierced.[29]

Perhaps the largest anti-kink police operation, and the most grotesque violation of consent, occurred on the night of April 10, 1976. A helicopter and at least sixty police officers descended on a Hollywood, California, bathhouse to arrest thirty-nine men and one woman at a mock slave auction, a fund-raiser organized by the Leather Fraternity and *Drummer* magazine for the Gay Community Services Center. The next day, the *Orange County Register*'s front-page headline read, "Police Free Gay Slaves." The bitter irony was that this "liberation" involved being handcuffed, arrested, imprisoned, taunted, and photographed. Mock captivity was met with real imprisonment and violence, and the headline suggested that the "gay slaves" had no right to object to their mistreatment. Even more absurd, the initial charges were based on an 1899 California law against slavery.[30] The police later claimed they were acting on an alleged link to a pandering conspiracy, though LAPD Chief Ed Davis's long-standing harassment of the gay community casts doubt upon that. Charges against thirty-six of the accused were dropped, and the remaining four (including *Drummer* owner John Embry) plead guilty to the misdemeanor of soliciting prostitution.[31]

Roughly a decade later, British police conducted "Operation Spanner," which led to the best-known legal case regarding sadomasochism. The story began in 1987, when a police raid seized a videotape that showed several identifiable men engaged in sadomasochistic acts. Fearing someone had been killed, the Greater Manchester police launched a murder investigation, named Operation Spanner by the media. The police arrested forty-two men, and eventually sixteen were charged with assault occasioning bodily harm and unlawful wounding. In a bizarre legal contortion, the recipients were charged with aiding and abetting actual bodily harm to themselves.[32]

In the light of public anxiety about child exploitation and snuff films, the police were determined to apply a narrative of victimizers and victims. The early reports of Operation Spanner referenced the Protection of Children Act, and implied that this was a child pornography or pedophile ring.[33]

By the conclusion of the trial[34] in 1990, it became clear that the men were adult voluntary members of a homosexual group that went as far back as 1978. The tapes were recorded at members' homes and distributed non-commercially to other members. The defense's argument that this was consensual and victimless was dismissed by the judge.[35] The sixteen men pleaded guilty and were convicted and sentenced to up to four and a half years in prison. The case revolved around fine distinctions of "actual bodily harm" and "grievous bodily harm."[36] Later, in the House of Lords, sadomasochism was condemned as "antipathetic to family and state, as potentially attractive to those not yet doing it, and as distinct from boxing, that 'manly diversion.'"[37] Three of the men arrested argued that their privacy had been violated to the European Commission on Human Rights in 1995, which ruled that the UK government was within its rights to intervene for the sake of "protection of health."[38] Sadomasochism could not be understood as a right.

The role of basic homophobia should not be overlooked in Operation Spanner: the Court of Appeal considered an incident of a man branding his initials on the buttocks of his wife to be "consensual activity in the privacy of the matrimonial home [and therefore] not a matter for criminal prosecution."[39]

Yet another police raid against kinky people came in July 2000 in Attleboro, Massachusetts. Local police entered an admission-by-donation party in a private home (literally across the street from the police station) without showing a warrant and found a BDSM play party. The host was arrested for a variety of charges including keeping a house of prostitution. One female guest was charged with assault for spanking the buttocks of another woman with a wooden spoon, and for possession of a dangerous weapon (that spoon).[40]

The kink community rallied to the defense of the two arrested in the incident informally known as "Paddleboro." The quickly organized Paddleboro Defense League raised $10,000 to pay for the host's legal fees. A dozen supporters with ribbons and spoon-shaped pins appeared at the pretrial hearing and spoke to reporters.[41] While the comparison to the Stonewall riots might be overdrawn, the community's swift and organized response to this attack was an early example of politicized BDSM. Kinky people were speaking for themselves in public.

The Paddleboro incident also meant the loss of the venue for educational events, which is where the BDSM community transmits knowledge about technique and safety, and grows social networks. Without such events, there's a consequent increase in risk of unsafe play.[42]

In these cases, we repeatedly see state agents intrude in situations where there are no victims and no complaints, where people were practicing their kinks "behind closed doors." For a long time, sadomasochists depended on privacy and secrecy for their security. There was no political representation of kinky people, no articulation of sadomasochism as a civil right. Even when courts allowed for the possibility of consent in situations that could result in injury, such as contact sports, they would not allow sadomasochism to be considered one of those exceptions.[43]

These prosecutions had definite negative effects on the BDSM community. In the wake of the Spanner trials, a submission to the Law Reform Commission stated:

> Sadomasochists have no ready access to safe sex literature or safe practice literature. It has also discouraged people from coming to our clubs and social spaces—the network of safety advice. . . . Some activities are simply

not safe to do alone. At least one person has died as a direct result of the "Brown" verdict. He was into breath restriction. . . . Following "Brown" he feared involving his partner in his activities and reverted to doing them alone. He was found dead. The current law endangers people rather than protects them. The best protection is sound safety information.[44]

As the Scene became larger and more publicly visible, such secrecy became more difficult. The police surveillance and raids that used to be exclusive to homosexuals expanded to include heterosexual kinksters. Repeated legal assaults on the sadomasochist community forced the creation of the NCSF and other legal advocacy organizations. These organizations talked back, creating the idea of a sadomasochistic person with rights instead of an unknowable and abject sexual deviant.

GOVERNMENT CENSORSHIP

A second front in the relations between the BDSM community and the state is over the issue of obscenity, and sadomasochistic media have been particularly vulnerable in this area.

In American law, the standard test for obscenity (not the same thing as indecency) is the so-called Miller test, which asks if the work under consideration is:

1. sexually explicit, and
2. patently offensive according to "local community standards," and
3. without any "serious literary, artistic, social, educational, or scientific value."

In the internet era, there is no way of applying "community standards" to a medium that covers the entire planet. Obscenity cases once involved the likes of D. H. Lawrence's novel *Lady Chatterley's Lover* and Allen Ginsberg's poem *Howl*. As pornography became big business, prosecutors shifted their attention to the "low-hanging fruit," small producers who made niche content likely to be off-putting to mainstream Americans, and who also had fewer resources to mount legal defenses or rally popular support. As representations of homosexuality became less likely to be considered obscene, the attention turned to nonnormative forms of sexuality, such as sadomasochism.

The posthumous exhibition tour of the work of photographer Robert Mapplethorpe, *The Perfect Moment*, in 1989 set off controversy over obscenity and the arts. Mapplethorpe had been the lover of *Drummer* magazine editor Jack Fritscher, and many of his works were portraits of people in the underground BDSM scene of the late 1960s and early 1970s. The exhibition included a self-portrait of Mapplethorpe in leather with the handle of a bullwhip self-inserted in his anus. The administration of the Corcoran Gallery of Art in Washington, D.C., along with several senators, objected to the content of the show. Groups such as the American Family Association opposed government support for such art. When the Corcoran rejected the exhibition, it was moved to the Washington Project for the Arts. The work of Mapplethorpe and other controversial artists like Andres Serrano were at issue when the funding and autonomy of the National Endowment for the Arts was being debated in the US legislature over 1989 and 1990. Senator Jesse Helms stated, "The American people . . . are disgusted with the idea of giving the taxpayers' money to artists . . . who will engage in whatever perversion it takes to win acclaim as an artist on the 'offending edge' and therefore entitled to taxpayer funding."[45]

In American law, obscenity prosecutions that did not involve children were a low priority for the Clinton administration.[46] However, the administration did approve the Communications Decency Act (CDA) of 1996. Born of cultural anxiety over the internet, the CDA criminalized the distribution of "any comment, request, suggestion, proposal, image, or other communication that, in context, depicts or describes, in terms patently offensive as measured by contemporary community standards, sexual or excretory activities or organs." In 1997, the case of Reno v. ACLU resulted in the US Supreme Court striking down the anti-indecency provisions of the act.

In the first summer of the George W. Bush administration, the NCSF knew that US Attorney General John Ashcroft had met with conservative organizations like the Christian Coalition and Concerned Women for America, who sent press releases about the new government's willingness to prosecute obscenity. To fight the CDA with a test case, the NCSF needed an artist who was willing to go up against the Justice Department.

Barbara Nitke had worked as a still photographer in the adult film industry in the 1980s, and later branched into documenting the BDSM and modern primitives subcultures, particularly in her 2003 photo book *Kiss of Fire: A Romantic View of Sadomasochism*, which went against the grain of most depictions of BDSM by focusing on moments of tenderness and intimacy between kinky people. "If two adults agree on what they're going to do in advance and find a couple of minutes of happiness, I can't imagine why anyone would begrudge them," she said.[47] As publishers and galleries were often wary of the content of her images, Nitke had to rely on her website for promotion, and found that the CDA could directly affect her. She had no way of controlling who would see her work.

Nitke worked with the NCSF to launch a lawsuit in 2001, *Nitke v. Ashcroft* (later *Nitke v. Gonzales*), using as a test case her website, which displayed her photographs. Whereas the Mapplethorpe controversy asked what the community standards of America as a whole were, the Nitke case asked if the community standards of an individual viewer could be determined, or if the most restrictive standards in America would apply nationwide. This would have a chilling effect on freedom of speech and violate Nitke's First Amendment rights.[48] The US Supreme Court finally decided the plaintiffs hadn't presented enough evidence in 2006.

The Bush administration's socially conservative backers urged the government to go after the adult entertainment business, but the focus on national security after 9/11 delayed that. A few years later, the prosecutions began with vigor. Under Bush, there were 361 defendants with obscenity charges, twice the number under Clinton.[49]

The newly appointed attorney general, Alberto Gonzales, created the Obscenity Prosecution Task Force in 2005. Defining "obscenity" had been a fraught issue in American law for decades, but the new task force would focus on "adult obscenity cases," which did not involve children or coercion in the creation of pornography. In practice, this meant something other than vanilla sex as produced by major porn companies and distributed by cable companies; in other words, kink.

However, task force leader Brent Ward soon found that other US attorneys had little interest in obscenity prosecutions. In one such conflict in 2006, the US attorney for Nevada, Daniel Bogden, refused to cooperate with Ward's task force, saying that not only was it a waste of resources, it was "small potatoes" to prosecute a husband for urinating on his wife in a video that an agent had viewed and considered obscene. Paul Charlton, US attorney for Arizona, likewise wanted nothing to do with the task force's prosecution. Later that year, Bogden and Charlton were two of nine US attorneys controversially dismissed by the Bush administration.[50]

Other US attorneys went ahead with obscenity prosecutions. Mary Beth Buchanan, US attorney for the Western District of Pennsylvania, made her name with *United States v. Fletcher* in 2006.[51] Karen Fletcher, indicted on six charges of distributing obscene materials on the internet, was a fifty-four-year-old agoraphobic grandmother who lived alone on disability. She wrote prose stories (without videos or images) of children under ten being molested and killed, and posted them on Rose Red, a members-only website with less than thirty subscribers. Fletcher considered her stories "catharsis" for her own history of abuse.

Despite the fact that there had not been a federal obscenity prosecution of text since 1973, Buchanan went ahead with the case. In interviews, Buchanan described Fletcher's stories as "the most disturbing, disgusting and vile material that I've ever viewed," and said the material "emboldens individuals who have an interest in sexually exploiting children."[52]

Fletcher pleaded guilty in exchange for five years probation, including six months of house arrest, and forfeiture of her computer. Buchanan pushed for the prosecution of Fletcher to rack up a victory for the prosecution and appease social conservatives.

Faced with a public largely indifferent to explicit media, prosecutors who thought their resources were better spent on other issues, and social conservatives who wanted the government to go after big media, the task force accomplished little.

Under President Obama, obscenity was a low priority again. By 2011, the task force was folded into the Child Exploitation and Obscenity section, indicating that the federal government was only interested in prosecutions in which minors were involved. The issue of obscenity in itself was largely ignored, and sadomasochism and fetish sexuality were safe from prosecution, for the moment.

RELIGIOUS PERSECUTION

Religiously based non-state organizations found their own uses for sadomasochism in the culture wars of the 2000s, taking it as a symbol of the depravity of homosexuals and of modern society in general.

In early 2002, Christian advocacy group Concerned Women for America allied with two other religious organizations, the American Family Association and the American Decency Association, to launch attacks on five different BDSM conventions in the Midwest, using sensationalized language to pressure the hotels to cancel the events. Two conferences were forced to relocate to other venues.[53] The next year, 2003, saw another wave of attacks on conferences.[54] CWA's press release used inflammatory language like "They advocate the gruesome practice of inserting objects, whipping and cutting each other to produce blood, and they demonstrate perverted techniques."[55] They had found perfect targets.

Named as a hate group by the Southern Poverty Law Center,[56] Americans for Truth about Homosexuality (AFTAH) is run by Peter LaBarbera. He was notorious for his photo exposés of leather events like the Folsom Street Fair, Up Your Alley, and International Mister Leather, relaying in shocked tones the supposed depravity and immorality. (These are called exposés, even though these public events are hardly secrets.) The overall goal was to demonize kinky gay men to represent all LGBTQ people as oversexed, immoral, and self-destructive.

His description of International Mister Leather:

> Once again, purveyors of leather-sex hawked their deviant wares and twisted pornography at IML, as the nights were filled with homosexual orgies so vile that it is difficult for the Average Joe to imagine such evil. (Then the poor hotel staff have to disinfect the rooms afterward.)[57]

AFTAH later added kinky non-homosexuals as targets. This was a crusade against the alleged "homosexual agenda," and straight kink, along with transgenderism and polyamory, were signs of the harmful influence of homosexuals on American society.[58]

LaBarbera would be a paper tiger except that he included in his bulletins a list of sponsors of and venues for kink organizations and events, including phone numbers to call and complain.[59] In 2009, AFTAH and a local radio station ran a smear campaign against the Winter Wickedness BDSM conference in Worthington, Ohio, describing it as "a freakish sadomasochistic perversion-fest." The bulletin also included workshop descriptions and the play party rules list, with the most inflammatory sections in bold. Other conservative Christian groups applied pressure to the hotel, and this attracted some local media attention. The Holiday Inn decided to maintain the reservation, and the event proceeded as planned, though under tighter scrutiny.[60]

LaBarbera blasted the Democratic Party for financially supporting the National Gay and Lesbian Task Force, citing the Leather Leadership awards given to leather educators and title-holders Guy Baldwin[61] and Race Bannon.[62]

Whether the actual target was marriage equality,[63] Planned Parenthood,[64] or Barack Obama,[65] any link to sadomasochism, no matter how tenuous, was a vulnerability to be exploited. LaBarbera intended his "exposés" to shock and disgust, as if this was a secret apocalyptic revelation, and inaction would lead to the Folsom Street Fair on every street in America, 365 days a year. "THIS is the depraved end game of the Sexual Revolution,"[66] he asserted.

Conservative Christian efforts against sexual minorities extended beyond observation and pressure. Starting on New Year's Eve 2008 and continuing through 2009, a militant radical Christianist group, Repent Amarillo, harassed the patrons of Route 66, a swingers club located in Amarillo, Texas. This was part of a campaign of "spiritual warfare" that targeted everything from gay bars to Islamic centers to Unitarian churches.

Before this, Route 66 kept a low profile; few Amarillo residents even knew it existed. Repent Amarillo's leader, David Grisham, said, "This is adultery. This is wrong. There's no telling how many venereal diseases get spread, how many abortions." Predictably, he used metaphors of uncleanness, disease, and the disruption of heteronormative reproduction. After attempts to get the city government to shut down the club for being a brothel or having fire safety violations, Repent turned to outing Route 66 members. They noted the license plates of parked cars, looked up the owners, and called their employers to try to get them fired.[67] Their harassment extended to a swinger party held at a private home.[68] Amarillo's authorities did not respond to either group's requests to shut the other down.

Repent Amarillo's tactics, a real-world version of internet doxing, exploited a key vulnerability of alternative sexual communities like swingers and kinksters. They have a strong ethos of secrecy and confidentiality, and breaching that hidden world by publicly identifying people is an effective form of intimidation.

Sadomasochists have also been drafted into the conflict over abortion and sex education. Pro-life organization Live Action maintained a website that criticized Planned Parenthood, including its links to educational resources on BDSM, which Live Action called "torture sex."[69] In 2014, it released a series of edited videos titled "SEXED: Dangerous Sex Advice for Kids." The organization sent young women, claiming to be fifteen years old, with hidden cameras into Planned Parenthood offices. There they recorded counselors giving beginners advice on BDSM. In a press release, Live Action president Lila Rose called this an "institutional ethos of promoting destructive sexual activity."[70] Links to these videos circulated through right-wing media channels. Live Action had used this tactic before in 2011, when it sent an investigator posing as a pimp into a clinic to get advice on secret abortions for underage prostitutes.

Live Action's SEXED program represented a new and disturbing development. Instead of gay BDSM being used to smear homosexuality in general, this was heterosexual BDSM specifically targeted as part of a campaign against reproductive freedom.

As observed previously (see chapter 2), a common tactic in wars of propaganda is associating enemies with sexual perversion. In modern conflicts over cultural issues like homosexuality and abortion, sadomasochists were dragged in for their shock value, with rhetoric that emphasizes bodily horror to disgust the reader. As sadomasochism depends on images of the body in extremis, it is an obvious target.

JACK MCGEORGE

Early in the post-9/11 era, one man's status as a sadomasochist became an issue in international politics. On Thanksgiving weekend in 2002, the *Washington Post* "revealed" that Harvey John "Jack" McGeorge,[71] a retired US Marine who worked for the UN mission to Iraq to search for weapons of mass destruction (UNMOVIC), was also a leader in the New England BDSM scene. The word "revealed" belongs in quotes because McGeorge's long-standing involvement in the BDSM scene was no secret, and anybody could have discovered that with a simple web search.

Post reporter John Grimaldi wrote three articles on McGeorge in the *Washington Post* in quick succession. This set off a wave of snide jokes in the media, like "A Taste of the Whip for Saddam,"[72] or a cartoon of a leatherman in full gear walking toward an Iraqi border gate. The UK *Telegraph* announced, "UN Weapons Inspector Is Leader of S&M Sex Ring."[73]

Grimaldi interviewed McGeorge by phone. McGeorge recalls, "When we started up the conversation, his stated reason for calling was not the thrust of his call, and that annoyed the hell out of me. He told me during the course of the conversation that I was to be the focus of an article, and that this article would have two thrusts. One, that the UNMOVIC, the organization I work for, the weapons inspection team, was obviously unqualified to do this job, because they hadn't done proper background investigations on the people, witness me, as he said. He said, 'You don't have any background to be doing what you're doing, and others more qualified were passed over.' And secondly, he felt that my S&M background certainly disqualified me from participation in an international endeavor like this."

McGeorge defended both his professional qualifications, learned as a bomb disposal expert in the US Marine Corps, and his right to work in this position. Years earlier, McGeorge had acquired and kept a security clearance, which allowed him to do consulting work for government agencies. In that time, he had always been up front with government officials and employers about his sexuality.

Around the same time as TES and the Society of Janus began in the early 1970s, he put his childhood interests in bondage into action with a fellow male Marine. "We tread most lightly," he recalls. While living in the all-male barracks with little privacy, he had few opportunities to pursue his interests, other than by buying bondage magazines published by House of Milan, and practicing self-bondage.

After leaving the service, McGeorge met a play partner through dating. "She asked me, 'Have you ever tied anybody up?' I just about crashed into a pole [while driving]. We talked. I said, 'Yes, I have.' She had not as strong a drive as I did in the area, but she was sure as hell interested. That began several years of very enjoyable time with her."

Through the sexuality special interest group in Mensa, he learned about and began attending BDSM groups in the early 1980s. They covered both techniques and discussions, though often without much to support their ideas. "It was a dozen people, sitting in somebody's living room, where the person giving the class was often times well meaning, but generally not well thought out or researched."

In 1987, he began attending meetings of PEP-DC, founded by Nancy Ava Miller, who later left the group to look after her ailing mother. "When Nancy disappeared, we looked around at each other and said, 'Okay, what do we do?' Lots of ideas were advanced. Ultimately we decided to make a transitional board of directors, which I was on, to come up with a course of action. 'Let's try and put an organization together on more sustainable grounds, not dependent on the energy and whim of one person.'" This eventually became Black Rose in late 1988 or early 1989.

When McGeorge interviewed with Dr. Hans Blix, leader of UN-MOVIC, in January 2001, he said, "'I come with baggage.' I explained my S&M interests, I explained my involvement in the community, I explained I've got lots of internet exposure on this topic. He told me, 'What you do, in the privacy of your bedroom, is not the business of the United Nations.' I said, 'Thank you very much.' I told him, at that time, that if this became a problem, that I would offer my resignation. He said, 'We'll cross that bridge when we come to it.'"

Right after the phone interview with Grimaldi, McGeorge informed his UNMOVIC superior, who told him to go to Dr. Blix. "I told him, 'Remember the discussion? Well, it just happened. Apparently, it's going to be in the *Washington Post* tomorrow.' He called in his political advisor. They listened. He said that the two of them needed to talk. I said, 'Do you want my resignation?' He said, 'No.' He interrupted me and he said, 'Let's make one thing clear. Is this preceding prosecution, or is this persecution?' I said, 'This is persecution. There's no prosecution in any way, shape, or form.' He said, 'Okay. Go back to work.'"

McGeorge stayed with UNMOVIC and went to Iraq. His unwanted reputation preceded him. "While I was in Iraq, I was on Iraqi television almost every day. We had a TV in the lunchroom. I'd be walking down the hall, and somebody from the lunchroom would call out, 'You're on again!' There's my picture with 'sex pervert' as the caption, or 'spy,' or many times 'CIA spy,' but 'sex pervert CIA spy' was not uncommon," McGeorge recalled, adding that this did not interfere with his work with his colleagues. "They were all, without exception, very professional and frankly very supportive of me. . . . Without them I would have been a basket case."

On returning from Iraq, McGeorge spent another year with UNMOVIC, while the Iraq War began, then applied to work at a consulting firm in Washington, D.C. He had been as transparent about his BDSM career as he had with previous employers. In his second week, he was summoned to HR. "No discussion, no reason. Just, 'We can, we are. You're out.'"

This put McGeorge into a major depression, followed by a heart condition. After a lengthy recovery, he continued with his dual careers. He said, "I also learned how you survive being made an object of public ridicule. This has happened to others, and no doubt will happen to others. I give a lecture on the subject; I call it 'Weathering the storm of public controversy.' I learned a lot about that. I learned a lot about the price to be paid, physically and mentally, for this."[74]

McGeorge wasn't attacked on the grounds he had harmed anyone, or broken any criminal, civil, or religious law. This was more personal. His identity as a practicing sadomasochist marked him as other, an abject person. It questioned his ability to do his job, to respect other cultures, because of his sexuality. His sexuality was characterized as deviant and uncontrollable, making him unsuitable for a sensitive position. Furthermore, his sexuality was deemed to be a public matter for discussion, not private.

By the early twenty-first century, queer people in developed Western nations have made astonishing gains in political and social equality. In part, this is based on the concept, going back to Krafft-Ebing, that instead of homosexual *acts*, there were homosexual *people*. That is, their sexuality was a fixed and unchanging aspect of their personality, and there was a distinct portion of the population that was homosexual, and always would be. Despite the complex and variable nature of gender and sexuality, most people have accepted the idea that LGBTQ people exist, and are entitled to political and social rights.

Kinky people have struggled along similar but divergent trajectories. Much as queer people were a few generations ago, kinky people are still partially entangled between the medical discourse, as in the diagnoses of "sexual sadism" and "sexual masochism" in the *Diagnostic and Statistical Manual*, and the legal discourse, as to the legality of consensual assault or sex in semi-public venues. This political struggle necessitated the BDSM subculture forming a political consciousness with organizations like the

National Coalition for Sexual Freedom. However, the sheer variety of sexual acts and interests grouped under the term BDSM, in its broadest definition, make it difficult to present a unified identity, not to mention find common cause across the boundaries of gay and straight, and bourgeois assimilation and bohemian divergence.

Admittedly, the heterosexual BDSM community in the early twenty-first century doesn't exactly look like an oppressed minority. Sadomasochists are not subject to the routine surveillance, harassment, and violence directed at LGBTQ people. It's easy for a heterosexual kinky couple to pass as "normal," unlike a gay or lesbian couple. Many kinky people are content to keep their sexuality a private matter, for the bedroom or the semi-private club, and see no need to engage in public politics. There has been no kinky equivalent of the Stonewall riots, and there may never be.

It is also clear that kinky people can no longer depend on secrecy for security. There is a struggle to be fought, but it will play out in courtrooms and conference rooms, not on barricades.

Conclusion

Without Contraries is no progression. Attraction and Repulsion, Reason and Energy, Love and Hate, are necessary to Human existence.

From these contraries spring what the religious call Good & Evil. Good is the passive that obeys Reason. Evil is the active springing from Energy.

Good is Heaven. Evil is Hell.

—William Blake, *The Marriage of Heaven and Hell*

Once upon a time, a man went up a mountain to kill his son. Instead, he spared his son and sacrificed a ram. The death of a human being was replaced by the death of an animal, the literal replaced by the symbolic.[1] Human beings are violent, sometimes even for its own sake, but we are also makers and users of symbols that can mediate that violence. Sadomasochism is the intersection of these two deep-seated human capacities.

This is not to say that sadomasochism is a human universal in the same way that sexuality is. Sadomasochism is historically contingent, the product of particular historical events: the changes in the view of the body in Christian thought, the impact of European colonialism and slavery, the application of science to human nature, the rise of consumer capitalism, and others. Had history unfolded in a slightly different way, sadomasochism as we know it today would not exist, though something else might resemble it.

Nonetheless, it does exist, as a subculture, a cultural style, an ethical system, and a mythology, comprised of disparate elements that came together in a process of bricolage, without a plan or a moment of inception; a rhizome, not a snowflake. In that regard, it is remarkable that over only a few decades, what existed as a fringe network of outsiders and deviants has grown into a worldwide subculture with political representation.

If the history of sadomasochism as a culture matters in the grand scheme of human affairs more than the history of, say, badminton, it is because sadomasochism has two things to offer the greater world.

First, it has exploded the definition of sex. The concept of homosexuality expanded sex beyond merely heterosexual coitus leading to conception, and uncoupled sex from reproduction. Sadomasochism has uncoupled pleasure from genital stimulation. This creates the possibility of new pleasures and experiences, new ways to use the human body. To return to Michel Foucault and what he said in a 1984 *Advocate* interview:

> [Sadomasochists] are inventing new possibilities of pleasure with strange parts of their body— through the eroticisation of the body. I think it's a kind of creation, a creative enterprise, which has as one of its main features what I call the desexualisation of pleasure. . . . The possibility of using our bodies as a possible source of very numerous pleasures is something that is important. For instance, if you look at the traditional constructions of pleasure, you see that bodily pleasure, or pleasures of the flesh, are always drinking, eating and fucking. And that seems to be the limit of our understanding of our body, our pleasures.[2]

Second, it has exploded not just sexual mores, but how we evaluate and manage bodily interactions entirely. Historically, sexual mores have been based on concepts of purity and social worth. Sadomasochists have developed an ethics of consent and pleasure, putting the power with the individuals directly involved and basing it on their own desires and choices. This potentially can be applied to other social interactions.

David Stein, who semi-accidentally formulated the principle of "Safe, sane and consensual," described a more detailed and complex theory of ethical BDSM:

> **Master principle: First, do no harm to oneself or others.** People engage in BDSM because it gives them pleasure or makes them happy, so why

elevate avoiding harm to the status of a master ethical principle, especially given that SM often involves hurting someone? Because *hurt* and *harm* are different: hurt is temporary, but harm is lasting—whether it's physical, like loss of a limb or function; psychological, like PTSD or reduced self-esteem; or spiritual, such as despair. What makes avoiding harm suitable as the master principle for BDSM (though not of *all* ethics) is precisely that it doesn't prescribe what people *should* find pleasurable or conducive to their happiness. Whatever your turn-ons and sources of satisfaction—and everyone's are different—**harm is lasting damage that diminishes your ability to enjoy life or pursue happiness**. In other words, the principle of avoiding harm helps us decide how far is *too* far to go with a clean conscience in BDSM play or relationships.[3]

Returning to Victor Turner's theory of ritual discussed in chapter 1, think of sadomasochism as a ritual zone of liminality, bounded in time and space, in which two or more people enter, knowing that the normal rules of life are suspended, and new and different rules are in effect. Actions that are socially unacceptable in regular time are allowed in this magic circle, and through them, the participants may experience the dissolution of the ego's usual boundaries and a connection to something greater, which Turner called *communitas*. However, liminality can be its own reward, without going on to experience communitas. It provides a heightened awareness and a sense of freedom. The ethical system of BDSM makes that possible.

NEW RITUALS FOR OLD

In other cultures, the closest we can see to modern BDSM is religious rituals. Modern Western culture has little in the way of liminal rituals. Instead, we have liminoid rituals, in which people step outside the normal social context and experience liminality, but then return to their former social status, instead of making the transition to a new social status. This allows people to experience liminality many times in many different ways, instead of just once in their lives or once per year.

Liminoid rituals are optional, instead of obligatory as liminal rituals are. Rituals that were once liminal have become liminoid, just another form of recreation. A wedding ceremony has become less the ritual of marking a radical shift in a person's social status and more a festival of extravagance.

What we see in modern sadomasochism was once part of religious practice. Nineteenth-century Europeans who saw the animistic religious practices of indigenous peoples, long suppressed in their own cultures, called the sacred objects fetishes. The word "fetish" comes from the Portuguese word *feitiço*, which means "magic," and is ultimately derived from the Latin word *factīcius*, meaning "made by art." Early sexologists, like Binet and Krafft-Ebing, looked at people fascinated and aroused by boots or gloves or flagellation and saw the same kind of primitive beliefs they saw in animistic religions, a divergence from the proper evolutionary path. For the people so discussed, these were indeed private religions. Sacher-Masoch's novel *Venus in Furs* functions as a rite of passage: Severin is renewed by his self-imposed ordeal with Wanda, and at the end says he is cured of his masochism. In reality, the author never completed his rite of passage. He stayed there, in the liminal state, playing out the same kind of scenario over and over again and never getting it right. Pauline Reage's *Story of O* is also structured as an initiation, but an endless one, in which O discovers ever-deeper levels of degradation from ever-harsher masters.

Arthur Munby wrote of Hannah Cullwick:

> [S]he was to become, and she *has* become, a noble and gentle woman, not only without the aid of technical helps, but in spite of ignorance and lowly isolation, and *by means* of that very toil and servile labour which is supposed to make a woman contemptible and vulgar. Physical degradation was to be the channel, and even the source of spiritual beauty. It has often been so, among religious women of old.[4]

Through a particular set of contingent historical events, certain acts, such as flagellation, were rejected from the mainstream religious discourse and fell into the discourse of sexuality, and a particularly underground, low-status discourse. A set of psychological needs and desires, which were once satisfied by religion, were instead condemned and forced into the cultural underground. In the heightened surveillance of individual behavior in the nineteenth century, these practices became visible to medical and legal authorities.

In one of many ironies, creating and reinforcing the boundary between the normal and the abnormal in law and medicine created the abnormal as an object of discourse, a thing in itself, which eventually produced its own discourses of self-validation. It existed as an ulterior subculture for most of the twentieth century, rose into visibility in the 1970s, and exploded in the 1990s. It was as if tiny private ritual cults had blossomed into a major faith with vast congregations in a matter of decades.

While sadomasochism lacks some of the characteristics of religion, such as a dogma or an eschatology or other grand narrative of the world, it provides some of the functions of religion: initiation, community, identity, the transformation of the self, experiences of physical and mental ecstasy. Modern mainstream religion has gradually shed the physical aspects of worship, making communion with the divine a cerebral affair. More peripheral faiths retain the physical practices. Donna Minkowitz, a lesbian and sadomasochist who wrote her book *Ferocious Romance* about exploring conservative Christian culture in America, described people seeking to escape themselves in ecstatic bodily worship at the Pentecostal service at the Toronto Airport Ministry:

> [T]wo women are dancing by themselves in the wide side aisle. One, a flush-faced fiftysomething, looks a little mad, twirling a pink streamer and scampering lightly on her feet like some sort of ecstatic elf. The other is a vigorous, Gray Pantherish old woman in a T-shirt and painter's pants, who looks as though she's just come back from painting signs for a peace demonstration. The Gray Panther gestures rapidly with a baby blue triangular flag, as though she were an airport worker signaling to a plane. They both look crazy, but I sort of envy them. At different times in my life, I too have wanted to be inhabited by gods and dance ecstatically; what's happening in this church is what I prayed would happen to me as a teenager (although I was a Dionysian, not a Christian, and I prayed that the spirit would enter me through eros, or through drugs).[5]

Minkowitz talks about her own ambivalent relationship with BDSM in quasi-religious terms, as a former true believer turned skeptic:

> S/M's method of redemption is quite close to Christianity's, although a bit more self-aware. The amazingly idealist notion that has won S/M so many converts in our time is that difficult things in the "real" world can be redeemed by their simulacra inside the "fake" world of sexuality. (The woman who wears a black hankie in her right pocket to celebrate her own

triumph over undesired pain is not too different from the churchgoer who kneels each week before a stylized image of a Roman torture device.)[6]

She sees this conflict of real versus fake, of violence versus symbol, as the fundamental paradox of BDSM:

> [T]he Platonic inquiry with which S/M is even more concerned is about the relation between reality and "simulacra," or as Plato preferred to think of it, between the world of appearances and the world of the spirit. Plato called the spirit real and the world of material reality a false and inferior "copy," and in their own way, S/M activists do the same. But what is being endlessly "copied" and transmuted in S/M land is violence, which is why S/M, unlike Plato, overtly privileges the fake over the real. Fake violence is indisputably "better," at least ethically.
>
> Deep down, though, sadomasochists are uneasily uncertain about what the relationship between "real" and "copied" violence really is, and how the two things should or shouldn't be brought together in their practice. The highly charged and contradictory relationship between violence in the world and violence in one's soul is itself the beating heart of S/M, the reason S/M porn is full of bragadocio to the effect that the sexual coercion between bottoms and tops is "real," while S/M cultural and political writing is simultaneously full of assurances that it is fake.[7]

THE TASTE OF MEAT

Liberal or feminist criticisms of sadomasochism, even if they accept the provision of negotiated consent and understand the interaction as a kind of game or theater, raise legitimate questions when they ask why sadomasochism is so preoccupied with violence and hierarchy. Does sadomasochism encourage or normalize beliefs that lead to abusive behavior? Must we avoid violence in all forms, even when contained by ritual? If we eschew violence and hierarchy, then do we also have to eschew a pleasurable form of expression based on those things (i.e., BDSM)? Phrased another way, is there a real difference between the violence of games and the violence of reality? And to give up the latter, must we also give up the former?

As a form of nonviolence, many Buddhists practice vegetarianism, in order to reduce the suffering of animals. Some Buddhists have developed vegetarian dishes that look, smell, and taste like meat as much as possible. If a person is vegetarian for *moral* reasons (not health or necessity), does the avoidance of violence (i.e., eating meat) necessitate the avoidance of the by-products of violence—that is, the pleasure of the taste of meat? A Christian might say "yes," while Buddhism does not have a problem with pleasure in itself, only in attachment to pleasurable things. In principle, there is no contradiction in eschewing the consumption of meat while still enjoying the consumption of meat substitutes.

In a similar way, contact sports, such as boxing and football, were once seen as excessively violent and incitements to social disruption. Now they are "tamed" by restriction to particular venues, and governed by rules and regulations, such as the Football Association's rules in 1863 and boxing's Queensbury rules drafted in 1865. The amateur versions are staples of educational institutions and the professional versions are massive, profitable businesses and even civic institutions. We imbue these practices with positive values: health, sportsmanship, self-discipline, teamwork, manliness, artistry, striving for excellence. In the Operation Spanner case, consensual sadomasochism was explicitly compared to contact sports such as boxing or association football, but denied the positive social worth applied to sports. Questions such as "which results in more fatalities or debilitating injuries, professional contact sports or sadomasochism?" were swept aside.

REDRAWING THE BORDERS

Since at least the 1940s, sadomasochists have slowly developed and disseminated a body of practice to ensure the physical and mental safety of practitioners. From the early 1970s, they have also advocated with legal and medical authorities for the destigmatization of those practices. Kinky people have worked very hard to create ways in which desires can be expressed in a positive way, not repressed. This work is still poorly understood and unappreciated by the mainstream, even when the imagery of sadomasochism is ubiquitous in popular media. The mainstream views the subculture of sadomasochism in such a way as to not see the ethical aspects, preferring to focus on the sensational, particularly in advertisements for everything from beer to furniture to breath mints.

As Gayle Rubin pointed out in her classic essay "Thinking Sex" (1984), vanilla sexuality is privileged above kinky sexuality. Even as BDSM has increased in visibility in the past few decades, it is still denied the privilege of full acceptance. Instead, the borders between "normal" and "abnormal" sexuality have subtly shifted.

Though savaged by critics, BDSM experts, and domestic violence advocates, the *Fifty Shades of Grey* romance trilogy by E. L. James (2011) and its film adaptations (2015, dir. Sam Taylor-Johnson; 2017 & 2018, dir. James Foley) were astonishing mainstream commercial successes, which broke book sale and box office records, and launched a wave of branded merchandise, including basic bondage toys.[8] The story concerns a naive literature student, Ana Steele, who falls for a brooding billionaire, Christian Grey. He insists that he only wants a dominant/submissive relationship and pressures her to sign a 24/7 contract, while she pleads with him for a romantic relationship. The sadomasochistic scenes are few and mild, and the story mostly follows the conventions of heterosexual romance.

The *Fifty Shades* phenomenon does not mean that the mainstream has embraced mainstream BDSM. Instead, the popularity indicates a redrawing of the borders between vanilla and kink. BDSM sexuality is acceptable to the mainstream as long as it is contained within a traditional monogamous heterosexual romance plot, reactionary gender roles, and a naked worship of wealth and privilege. The trilogy's blatant misunderstanding of consent shows that the mainstream wants the toys and the glamour of BDSM, but not the ethos of negotiated roles. Those who can position themselves on the "normal" side of the border remain privileged. Those on the other side are visible, but silenced.

Fifty Shades can be compared with another successful mainstream romance film with sadomasochistic themes, *Secretary* (2002, dir. Steven Shainberg, based on a short story by Mary Gaitskill), for how the two texts make BDSM acceptable to the mainstream. The film concerns Lee, a woman with a history of self-injury, who becomes the secretary of a withdrawn lawyer, not coincidentally named Mr. Grey. The secretary and her employer gradually shift into a sadomasochistic relationship, in which she happily performs her work while in bondage. This alleviates her urge to self-injure. Their relationship leads to marriage and happily ever after in the suburbs.

Margot Weiss wrote that "popular images of SM promote the acceptance and understanding of sexual minorities through two mechanisms: *acceptance via normalization*, and *understanding via pathologizing*. Rather than challenging the privileged status of normative sexuality, these mechanisms reinforce boundaries between protected/privileged and policed/pathological sexualities."[9]

> In the former mechanism, SM is acceptable only when it falls under the rubric of normative American sexuality. In the latter mechanism, SM is understandable only when it is the symptom of a deviant type of person with a sick, damaged core. Both mechanisms offer a form of acceptance or understanding, but these forms do not further the cause of sexual freedom. They allow the mainstream audience to flirt with danger and excitement, but ultimately reinforce boundaries between protected and privileged normal sexuality, and policed and pathological not normal sexuality.[10]

> An analysis of critical and interview responses to the film *Secretary* indicates that increasingly mainstream depictions yield both acceptance and understanding of BDSM. . . . *Secretary* depicts SM as exotic, sexy, and other *and* conventional, mainstream, and normal. However, the form of acceptance that these mainstream representations promote is predicated on conformity to normative American sexuality (acceptance through normalization). Similarly, the form of understanding that these mainstream representations promote is reliant on the classification as an abnormal, damaged type (understanding through pathologizing). Both mechanisms reinforce boundaries between normal, protected, and privileged sexuality, and abnormal, policed, and pathological sexuality. Together, these dual mechanisms diminish any positive political outcome of the mainstreaming of BDSM.[11]

Secretary and *Fifty Shades* follow the tried-and-true romance plot: meet, struggle, crisis, resolution, happily ever after. The BDSM provides a flirtation with exoticism without breaking out of the romantic ideals.

> Like representations of the native other, the dark other, or the dangerous other, the sexual other is tied to a long practice of distanced consumption. This mode of viewership enables the privileged use of the other in a way that gives the normative audience familiarity, knowledge, and even intimacy of the other, all the while shoring up a basic power differential that maintains the one's power, and the other's essential alterity. . . . These

representations reinforce boundaries between normal and not normal by allowing the viewer to consume a bit of the kinky other while buttressing the privilege, authority, and essential normalcy of the self.[12]

Secretary's twist on the romance formula relied on the preconception in the mainstream viewers that BDSM could only be rough and without intimacy. In the end, however, the relationship of the two leads is shown as excruciatingly normal: a suburban husband and wife. BDSM is acceptable as a means to conventional views of relationships and intimacy, not as an end in itself.

> These images do not challenge normative sexuality and relationships; rather they flirt with exoticism and excitement while reinforcing the borders between normal and not normal sexuality. Rather than being a clearly positive first step, this form of acceptance is quite politically dangerous. The dynamic of acceptance via normalization means that BDSM is acceptable to the mainstream only when it turns out to be not SM at all.[13]

The other dynamic in mainstream depiction, understanding by pathologizing, makes kinkiness a sickness, a problem to be solved. Even before Lee, the protagonist of *Secretary*, meets Mr. Grey, she is depicted as childlike and vulnerable, discharged from a mental institution and still struggling with compulsive self-cutting.[14] Her masochism influences her entire personality to the point that she cannot function as an adult. It makes masochism something a specific type of person does, rather than a practice that even "normal" people could participate in. Mr. Grey, the male lead, is riddled with compulsive tics and unable to connect to people, in need of fixing. Like the other Mr. Grey, he is far more interested in BDSM scenes than conventional sexual intercourse or romance.

> Presenting SM as a (pathological) identity rather than a practice works to shore up boundaries between normal and abnormal. Offering understanding through pathologizing, this representation reinforces boundaries between the person who might take a slightly kinky trip to Good Vibrations (a San Francisco sex store) and the full-on pervert with a sick core. It allows the normative viewer access and understanding to BDSM through a pathologizing, stigmatizing gaze.[15]

In *Fifty Shades*, the stigma of abnormality is placed on Christian (and by extension his former dominant Elena and Christian's other submissives). Ana is presented as normal, the viewpoint character the reader and viewer should identify with, even though she is very naive and, until she meets Christian, asexual. The narrative of the *Fifty Shades* novels ends with the usual happily-ever-after marriage and children for Ana and Christian, which includes at least some BDSM play. But even as Ana is bound and flogged by Christian, she still doesn't think of herself as kinky. She is "normal" and healthy and deserving of Christian's love, and her definition of "normal" has slightly expanded to include the things she wants to do. All the other women in Christian's life are "abnormal" and unworthy of Christian, and they remain in the pathological category. BDSM is acceptable as long as it remains subordinate to the demands of heterosexual romance conventions.

Many of the viewers and critics of *Secretary* described it as disappointing, that the BDSM depicted was too soft and tame, and there were similar criticisms against *Fifty Shades of Grey*. This is the unresolvable dilemma of the mainstreaming of kink. For BDSM to appear in the beer commercial or the Hollywood romance, it must, by definition, have lost nearly all of its transgressive, authentic edge. Only by staying in the netherworld, without full sanction of legal/medical authorities, can it remain authentic.

> As the U.S. popular cultural landscape becomes increasingly beholden to sex-as-spectacle, sex-as-consumption, these mainstream representations will always fail. SM promises a taste of something real and authentic, something deep and satisfying, and when these representations dissatisfy (as, of course, they must), viewers experience boredom.[16]

Perhaps BDSM can never live up to its own hype, but the disappointment and boredom with which some critics responded to *Fifty Shades of Grey* is symptomatic of an unsatisfied desire for freedom, authenticity, and transgression.

BDSM offers the possibility that we can accept the sadistic or masochistic aspects of human nature and, instead of repressing them, give them a way to run free within limits and not have society disintegrate into total chaos.

It's a way out of the deep-seated binary oppositions of Western thought: pleasure and virtue, flesh and spirit. This opens up new frontiers of human experience, new pleasures and new intimacies that cannot be reached any other way. Like all Utopian projects, it is aspirational, life-affirming in its audacity, regardless of how much it falls short of its goals. It's the union of Rousseau and Sade, or, to borrow a phrase from William Blake, the marriage of heaven and hell.

Notes

INTRODUCTION

1. Michel Foucault, *Madness and Civilization: A History of Insanity in the Age of Reason* (London: Routledge, 2001), 199.
2. From T. S. Eliot's poem "Gerontion" (1920).
3. Anna Freud, "Beating Fantasies and Daydreams," in *Essential Papers on Masochism*, ed. Margaret Ann Fitzpatrick Hanly (New York: NYU Press, 1995), 286–99.
4. Freud, "Beating Fantasies," 291.
5. Freud, "Beating Fantasies," 292.
6. Terry Pratchett, *Eric* (New York: HarperCollins, 2002).
7. Roger Callois, *Man, Play and Games*, trans. Meyer Barash (Chicago: University of Chicago Press, 1961).
8. John R. Clarke and Michael Larvey, *Roman Sex: 100 B.C. to 250 A.D.* (New York: Harry N. Abrams, 2003), 12.
9. Walter M. Kendrick, *The Secret Museum: Pornography in Modern Culture* (New York: Viking, 1987), 136.
10. Mel Gordon, *Voluptuous Panic: The Erotic World of Weimar Berlin* (Port Townsend, WA: Feral House, 2006), 212.
11. David Kunzle, *Fashion and Fetishism: Corsets, Tight-Lacing and Other Forms of Body-Sculpture* (Stroud, UK: Sutton, 2004), xiii.
12. Ian Gibson, *The English Vice: Beating, Sex, and Shame in Victorian England and After* (London: Duckworth, 1978), 243–44.
13. Ian Gibson, *The Erotomaniac: The Secret Life of Henry Spencer Ashbee* (London: Faber, 2002), 109.
14. See also John Preston's "Network" novels, "the Club" of Anne Rice's novel *Exit to Eden* (1984), and Laura Antoniou's "Markeplace" novels.

15. Twisted Monk, "The Obligatory Birthday Post," August 10, 2006, accessed January 8, 2015, http://twistedmonk.blogspot.ca/2006/08/obligatory-birthday-post-so-today.html.

CHAPTER ONE

1. Thomas E. Mails, *Sundancing: The Great Sioux Piercing Ritual* (Tulsa, OK: Council Oak Books, 1998), 133–44.
2. "Thaipusam," *Wikipedia*, accessed December 20, 2011, https://en.wikipedia.org/wiki/Thaipusam; J. Gordon Melton, *The Encyclopedia of Religious Phenomena* (Detroit: Visible Ink, 2007), 332.
3. "Tatbir," *Wikipedia*, accessed December 20, 2011, https://en.wikipedia.org/wiki/Tatbir.
4. P. R. McKenzie, *Hail Orisha! A Phenomenology of a West African Religion in the Mid-Nineteenth Century* (Leiden: Brill, 1997), 242–45.
5. Plutarch, *Life of Caesar*, LXI.
6. John R. Clarke and Michael Larvey, *Roman Sex: 100 B.C. to 250 A.D.* (New York: Harry N. Abrams, 2003).
7. Victor W. Turner, *The Ritual Process: Structure and Anti-Structure* (New York: Aldine de Gruyter, 1995), 95.
8. Turner, *The Ritual Process*, 138–39.
9. Turner, *The Ritual Process*, 154.
10. Ariel Glucklich, *Sacred Pain: Hurting the Body for the Sake of the Soul* (Oxford: Oxford University Press, 2001), 207.
11. Glucklich, *Sacred Pain*, 152.
12. Turner, *The Ritual Process*, 176.
13. Proverbs 3:12 (King James Version).
14. Proverbs 13:24 (KJV).
15. Proverbs 23:14 (KJV).
16. David Morgan, *Visual Piety: A History and Theory of Popular Religious Images* (Berkeley: University of California Press, 1998), 63.
17. Niklaus Largier, *In Praise of the Whip: A Cultural History of Arousal* (New York: Zone Books, 2007), 30.
18. Cited in Vern Bullough, Dwight Dixon, and Joan Dixon, "Sadism, Masochism, and History, or When Is Behaviour Sado-Masochistic?," in *Sexual Knowledge, Sexual Science: The History of Attitudes to Sexuality*, ed. Roy Porter and Mikuláš Teich (Cambridge: Cambridge University Press, 1994), 54.
19. Rachel Fulton, *From Judgment to Passion: Devotion to Christ and the Virgin Mary, 800–1200* (New York: Columbia University Press, 2002), 96.

20. Fulton, *From Judgment to Passion*, 98.

21. Fulton, *From Judgment to Passion*, 101.

22. Morgan, *Visual Piety*, 67.

23. Goswin of Bossut, *Send Me God: The Lives of Ida the Compassionate of Nivelles, Nun of La Ramée, Arnulf, Lay Brother of Villers, and Abundus, Monk of Villers* (University Park: Pennsylvania State University Press, 2006), xli.

24. Goswin, *Send Me God*, xlii.

25. Bullough et al., "Sadism, Masochism, and History," 55.

26. Fulton, *From Judgment to Passion*, 99–101.

27. Largier, *In Praise of the Whip*, 108.

28. Brian Moynahan, *The Faith: A History of Christianity* (New York: Doubleday, 2002), 288–94.

29. Geoffrey Barraclough, *The Christian World: A Social and Cultural History* (New York: Harry N. Abrams, 1981), 164; Norman Rufus Colin Cohn, *The Pursuit of the Millennium: Revolutionary Millenarians and Mystical Anarchists of the Middle Ages* (London: Pimlico, 1993), 140–41.

30. Largier, *In Praise of the Whip*, 156–57.

31. Morgan, *Visual Piety*, 71.

32. Moynahan, *The Faith*, 288–94.

33. Nicholas Terpstra, *Lay Confraternities and Civic Religion in Renaissance Bologna* (Cambridge: Cambridge University Press, 1995), 5, 62–64.

34. Lisa Silverman, *Tortured Subjects: Pain, Truth, and the Body in Early Modern France* (Chicago: University of Chicago Press, 2001).

35. Morgan, *Visual Piety*, 63–65.

36. Gabriele Finaldi and Susanna Avery-Quash, *The Image of Christ* (London: National Gallery, 2000), 106.

37. Finaldi and Avery-Quash, *The Image of Christ*, 122.

38. Finaldi and Avery-Quash, *The Image of Christ*, 136.

39. Martha Easton, "Pain, Torture and Death in the Huntington Library *Legenda aurean*, in *Gender and Holiness: Men, Women and Saints in Late Medieval Europe*, ed. Samantha J. E. Riches and Sarah Salih (London: Routledge, 2002), 49–64.

CHAPTER TWO

1. The Sacred Arts, accessed September 7, 2017, http://thesacredarts.org/newsite/knowledge-base/from-the-holy-see/105-the-council-of-trent-on-the-invocation-veneration-and-relics-of-saints-and-on-sacred-images-1563.

2. Teresa of Ávila, *Life of St. Teresa*, XXIX, 17.

3. Franco Mormando, *Bernini: His Life and His Rome* (Chicago: University of Chicago Press, 2011), 161–62.

4. Robert Mills, "Ecce Homo," in *Gender and Holiness: Men, Women and Saints in Late Medieval Europe*, ed. Samantha J. E. Riches and Sarah Salih (London: Routledge, 2002), 163. The original Latin uses the word *persona*, making the gender ambiguous.

5. Mills, "Ecce Homo," 163.

6. David Morgan, *Visual Piety: A History and Theory of Popular Religious Images* (Berkeley: University of California Press, 1998), 73.

7. Ian Gibson, *The English Vice: Beating, Sex, and Shame in Victorian England and After* (London: Duckworth, 1978), 2–3.

8. Gibson, *The English Vice*, 2–3.

9. Gibson, *The English Vice*, 3.

10. Carolyn E. Brown, "Erotic Religious Flagellation and Shakespeare's Measure for Measure," *English Literary Renaissance* 16, no. 1 (1986): 141.

11. Brown, "Erotic Religious Flagellation," 143.

12. Shakespeare, *Measure for Measure*, 3.2.105.

13. Shakespeare, *Measure for Measure*, 1.4.60.

14. Brown, "Erotic Religious Flagellation," 153.

15. Shakespeare, *Measure for Measure*, 1.4.1.

16. Brown, "Erotic Religious Flagellation," 150–51.

17. Shakespeare, *Measure for Measure*, 2.4.159–60.

18. Shakespeare, *Measure for Measure*, 2.4.100-103.

19. Gibson, *The English Vice*, 4–5.

20. Boileau, 294–95, quoted in Gibson, *The English Vice*, 7.

21. Gibson, *The English Vice*, 8–9.

22. Gibson, *The English Vice*, 9.

23. Julie Peakman, *Mighty Lewd Books: The Development of Pornography in Eighteenth-Century England* (Houndmills, Basingstoke, UK: Palgrave Macmillan, 2003), 126–28.

24. Richard Hofstadter, *The Paranoid Style in American Politics* (1952; reprinted New York: Vintage, 2008), 21.

25. Note the resemblance to the affair of Peter Abelard and Heloise.

26. Peakman, *Mighty Lewd Books*, 143.

27. Peakman, *Mighty Lewd Books*, 144–45.

28. Anti-Catholic erotica also appeared in German. "Giovanni Frusta" (a pseudonym for Karl August Fetzer) wrote *Der Flagellantismus und die Jesuitenbeichte* in 1834, an anti-flagellation and anti-Jesuit book that included a fictionalized version of the Girard-Cadiere story. Set in the sixteenth century,

it tells of Brother Cornelis Adriensen, a lascivious monk who tried to seduce a young woman named Calleken Peter. Calleken met two other women who were instructed in discipline by Cornelis, for whom confession, instead of being a holy act, is a means of seduction. There was lots of doubletalk about overcoming shame and inner hypocrisy. Calleken eventually questions Cornelis's teachings. She educates herself via reading the Bible, finding nothing in it about flagellation. Eventually she becomes a good Protestant girl. The pornographic content was excused and camouflaged by the anti-Catholic message. See Niklaus Largier, *In Praise of the Whip: A Cultural History of Arousal* (New York: Zone Books, 2007).

29. Peakman, *Mighty Lewd Books*, 131.

30. Robert Darnton, *The Forbidden Best-Sellers of Pre-Revolutionary France* (New York: W.W. Norton, 1995), 95.

31. Darnton, *The Forbidden Best-Sellers*.

32. This novel was, in turn, referenced in one of the Marquis de Sade's novels. However, *Thérèse* was a much more humanist and Romantic (in a philosophical sense) work than Sade's nihilistic and Gothic works.

33. Peakman, *Mighty Lewd Books*, 129.

34. Peakman, *Mighty Lewd Books*, 17–20.

35. Frances E. Dolan, "Why Are Nuns Funny?" *Huntington Library Quarterly* 70, no. 4 (2007): 510.

36. Dolan, "Why Are Nuns Funny?" 512.

37. Dolan, "Why Are Nuns Funny?" 528.

38. Patrick R. O'Malley, *Catholicism, Sexual Deviance, and Victorian Gothic Culture* (Cambridge: Cambridge University Press, 2006), 91.

39. This was not the only example of the Protestant Electoral Union dealing in a combination of sex and violence. In 1866, the union published a circular with a column called "Facts Worth Considering," which included an allegedly true story from "the French paper" about seven priests ritually murdering a young female cleaner of a French chapel. A bystander reported the seven knife-wielding priests descending into a secret cell under the altar, where the bloody deed was done over the protests of the young girl. Diana Peschier, "Religious Sexual Perversion in Nineteenth-Century Anti-Catholic Literature," in *Sexual Perversions, 1670–1890*, ed. Julie Peakman (Basingstoke, UK: Palgrave Macmillan, 2009), 204–5.

40. O'Malley, *Catholicism, Sexual Deviance, and Victorian Gothic Culture*, 74–75.

41. Walter M. Kendrick, *The Secret Museum: Pornography in Modern Culture* (New York: Viking, 1987), 120–22.

42. Tracy Fessenden, "The Convent, the Brothel, and the Protestant Woman's Sphere," *Signs* 25, no. 2 (2000): 460.

43. Donna Dennis, *Licentious Gotham: Erotic Publishing and Its Prosecution in Nineteenth-Century New York* (Cambridge, MA: Harvard University Press, 2009).

44. Rebecca Theresa Reed, Nancy Lusignan Schultz, and Maria Monk, *A Veil of Fear: Nineteenth-Century Convent Tales by Rebecca Reed and Maria Monk* (West Lafayette, IN: Notabell, 1999), 24–25.

45. Reed et al., *A Veil of Fear*, 114–16, passim.

46. Reed et al., *A Veil of Fear*, 25, 49.

47. Peschier, "Religious Sexual Perversion in Nineteenth-Century Anti-Catholic Literature."

48. Dennis, *Licentious Gotham*, 2009.

49. Charles Bernheimer, *Figures of Ill Repute: Representing Prostitution in Nineteenth-Century France* (Cambridge, MA: Harvard University Press, 1989), 196.

50. Oscar Wilde, *The Picture of Dorian Gray*, ch.11.

51. These same patterns appear in the satanic ritual abuse moral panics of the 1980s, and the theme of "Illuminati mind control sex slaves" in conspiracy theory literature beginning in the 1990s. Michael Barkun, *Culture of Conspiracy: Apocalyptic Visions in Contemporary America* (Berkeley: University of California Press, 2013), 76–78, 133–34.

CHAPTER THREE

1. Lawrence Stone, "Libertine Sexuality in Post-Restoration England: Group Sex and Flagellation among the Middling Sort in Norwich in 1706–07," *Journal of the History of Sexuality* 2, no. 4 (1992): 511–26.

2. Ian Gibson, *The English Vice: Beating, Sex, and Shame in Victorian England and After* (London: Duckworth, 1978), 12.

3. Fergus Linnane, *London: The Wicked City; A Thousand Years of Vice in the Capital* (London: Robson, 2003), 105.

4. See Dan Cruickshank, *London's Sinful Secret: The Bawdy History and Very Public Passions of London's Georgian Age* (New York: St. Martin's Press, 2010) for details on the link between Hogarth's art-stories and religious art depicting the life of Virgin Mary and of Christ.

5. Katie Hickman, *Courtesans: Money, Sex, and Fame in the Nineteenth Century* (New York: Morrow, 2003), 86.

6. Neil Philip, *Working Girls: An Illustrated History of the Oldest Profession* (London: Bloomsbury, 1991), 110–12, citing Ann Sheldon's *Authentic and Interesting Memoirs of Miss Ann Sheldon*, privately printed, 1787–1788.

7. Project Gutenberg edition. Rousseau was a little off in his dates; he would have been eleven and Mlle. Lambercier forty. Gibson, *The English Vice*, 19.

8. Gibson, *The English Vice*, 22n23, referring to Binet's "Le fetichisme dans l'amour."

9. G. J. Barker-Benfield, *The Culture of Sensibility: Sex and Society in Eighteenth-Century Britain* (Chicago: University of Chicago Press, 1996).

10. Locke, *Essay*, 2.7.4.

11. Edmund Burke, *A Philosophical Inquiry into the Origin of Our Ideas of The Sublime and Beautiful*, part 1, sec. 7, part 1, sec. 17.

12. R. F. Brissenden, *Virtue in Distress: Studies in the Novel of Sentiment from Richardson to Sade* (New York: Barnes and Noble, 1974), 74–75.

13. Barker-Benfield, *The Culture of Sensibility*, 183.

14. Barker-Benfield, *The Culture of Sensibility*, 304.

15. Marcus Wood, *Slavery, Empathy, and Pornography* (Oxford: Oxford University Press, 2002), 12.

16. Brissenden, *Virtue in Distress*, 97.

17. R. P. T. Davenport-Hines, *Gothic: Four Hundred Years of Excess, Horror, Evil, and Ruin* (New York: North Point Press, 1999), 121.

18. Davenport-Hines, *Gothic*, 121–22.

19. Patrick R. O'Malley, *Catholicism, Sexual Deviance, and Victorian Gothic Culture* (Cambridge: Cambridge University Press, 2006), 10.

20. J. V. Ridgely, "George Lippard's *The Quaker City*: The World of the American Porno-Gothic," *Studies in the Literary Imagination* 7, no. 1 (1974): 88–89.

21. Ann Ward Radcliffe, *The Mysteries of Udolpho* (1794) Project Gutenberg edition, https://www.gutenberg.org/ebooks/3268, accessed March 11, 2018.

22. M.G. Lewis, *The Monk: A Romance* (1796) Project Gutenberg edition, https://www.gutenberg.org/ebooks/601, accessed March 11, 2018.

23. Brissenden, *Virtue in Distress*, 279.

24. Francine du Plessix Gray, *At Home with the Marquis de Sade: A Life* (New York: Simon & Schuster, 1998), 282, quoting Sade to M. de Crosne, lieutenant general of police, September 1785.

25. Gray, *At Home with the Marquis de Sade*, 264–66.

26. Gray, *At Home with the Marquis de Sade*, 316–19.

27. Gray, *At Home with the Marquis de Sade*, 357–60.

28. Gray, *At Home with the Marquis de Sade*, 377–80.

29. Mario Praz, *The Romantic Agony* (New York: Meridian Books, 1956), 128.

30. O'Malley, *Catholicism*, 4.

CHAPTER FOUR

1. Irvin C. Schick, *The Erotic Margin: Sexuality and Spatiality in Alteritist Discourse* (London: Verso, 1999), 53–54.
2. Rana Kabbani, *Imperial Fictions: Europe's Myths of the Orient* (London: Saqi, 2008), 24
3. İrvin C. Schick, *The Erotic Margin: Sexuality and Spatiality in Alteritist Discourse* (London: Verso, 1999), 59.
4. Schick, *The Erotic Margin*, 66–67.
5. Joan DelPlato, *Multiple Wives, Multiple Pleasures Representing the Harem, 1800–1875* (Madison, NJ: Fairleigh Dickinson University Press, 2002), 29.
6. Robert C. Davis, *Christian Slaves, Muslim Masters: White Slavery in the Mediterranean, the Barbary Coast, and Italy, 1500–1800* (London: Palgrave Macmillan, 2004), 5–6.
7. Stephen Clissold, *The Barbary Slaves* (Totowa, NJ: Rowman & Littlefield, 1977), 2.
8. Davis, *Christian Slaves, Muslim Masters*, 52.
9. Davis, *Christian Slaves, Muslim Masters*, 55.
10. Davis, *Christian Slaves, Muslim Masters*, 59.
11. Davis, *Christian Slaves, Muslim Masters*, 59–60.
12. Schick, *The Erotic Margin*, 211.
13. Schick, *The Erotic Margin*, 220.
14. Davis, *Christian Slaves, Muslim Masters*, 61.
15. Davis, *Christian Slaves, Muslim Masters*, 105–6.
16. Clissold, *The Barbary Slaves*, 43.
17. Clissold, *The Barbary Slaves*, 43.
18. Clissold, *The Barbary Slaves*, 89–90.
19. Davis, *Christian Slaves, Muslim Masters*, 125.
20. Clissold, *The Barbary Slaves*, 44.
21. Clissold, *The Barbary Slaves*, 45.
22. Clissold, *The Barbary Slaves*, 43–44.
23. Clissold, *The Barbary Slaves*, 47.
24. Schick, *The Erotic Margin*, 218, quoting Aaron Hill, *A Full and Just Account of the Present State of the Ottoman Empire* (London: John Mayo, 1709), 103 (emphasis in original).
25. Clissold, *The Barbary Slaves*, 90.
26. Davis, *Christian Slaves, Muslim Masters*, 36.
27. Clissold, *The Barbary Slaves*, 8.
28. Clissold, *The Barbary Slaves*, 40.

29. Davis, *Christian Slaves, Muslim Masters*, 182–84.
30. Clissold, *The Barbary Slaves*, 110, 115, 116.
31. Davis, *Christian Slaves, Muslim Masters*, 181.
32. Davis, *Christian Slaves, Muslim Masters*, 176.
33. Davis, *Christian Slaves, Muslim Masters*, 132.
34. Davis, *Christian Slaves, Muslim Masters*, 126–27.
35. Davis, *Christian Slaves, Muslim Masters*, 156.
36. Davis, *Christian Slaves, Muslim Masters*, 174.
37. Schick, *The Erotic Margin*, 132, 153–54.
38. Philippe Jullian, *The Orientalists: European Painters of Eastern Scenes* (Oxford: Phaidon, 1977), 28.
39. Schick, *The Erotic Margin*, 224–25.
40. DelPlato, *Multiple Wives, Multiple Pleasures*, 75.
41. DelPlato, *Multiple Wives, Multiple Pleasures*, 73.
42. DelPlato, *Multiple Wives, Multiple Pleasures*, 22.
43. DelPlato, *Multiple Wives, Multiple Pleasures*, 86.
44. Charles D. Martin, *The White African American Body: A Cultural and Literary Exploration* (New Brunswick, NJ: Rutgers University Press, 2002), 103–4.
45. Martin, *The White African American Body*, 104.
46. William Beckford's novel *Vathek* (1786) is a Gothic novel in the fictional, eastern land of Samarah, serving as a link between the Gothic and the Oriental.
47. Robert Hughes, *American Visions: The Epic History of Art in America* (New York: Alfred A. Knopf, 1997), 216–17.
48. Oliver W. Larkin, *Art and Life in America* (New York: Holt, Rinehart and Winston, 1960), 181.
49. There is no evidence that Palmer directly based it on Powers's statue, though they worked in the same tradition and Palmer had likely seen the famous *Greek Slave* on exhibition. James C. Webster, *Erastus D. Palmer: Sculpture—Ideas* (Newark: University of Delaware Press, 1983), 100–104.
50. Mitchell Robert Breitwieser, *American Puritanism and the Defense of Mourning: Religion, Grief, and Ethnology in Mary White Rowlandson's Captivity Narrative* (Madison: University of Wisconsin Press, 1990), 133.

CHAPTER 5

1. Walter Johnson, *Soul by Soul: Life inside the Antebellum Slave Market* (Cambridge, MA: Harvard University Press, 1999), 113–14.
2. Marcus Wood, *Slavery, Empathy, and Pornography* (Oxford: Oxford University Press, 2002), 22.

3. This parody of Botticelli's *Venus on the Half-Shell* was published in the second book of the third edition of *The History, Civil and Commercial, of the British Colonies in the West Indies*, by Bryan Edwards, in 1801.

4. James Oliver Horton and Lois E. Horton, *Slavery and the Making of America* (Oxford: Oxford University Press, 2005), 31.

5. Susan D. Amussen, "Violence, Gender and Race in the Seventeenth Century Mid-Atlantic," in *Masculinities, Childhood, Violence: Attending to Early Modern Women—and Men*, ed. Amy E. Leonard, Karen L. Nelson, Sarah R. Cohen, Alexandra Shepard, and Margaret Ferguson (Newark: University of Delaware Press, 2011), 283–85.

6. Srinivas Aravamudan, *Tropicopolitans: Colonialism and Agency, 1688–1804* (Durham, NC: Duke University Press, 1999), 38.

7. Catherine Molineux, "Hogarth's Fashionable Slaves: Moral Corruption in Eighteenth-Century London," *English Literary History* 72 (2005): 495–520.

8. Wood, *Slavery, Empathy, and Pornography*, 12.

9. Wood, *Slavery, Empathy, and Pornography*, 160.

10. Wood, *Slavery, Empathy, and Pornography*, 261.

11. Wood, *Slavery, Empathy, and Pornography*, 237.

12. Walt Whitman, *Leaves of Grass*, section 33.

13. David S. Reynolds, *Mightier Than the Sword: Uncle Tom's Cabin and the Battle for America* (New York: W.W. Norton, 2012), 33.

14. Thomas F. Gossett, *Uncle Tom's Cabin and American Culture* (Dallas, TX: Southern Methodist University Press, 1985), 15–16.

15. Reynolds, *Mightier Than the Sword*, 65.

16. Diane Roberts, *The Myth of Aunt Jemima: Representations of Race and Region* (London: Routledge, 1994), 29–30.

17. Roberts, *The Myth of Aunt Jemima*, 31.

18. Stowe, incidentally, had an unlikely crush on Lord Byron when she was a young woman, so she might have been influenced by Byron's Orientalist writings, such as *Don Juan* and *Sardanapalus*, which also influenced Hannah Cullwick.

19. Wood, *Slavery, Empathy, and Pornography*, 175.

20. Kathryn Hughes, *The Short Life and Long Times of Mrs. Beeton* (London: Fourth Estate, 2005), 93.

21. Harriet Beecher Stowe, letter of 27 September 1852, quoted in Maurie Dee McInnis, *Slaves Waiting for Sale: Abolitionist Art and the American Slave Trade* (Chicago: University of Chicago Press, 2011), emphasis in original.

22. Wood, *Slavery, Empathy, and Pornography*, 184.

23. Roberts, *The Myth of Aunt Jemima*, 63.

24. The issue of sexual liaisons between slave men and slaveholding women was a complex and taboo one. During the Civil War, abolitionists testified before

the American Freedman's Inquiry Commission (AFIC) that it was much more common than thought. They told anecdotes of slaveholding women carrying on affairs with their male slaves and bearing mixed-race children. According to a secondhand account, a black male servant would attend a white woman in her room. She would thrust out her foot and ask him to tie her boot, and he would say, "What a pretty foot!" This testimony should be taken with reservations, as filtered through white Northern perceptions of the alleged sexual depravity of the slave South. The reports to the AFIC were suppressed. Martha Elizabeth Hodes, *White Women, Black Men: Illicit Sex in the Nineteenth-Century South* (New Haven, CT: Yale University Press, 1997), 126–32.

25. Harriet Jacobs, *Incidents in the Life of a Slave Girl*, ch. 5.

26. Jacobs, *Incidents in the Life of a Slave Girl*, ch. 6.

27. Jacobs, *Incidents in the Life of a Slave Girl*, ch. 9.

28. Jacobs, *Incidents in the Life of a Slave Girl*, ch. 40.

29. Colette Colligan, "Anti-Abolition Writes Obscenity: The English Vice, Transatlantic Slavery, and England's Obscene Print Culture," in *International Exposure: Perspectives on Modern European Pornography, 1800–2000*, ed. Lisa Z. Sigel (New Brunswick, NJ: Rutgers University Press, 2005), 78–79.

30. Charles Carrington, *The Memoirs of Dolly Morton: The Story of a Woman's Part in the Struggle to Free the Slaves* (Paris: Charles Carrington, 1890), 4.

31. Carrington, *The Memoirs of Dolly Morton*, 64.

32. Colligan, "Anti-Abolition Writes Obscenity," 2005.

33. Toni Morrison, *Playing in the Dark: Whiteness and the Literary Imagination* (New York: Vintage Books, 1992), 66, quoted in Roberts, *The Myth of Aunt Jemima*, 27.

34. Biman Basu, *The Commerce of Peoples: Sadomasochism and African American Literature* (Lanham, MD: Lexington Books, 2012), 42–43.

35. Basu, *The Commerce of Peoples*, 47.

36. Basu, *The Commerce of Peoples*, 48.

37. Michael Hiley and Arthur Joseph Munby, *Victorian Working Women: Portraits from Life* (Boston: D. R. Godine, 1980), 24.

38. Derek Hudson and Arthur Joseph Munby, *Munby, Man of Two Worlds: The Life and Diaries of Arthur J. Munby, 1828–1910* (London: J. Murray, 1972), 112.

39. Hudson and Munby, *Munby, Man of Two Worlds*, 117–18.

40. Hannah Cullwick and Liz Stanley, *The Diaries of Hannah Cullwick, Victorian Maidservant* (New Brunswick, NJ: Rutgers University Press, 1984), 40.

41. Pamela Horn, *The Rise and Fall of the Victorian Servant* (Stroud, UK: Sutton, 2004), 113.

42. Horn, *The Rise and Fall of the Victorian Servant*, 112–13.

43. Ann McClintock, *Imperial Leather: Race, Gender, and Sexuality in the Colonial Contest* (New York: Routledge, 1995), passim.

44. Horn, *The Rise and Fall of the Victorian Servant*, 11–12.

45. Cullwick and Stanley, *The Diaries of Hannah Cullwick*, 139.

46. Hudson and Munby, *Munby, Man of Two Worlds*, 55, 62; Hiley and Munby, *Victorian Working Women*, 20.

47. Barry Reay, *Watching Hannah: Sexuality, Horror and Bodily Deformation in Victorian England* (London: Reaktion, 2002), 148, citing Hiley and Munby, *Victorian Working Women*, 24; Hudson and Munby, *Munby, Man of Two Worlds*, 86–89.

48. Diane Atkinson, *Love and Dirt: The Marriage of Arthur Munby and Hannah Cullwick* (London: Macmillan, 2003), 29–34, 309, 323.

49. Cullwick and Stanley, *The Diaries of Hannah Cullwick*, 47.

50. Cullwick and Stanley, *The Diaries of Hannah Cullwick*, 66.

51. Hudson and Munby, *Munby, Man of Two Worlds*, 51–52.

52. Cullwick and Stanley, *The Diaries of Hannah Cullwick*, 85.

53. Cullwick and Stanley, *The Diaries of Hannah Cullwick*, 61.

54. Cullwick and Stanley, *The Diaries of Hannah Cullwick*, 167.

55. Cullwick and Stanley, *The Diaries of Hannah Cullwick*, 170; Reay, *Watching Hannah*, 72, shows that Munby did write about their switching.

56. Cullwick and Stanley, *The Diaries of Hannah Cullwick*, 170.

57. Hudson and Munby, *Munby, Man of Two Worlds*, 134.

58. Hudson and Munby, *Munby, Man of Two Worlds*, 133–34.

59. Hudson and Munby, *Munby, Man of Two Worlds*, 334–35.

60. Cullwick and Stanley, *The Diaries of Hannah Cullwick*, 274.

61. Hudson and Munby, *Munby, Man of Two Worlds* 431–32.

62. Hiley and Munby, *Victorian Working Women*, 32.

CHAPTER SIX

1. Michael Mason, *The Making of Victorian Sexuality* (Oxford: Oxford University Press, 1994), 9–10.

2. Peter Gay, *Education of the Senses* (New York: Oxford University Press, 1984).

3. Ian Gibson, *The English Vice: Beating, Sex, and Shame in Victorian England and After* (London: Duckworth, 1978), 142–43.

4. Gibson, *The English Vice*, 247.

5. According to a letter written by Hankey to Swinburne and printed in Ashbee's *Index*.

6. Gibson, *The English Vice*, 249.

7. Gibson, *The English Vice*, 254.

8. Gibson, *The English Vice*, 260.

9. Gibson, *The English Vice*, 260.

10. Trevor Fisher, *Prostitution and the Victorians* (Stroud, UK: Sutton, 1997), 48.

11. Fisher, *Prostitution and the Victorians*, 56–57. In James Joyce's *Ulysses* (1904), the episode in which Bloom visits a brothel is called "Circe."

12. Katie Hickman, *Courtesans: Money, Sex, and Fame in the Nineteenth Century* (New York: Morrow, 2003), 248.

13. Émile Zola, *Nana*, chap. 9.

14. Rachilde, *The Marquise de Sade*, trans. Liz Heron (Sawtry, UK: Dedalus, 1994), 237–38.

15. Alain Corbin, *Women for Hire: Prostitution and Sexuality in France after 1850* (Cambridge, MA: Harvard University Press, 1990), 124–25.

16. Corbin, *Women for Hire*, 127.

17. Valerie Steele, *The Corset: A Cultural History* (New Haven, CT: Yale University Press, 2001), 121–23.

18. Steele, *The Corset*, 129.

19. Steele, *The Corset*, 129.

20. See Steele, *The Corset*; and David Kunzle, *Fashion and Fetishism: Corsets, Tight-Lacing and Other Forms of Body-Sculpture* (Stroud, UK: Sutton, 2004).

21. Kunzle, *Fashion and Fetishism*, 313.

22. Gibson, *The English Vice*, 99.

23. Gibson, *The English Vice*, 67–68. The beating of girls was apparently much less common, at least in schools for the upper classes. Girls' reformatory and industrial schools were another matter, with the birch, cane, and tawse in regular use, though mainly on the hands or shoulders, and in private (79–82).

24. Gibson, *The English Vice*, 48–50.

25. Gibson, *The English Vice*, 73–74.

26. Tamar Heller, "Flagellating Feminine Desire: Lesbians, Old Maids, and New Women in 'Miss Coote's Confession,' a Victorian Pornographic Narrative," *Victorian Newsletter*, Fall 1997, 9.

27. Heller, "Flagellating Feminine Desire," 10.

28. Heller, "Flagellating Feminine Desire," 10. The name may also be a joking reference to Angela Burdett-Coutts, a wealthy heiress and philanthropist associated with charitable endeavors.

29. Heller, "Flagellating Feminine Desire," 12.

30. Heller, "Flagellating Feminine Desire," 13, quoting page 226 of *Miss Coote's Confession*.

31. Heller, "Flagellating Feminine Desire," 14.

32. "Etonensis," *Mysteries of Verbena House*, 2.53.

33. "The Mysteries of Verbena House," *The Birch Grove* (blog), accessed July 2, 2013, http://birchgrovepress.blogspot.ca/2010/07/mysteries-of-verbena-house.html.

34. "Experimental Lecture by Colonel Spanker," *The Birch Grove* (blog), accessed July 2, 2013, http://birchgrovepress.blogspot.ca/2010/08/experimental-lecture-by-colonel-spanker.html.

35. "Experimental Lecture Introduction," Google Docs, accessed July 2, 2013, https://docs.google.com/document/edit?id=1dX6OuPnCppCXXhWM3qHulVlD_P3CsNv3Qzi_PdGIY3A&hl=en&authkey=CMfa2owM.

36. Donald Thomas, *Swinburne, the Poet in His World* (New York: Oxford University Press, 1979), 109.

37. Gibson, *The English Vice*, 198–209.

38. Hughes attributes this, in part, to Beeton being afflicted with tertiary-stage syphilis, which can cause personality changes and dementia. Hughes presents some circumstantial evidence that Beeton had contracted syphilis as a "gay" youth ("gay" meaning involved in the demimonde of prostitutes and clients), which would also explain the Beetons' long struggle to have healthy children. Kathryn Hughes, *The Short Life and Long Times of Mrs. Beeton* (London: Fourth Estate, 2005).

39. Sharon Marcus, *Between Women: Friendship, Desire, and Marriage in Victorian England* (Princeton, NJ: Princeton University Press, 2009), 138.

40. *Englishwoman's Domestic Magazine Supplement*, April 1870, 2–3, quoted in Peter Farrer, "In Female Attire: Male Experiences of Cross-Dressing—Some Historical Fragments," in *Blending Genders: Social Aspects of Cross-Dressing and Sex-Changing*, ed. Richard Ekins and Dave King (London: Routledge, 2002), 10–11.

41. *Daily Telegraph*, January 18, 1869.

42. Margaret Beetham and Kay Boardman, *Victorian Woman's Magazines: An Anthology* (Manchester: Manchester University Press, 2001), 170, quoting *Lady's Own Paper* 5 (1870): 369.

43. Steele, *The Corset*, 88–94.

44. Gibson, *The English Vice*, 206.

45. Stewart P. Evans and Keith Skinner, *Jack the Ripper: Letters from Hell* (Stroud, UK: Sutton, 2001).

46. Jean Overton Fuller, *Swinburne* (London: Chatto and Windus, 1971), 64.

CHAPTER SEVEN

1. Harry Oosterhuis, *Stepchildren of Nature: Krafft-Ebing, Psychiatry, and the Making of Sexual Identity* (Chicago: University of Chicago Press, 2000), 45.
2. Derek Hudson and Arthur Joseph Munby, *Munby, Man of Two Worlds: The Life and Diaries of Arthur J. Munby, 1828–1910* (London: J. Murray, 1972), 161.
3. Ian Gibson, *The English Vice: Beating, Sex, and Shame in Victorian England and After* (New York: Schocken Books, 1978), 123–25.
4. Jean Overton Fuller, *Swinburne* (London: Chatto and Windus, 1968), 64.
5. Donald Thomas, *Swinburne: The Poet in His World* (New York: Oxford University Press, 1979), 100–101.
6. Thomas, *Swinburne: The Poet in His World*, 98.
7. Fuller, *Swinburne*, 272.
8. Hudson and Munby, *Munby, Man of Two Worlds*, 25.
9. Fuller, *Swinburne*, 67.
10. Ian Gibson, *The Erotomaniac: The Secret Life of Henry Spencer Ashbee* (London: Faber, 2002), passim.
11. Gibson, *The Erotomaniac*, 105.
12. Gibson, *The Erotomaniac*, 150–54.
13. Gibson argues in *Erotomaniac* that Ashbee wrote *My Secret Life*, or more likely compiled various anecdotes and stories in it.
14. Steven Marcus, *The Other Victorians: A Study of Sexuality and Pornography in Mid-Nineteenth-Century England* (New York: Basic Books, 1966), 136–38.
15. Marcus, *The Other Victorians*, 151, 152.
16. Sacher-Masoch, *Venus in Furs*.
17. James Cleugh, *The First Masochist: A Biography of Leopold von Sacher-Masoch* (New York: Stein and Day, 1967), 10.
18. Cleugh, *The First Masochist*, 15.
19. Cleugh, *The First Masochist*, 13–14.
20. Cleugh, *The First Masochist*, 10, 19.
21. Cleugh, *The First Masochist*, 122–25.
22. Gilles Deleuze, *Masochism: Coldness and Cruelty* (New York: Zone Books, 1991), 84–85.
23. Wanda von Sacher-Masoch, *The Confessions of Wanda von Sacher-Masoch*, trans. Marian Phillips, Caroline Hébert, and V. Vale (San Francisco: Re/Search Publications, 1990), 102.
24. Cleugh, *The First Masochist*, 96.
25. Sacher-Masoch, *The Confessions of Wanda*, 32.

26. Sacher-Masoch, *The Confessions of Wanda*, 106–7.
27. Cleugh, *The First Masochist*.
28. Oosterhuis, *Stepchildren of Nature*, 49–50.
29. Oosterhuis, *Stepchildren of Nature*, 122–23.
30. Emily S. Apter, *Feminizing the Fetish: Psychoanalysis and Narrative Obsession in Turn-of-the-Century France* (Ithaca, NY: Cornell University Press, 1991), 23.
31. Oosterhuis, *Stepchildren of Nature*, 44.
32. Apter, *Feminizing the Fetish*, 19. Psychologist Alfred Binet argued they were actually caused by early traumatic experiences.
33. Richard von Krafft-Ebing, *Psychopathia Sexualis*, trans. Domino Falls (London: Velvet Publications, 1997), 58–59; see Internet Archive, accessed March 9, 2015, https://archive.org/stream/psychopathiasexu00krafuoft/psychopathiasexu00krafuoft_djvu.txt.
34. Krafft-Ebing, *Psychopathia Sexualis*, 84.
35. Sigmund Freud, *The Standard Edition of the Complete Psychological Works of Sigmund Freud*, vol. 17, trans. Josef Breuer and Angela Richards (London: Hogarth Press, 1917–1919), 180.
36. Oosterhuis, *Stepchildren of Nature*, 184.
37. Oosterhuis, *Stepchildren of Nature*, 175.
38. Oosterhuis, *Stepchildren of Nature*, 190–91.
39. Oosterhuis, *Stepchildren of Nature*, 153–54.
40. Oosterhuis, *Stepchildren of Nature*, 157.
41. Oosterhuis, *Stepchildren of Nature*, 174.
42. Krafft-Ebing, *Psychopathia Sexualis*, 84.
43. Oosterhuis, *Stepchildren of Nature*, 14.
44. Oosterhuis, *Stepchildren of Nature*, 204.
45. Oosterhuis, *Stepchildren of Nature*, 204–6.
46. Oosterhuis, *Stepchildren of Nature*, 206.
48. Katie Hickman, *Courtesans: Money, Sex, and Fame in the Nineteenth Century* (New York: Morrow, 2003) 309–10.

CHAPTER EIGHT

1. Michael Fuchs, "Of Blitzkriege and Hardcore BDSM: Revisiting Nazi Sexploitation Camps," in *Nazisploitation! The Nazi Image in Low-Brow Cinema and Culture*, ed. Daniel H. Magilow, Elizabeth Bridges, and Kristin T. Vander Lugt (New York: Continuum, 2012), 281.

2. Bernardo Bertolucci's film *The Conformist* (1970) inverted this paradigm by linking fascist Italy with sterile bourgeois heterosexuality and democratic France with free-flowing queer sexuality.

3. Interview with Michel Foucault, *Cahiers du cinéma*, nos. 251–52, July–August 1974, 33. Quoted in Saul Friedländer, *Reflections of Nazism: An Essay on Kitsch and Death* (Bloomington: Indiana University Press, 1993), 74.

4. Laura Catherine Frost, *Sex Drives: Fantasies of Fascism in Literary Modernism* (Ithaca, NY: Cornell University Press, 2002), 32.

5. Leo Bersani, *Homos* (Cambridge, MA: Harvard University Press, 1996), 88.

6. Poster by H. R. Hopps, circa 1917, in Adam Parfrey, *It's a Man's World: Men's Adventure Magazines, the Postwar Pulps* (Los Angeles, CA: Feral House, 2003), 40.

7. Frost, *Sex Drives*, 26.

8. Régine Deforges and Pauline Réage, *Confessions of O: Conversations with Pauline Réage* (New York: Viking Press, 1979), 118–19.

9. Susan Brownmiller, *Against Our Will: Men, Women and Rape* (New York: Simon and Schuster, 1975), 311.

10. Daniel H. Magilow, "Introduction," in Magilow et al., *Nazisploitation*, 18n27. Roehm was later executed in the "Night of the Long Knives."

11. Michael D. Richardson, "Sexual Deviance," in Magilow et al., *Nazisploitation*, 42.

12. Richardson, "Sexual Deviance," 42.

13. Wilhelm Reich, *The Mass Psychology of Fascism* (New York: Orgone Institute Press, 1946), 25.

14. Edward Dmytryk (dir.), Emmet Lavery, and Gregor Ziemer (wri.), *Hitler's Children,* RKO Radio Pictures, 1943.

15. John Cromwell (dir.), Erich Maria Remarque, and Talbot Jennings (wri.), *So Ends Our Night*, David L. Loew-Albert Lewin, 1941.

16. Parfrey, *It's a Man's World*, 178–79.

17. Parfrey, *It's a Man's World*, 178.

18. Parfrey, *It's a Man's World*, 7.

19. Amit Pinchevski and Roy Brand, "Holocaust Perversions: The Stalags Pulp Fiction and the Eichmann Trial," *Critical Studies in Media Communication* 24, no. 5 (2007): 390.

20. M. Baden, *Stalag 13* (Tel Aviv: Yam Suf, 1961), 60.

21. Pinchevski and Brand, "Holocaust Perversions," 389.

22. Pinchevski and Brand, "Holocaust Perversions," 393.

23. Pinchevski and Brand, "Holocaust Perversions," 396.

24. Pinchevski and Brand, "Holocaust Perversions," 394.

25. Liliana Cavani (dir.), Liliana Cavani and et al. (wri.) *The Night Porter*, Lotar Film Productions, 1974.

26. Don Edmonds (dir.), Jonah Royston, and John C. W. Saxton (wri.), *Ilsa: She-Wolf of the SS*, Aeteas Filmproduktions, 1975.

27. Magilow, "Introduction," in Magilow et al., *Nazisploitation*, 10–11.

28. Lynn Rapaport, "Holocaust Pornography: Profaning the Sacred in *Ilsa, She-Wolf of the SS*," in *Monsters in the Mirror: Representations of Nazism in Post-War Popular Culture*, ed. Sara Buttsworth and Maartje Abbenhuis (Santa Barbara, CA: Praeger Publishers, 2010), 105.

29. Gualtiero Jacopetti and Franco Prosperi (dir., wri.), *Goodbye Uncle Tom*. Euro International Film (EIA), 1971.

30. Don Edmonds (dir.) and Langston Stafford (wri.), *Ilsa, Harem Keeper of the Oil Sheiks*, Mount Everest Enterprises Ltd, 1976.

31. Jess Franco (dir., wri.) and Erwin C. Dietrich (wri), *Wanda, the Wicked Warden* (aka *Ilsa, the Wicked Warden*), Cinépix, Elite Film, 1977.

32. Jean LaFleur (dir.) and Marven McGara (wri.), *Ilsa the Tigress of Siberia*, Mount Everest Enterprises Ltd, 1977.

33. Pier Paolo Pasolini (dir., wri.), *Salò, or the 120 Days of Sodom*, Produzioni Europee Associate (PEA), Les Productions Artistes Associés, 1975.

34. Tinto Brass (dir.) and Antonio Colantuoni et al. (wri.), *Salon Kitty*, Coralta Cinematografica, Cinema Seven Film, Les Productions Fox Europa, 1976.

35. Kantrowitz, "Swastika Toys," in *Leatherfolk: Radical Sex, People, Politics, and Practice*, ed. Mark Thompson (Boston: Alyson Publications, 1991), 193.

36. Arnie Kantrowitz. "Swastika Toys," 194.

37. Jack Fritscher, *Gay San Francisco: Eyewitness, Vol. 4—The Rise and Fall of Drummer Magazine*, chapter 5, 16–21, accessed November 14, 2013, http://www.jackfritscher.com/PDF/Drummer/Vol%204/SalonChapter-5_2013-06-05%20Final-Web.pdf.

38. Richard Goldstein, "S&M: The Dark Side of Gay Liberation," *Village Voice*, July 7, 1975, 10–13.

39. *Drummer* editor Jack Fritscher describes Goldstein's article as a "smear-campaign manifesto" that "ignorantly slandered gay S&M sex, and leather uniforms, by connecting our erotic disciplines to Nazi punishments." Fritscher, *Gay San Francisco: Eyewitness Vol. 4*, chapter 15, 2.

40. Susan Sontag, *Under the Sign of Saturn* (New York: Farrar, Straus & Giroux, 1980), 91.

41. Sontag, *Under the Sign of Saturn*, 101–2.

42. Sontag, *Under the Sign of Saturn*, 103–4.

43. Sontag, *Under the Sign of Saturn*, 104.

44. Sontag, *Under the Sign of Saturn*, 105.

45. Robin Ruth Linden, Darlene R. Pagano, Diana E. H. Russell, and Susan Leigh Star, *Against Sadomasochism: A Radical Feminist Analysis* (East Palo Alto, CA: Frog in the Well, 1982).

46. Linden, "Introduction," in Linden et al., *Against Sadomasochism*, 7–8.

47. Linden, "Introduction," in Linden et al., *Against Sadomasochism*, 10.

48. Sarah Lucia Hoagland, "Sadism, Masochism and Lesbian-Feminism," in Linden et al., *Against Sadomasochism*, 155.

49. Susan Leigh Star, "Swastikas: The Street and the University," in Linden et al., *Against Sadomasochism*, 132.

50. Star, "Swastikas," in Linden et al., *Against Sadomasochism*, 133–35.

51. Sheila Jeffreys, *The Lesbian Heresy: A Feminist Perspective on the Lesbian Sexual Revolution* (London: Women's Press, 1994).

52. Jeffreys, *The Lesbian Heresy*, 176.

53. Jeffreys, *The Lesbian Heresy*, 178.

54. Jeffreys, *The Lesbian Heresy*, 179.

55. Jeffreys, *The Lesbian Heresy*, 180.

56. Irene Reti and Pat Parker, eds., *Unleashing Feminism: Critiquing Lesbian Sadomasochism in the Gay Nineties* (Santa Cruz, CA: HerBooks, 1993).

57. Jamie Lee Evans, "Rodney King, Racism and the S/M Culture of America," in Reti and Parker, *Unleashing Feminism*, 74.

58. Evans, "Rodney King, Racism and the S/M Culture of America," 76, emphasis in original.

59. Irene Reti, "Remember the Fire: Lesbian Sadomasochism in a Post Nazi Holocaust World," in Reti and Parker, *Unleashing Feminism*, 81–82.

60. Irene Reti, "Remember the Fire," 81–82.

61. D. A. Clarke, "Consuming Passion: Some Thoughts on History, Sex and Free Enterprise," in Reti and Parker, *Unleashing Feminism*, 145.

62. Fuchs, "Of Blitzkriege and Hardcore BDSM," 291.

63. Frost, *Sex Drives*, 33–34.

64. Frost, *Sex Drives*, 34.

CHAPTER NINE

1. Robert V. Bienvenu, "The Development of Sadomasochism as a Cultural Style in the Twentieth-Century United States" (PhD diss., Indiana University, 1998), 236–38, 243.

2. Bienvenu, "The Development of Sadomasochism," 243–44 (ellipses in original), quoting Gregory Sprague's interview with Samuel Steward, May 20, 1982 (LA&M).

3. Samuel M. Steward, "Dr. Kinsey Takes a Peek at S/M: A Reminiscence," in *Leatherfolk: Radical Sex, People, Politics, and Practice*, ed. Mark Thompson (Boston: Alyson Publications, 1991), 83.

4. Justin Spring, *Secret Historian: The Life and Times of Samuel Steward, Professor, Tattoo Artist, and Sexual Renegade* (New York: Farrar, Straus and Giroux, 2010), 102–3.

5. Spring, *Secret Historian*, 189.

6. Steward, "Dr. Kinsey Takes a Peek at S/M," 85–89.

7. Spring, *Secret Historian*, 139.

8. Bienvenu, "The Development of Sadomasochism," 244.

9. Spring, *Secret Historian*, 288–89.

10. Spring, *Secret Historian*, 302.

11. Thom Magister, "One Among Many: The Seduction and Training of a Leatherman," in Thompson, *Leatherfolk*, 96–97.

12. slave david stein, "From S&M to M/s: How Consensual Slavery Became Visible in the Gay Leather Community, 1950 to 1999," in Peter Tupper, ed., *Our Lives, Our History: Consensual Master/slave Relationships from Ancient Times to the 21st Century* (New York: Perfectbound Press, 2016), 77.

13. Len G., e-mail to slave david stein, dated October 19, 2014, quoted in stein, "From S&M to M/s," 79–80. Ellipsis in original.

14. Shaun Cole, *Don We Now Our Gay Apparel: Gay Men's Dress in the Twentieth Century* (Oxford: Berg, 2000), 3.

15. Cole, *Don We Now Our Gay Apparel*, 15–16.

16. British Fascist newspaper *The Blackshirt*, 1934, quoted in J. R. Harvey, *Men in Black* (Chicago: University of Chicago Press, 1996), 240.

17. Harvey, *Men in Black*, 113.

18. Harvey, *Men in Black*, 245.

19. Marvin J. Taylor, "Looking for Mr. Benson: The Black Leather Motorcycle Jacket and Narratives of Masculinities," in *Fashion in Popular Culture: Literature, Media and Contemporary Studies*, ed. Joseph Hancock, Toni Johnson-Woods, and Vicki Karaminas (Bristol, UK: Intellect, 2013), 124.

20. Mick Farren, *The Black Leather Jacket* (New York: Abbeville Press, 1985), 18–38.

21. Taylor, "Looking for Mr. Benson," 125.

22. Hunter S. Thompson, *Hell's Angels: A Strange and Terrible Saga* (New York: Ballantine, 1967), 81–82, 84–86.

23. Farren, *The Black Leather Jacket*, 44–48.

24. Cole, *Don We Now Our Gay Apparel*, 107.

25. Cole, *Don We Now Our Gay Apparel*, 112.

26. Taylor, "Looking for Mr. Benson," 125–26.

27. Valentine Hooven III, "Tom of Finland: A Short Biography," Tom of Finland Foundation, accessed November 27, 2013, http://tomoffinlandfoundation.org/foundation/touko.html.

28. Taylor, "Looking for Mr. Benson," 129–33.

29. Ambrosio, *Marginalia on the Old Guard, Leather Traditions, and BDSM History*, Version 1.05, September 1, 2006, accessed November 29, 2013, http://www.evilmonk.org/a/notetrad.cfm.

30. Joseph W. Bean, "Old Guard? If You Say So," accessed November 29, 2013, http://www.evilmonk.org/a/jwbean.cfm.

31. Paul Welch, Paul with photography by Bill Eppridge, "Homosexuality in America," *Life,* June 25, 1964, 68–69, accessed November 26, 2013, http://thornyc.livejournal.com/484117.html; and http://thornyc.livejournal.com/484888.html.

32. David Stein, "S/M's Copernican Revolution: From a Closed World to the Infinite Universe," in Thompson, *Leatherfolk*, 147–48.

33. Jay A. Gertzman, "1950s Sleaze and the Larger Literary Scene: The Case of Times Square Porn King Eddie Mishkin," *eI15* 3, no. 4 (August 2004), accessed November 26, 2013, http://efanzines.com/EK/eI15/; Brittany A. Daley and Stephen J. Gertz, *Sin-A-Rama: Sleaze Sex Paperbacks of the Sixties* (Los Angeles: Feral House, 2005).

34. Richard Pérez Seves, *Charles Guyette: Godfather of American Fetish Art* (Richard Pérez Seves, 2017), 111–42.

35. Bienvenu, "The Development of Sadomasochism," 91.

36. Tim Pilcher and Gene Kannenberg, *Erotic Comics: A Graphic History from Tijuana Bibles to Underground Comix* (New York: Abrams, 2008), 121–23.

37. Bienvenu, "The Development of Sadomasochism," 96–97.

38. Gloria Leonard, "Interview with Paula Klaw," *High Society*, 1980, accessed November 23, 2013, http://www.americansuburbx.com/2013/05/interview-about-irving-klaw-interview-with-paula-klaw.html.

39. Bienvenu, "The Development of Sadomasochism," 117.

40. Bienvenu, "The Development of Sadomasochism," 107–8.

41. Bienvenu, "The Development of Sadomasochism," 152.

42. Bienvenu, "The Development of Sadomasochism," 109–10.

43. Richard Pérez, "Eric Stanton, aka Ernest Stanten . . . ," accessed November 26, 2013, http://permanentobscurity.com/perm-obsc-stanton-klaw.htm.

44. Eric Stanton, *The Dominant Wives and Other Stories* (Köln: Taschen, 1998), 6–9.

45. Pilcher and Kannenberg, *Erotic Comics*, 124–27.

46. Jim Linderman, "Gene Bilbrew African-American Artist of Vintage Sleaze (part two)" and "Gene Bilbrew African-American Artist of Vintage Sleaze

(part three)," *Dull Tool Dim Bulb* (blog), March 2009, accessed November 26, 2013, http://dulltooldimbulb.blogspot.ca/2009/03/eugene-bilbrew-african-amer ican-artist.html and http://dulltooldimbulb.blogspot.ca/2009/03/gene-bilbrew -african-american.html.

47. Bienvenu, "The Development of Sadomasochism," 180–81.
48. Bienvenu, "The Development of Sadomasochism," 179.
49. Bienvenu, "The Development of Sadomasochism," 190–94.
50. Richard Pérez, "Leonard Burtman, Selbee Associates, and the Reinvention of Sexploitation/fetish Magazines," PermanentObscurity.com, accessed November 27, 2013, http://permanentobscurity.com/perm-obsc-lenny -burtman.htm.
51. Bienvenu, "The Development of Sadomasochism," 207–10.
52. Kenneth Turan and Stephen F. Zito, *Sinema: American Pornographic Films and the People Who Make Them* (New York: Praeger, 1974), 19–25.
53. Anne-Laure Quilleriet, *The Leather Book* (Paris: Editions Assouline, 2003), 216–26.
54. Jonny Trunk and Damon Murray, *Dressing for Pleasure in Rubber, Vinyl and Leather: The Best of Atomage, 1972–1980* (London: FUEL, 2010), 7–8.
55. Michael Leigh and Louis Berg, *The Velvet Underground* (New York: Macfadden, 1963), 21.
56. Bienvenu, "The Development of Sadomasochism," 124.
57. Leigh and Berg, *The Velvet Underground*, 45, 50–51.
58. Leigh and Berg, *The Velvet Underground*, 13–14.

CHAPTER TEN

1. David Stein, "S/M's Copernican Revolution," in *Leatherfolk: Radical Sex, People, Politics, and Practice*, ed. Mark Thompson (Boston: Alyson Publications, 1991), 147.
2. S. Veit, "Sexual Minorities Report: Eulenspiegel? What's That?" *Pro-Me-Thee-Us*, Special Introductory Issue, 1973.
3. S. Veit, "Sexual Minorities Report."
4. S. Veit, "Sexual Minorities Report."
5. Todd H., *Society of Janus: 25 Years* (San Francisco: Society of Janus, 1999), 43.
6. Jack Fritscher, "The Janus Society: Kiss and Don't Tell: Cynthia Slater and the Catholic Priest," *Drummer*, February 27, 1979, accessed November 29, 2013, http://jackfritscher.com/Drummer/Issues/027/Janus%20Society.html.

7. Jay Wiseman, "An Essay about 'The Old Days' (Essay # 1)," Jaywiseman.com, 2008, accessed December 3, 2008, http://www.jaywiseman.com/SEX_BDSM_Old_Guard_1.php.

8. H., *Society of Janus*, 14.

9. H., *Society of Janus*, 13.

10. H., *Society of Janus*, 14.

11. H., *Society of Janus*, 18–19.

12. H., *Society of Janus*, 19.

13. Gayle Rubin, "Elegy for the Valley of the Kings: AIDS and the Leather Community in San Francisco, 1981–1996," in *In Changing Times: Gay Men and Lesbians Encounter HIV/AIDS*, ed. Martin P. Levine, Peter M. Nardi, and John H. Gagnon (Chicago: University of Chicago Press, 1997), 110–12.

14. Rubin, "Elegy for the Valley," 114, quoting Shilts (1987), 89.

15. Rubin, "Elegy for the Valley," 116–18.

16. Rubin, "Elegy for the Valley," 124.

17. Rubin, "Elegy for the Valley," 131–33.

18. Nancy Ava Miller, *Pervert: Notes from the Sexual Underground* (n.p.: Peplove Press, 2009), 129.

19. Miller, *Pervert*, 106.

20. Miller, *Pervert*, 9, 108.

21. Miller, *Pervert*, 116.

22. Miller, *Pervert*, 297.

23. See Margot Danielle Weiss, *Techniques of Pleasure: BDSM and the Circuits of Sexuality* (Durham, NC: Duke University Press, 2011).

24. Anna Robinson, "Passion, Politics, and Politically Incorrect Sex: Towards a History of Lesbian Sadomasochism in the USA 1975–1993" (master's thesis, Central European University, Budapest, 2015), 47.

25. Lynda Hart, *Between the Body and the Flesh: Performing Sadomasochism* (New York: Columbia University Press, 1998), 52.

26. As Anna Robinson put it, "Lesbian SM surely existed before 1975," and adds an anecdote in a footnote: "[Patrick] Califia even recalls a story of a couple who cruised in gay men's leather bars in the early 1960s looking for partners—but organised groups and published work did not." Robinson, "Passion, Politics, and Politically Incorrect Sex," 7.

27. In 1972, *Echo of Sappho* published a seven-page interview with Beverly, a member of the recently founded Eulenspiegel society. Beverly described herself as lesbian and often co-topped a male submissive with another lesbian. However, she also said she refused to dominate another woman on feminist grounds. Alex Ellis Warner, "'Where Angels Fear to Tread': Feminism, Sex and the Problem of SM, 1969–1993" (master's thesis, Rutgers, 2011), 54, http://hdl.rutgers.edu/1782.1/rucore10001600001.ETD.000061536.

28. Warner, "'Where Angels Fear to Tread,'" 27–29, quoting Karla Jay, "The Spirit Is Feminist but the Flesh Is?" *Lesbian Tide*, October 1974, 1.

29. Jay, "The Spirit Is Feminist," 15.

30. That Jay used a paraphrase of Matthew 26:41 in the Christian Bible ("Watch and pray so that you will not fall into temptation. The spirit is willing, but the flesh is weak.") is almost prophetic, as much of the "lesbian sex wars" paralleled Judeo-Christian themes concerning the body and the soul.

31. Robinson, "Passion, Politics, and Politically Incorrect Sex," 65.

32. Warner, "'Where Angels Fear to Tread,'" 33–36.

33. Warner, "'Where Angels Fear to Tread,'" 37.

34. Jeanne Cordova, "Towards a Feminist Expression of Sado-Masochism," *Lesbian Tide*, November–December 1976, 14–17.

35. Califia quoted in Thomas S. Weinberg, *S & M: Studies in Dominance and Submission* (Amherst, NY: Prometheus Books, 1995).

36. Pat Califia, *Public Sex: The Culture of Radical Sex* (Pittsburgh, PA: Cleiss Press, 1994), 12.

37. Califia, *Public Sex*, 157.

38. Gayle Rubin, "The Leather Menace, Comments on Politics and S/M," in *Coming to Power: Writings and Graphics on Lesbian S/M*, ed. Samois (Boston: Alyson Publications, 1987), 222.

39. Califia, "A Personal View of the History of the Lesbian S/M Community and Movement in San Francisco," in *Coming to Power*, 248.

40. Anonymous, "History of Our Leather Women's Group in San Francisco," The Exiles, accessed May 10, 2015, http://theexiles.org/history-new/.

41. Rubin, "The Leather Menace," 222.

42. Katherine Davis, "Introduction: What We Fear We Try to Keep Contained," in Samois, *Coming to Power*, 9.

43. Warner, "'Where Angels Fear to Tread,'" 75–77.

44. Gayle Rubin, "The Outcasts: A Social History," in *The Second Coming*, ed. Pat Califia and Robin Sweeney (Boston: Alyson, 1996), 339–44.

45. Dorothy Allison, "Public Silence, Private Terror," in *Skin: Talking about Sex, Class and Literature* (New York: Open Road Integrated Media, 2013).

46. Anonymous, "Lesbian Sex Mafia," in Califia and Sweeney, *The Second Coming*, 338.

47. Califia, "A Personal View," 248.

48. Carole S. Vance, *Pleasure and Danger: Exploring Female Sexuality* (Boston: Routledge & K. Paul, 1984), 61–62.

49. Robin Ruth Linden, *Against Sadomasochism: A Radical Feminist Analysis* (East Palo Alto, CA: Frog in the Well, 1982), 91 (emphasis in original).

50. Linden, *Against Sadomasochism*, 91.

51. Linden, *Against Sadomasochism*, 92.
52. Warner, "'Where Angels Fear to Tread,'" 29–31.
53. Susan Brownmiller, *Against Our Will: Men, Women and Rape* (New York: Simon & Schuster, 1975), 263.
54. Warner, "'Where Angels Fear to Tread,'" 32.
55. Warner, "'Where Angels Fear to Tread,'" 41–42, 99.
56. Gayle Rubin, "Blood under the Bridge: Reflections on 'Thinking Sex,'" in *Deviations: A Gayle Rubin Reader* (Durham, NC: Duke University Press, 2011), 206–12.
57. Hart, *Between the Body and the Flesh*.
58. Catherine A. Pomerleau, "Among and between Women: Califia Community, Grassroots Feminist Education, and the Politics of Difference, 1975–1987" (PhD diss., University of Arizona, 2004), 228–45.
59. Califia, "A Personal View," 248.
60. Califia, "A Personal View," 248.
61. *Advocate*, no. 315, April 16, 1981, 9, Hart, *Between the Body and the Flesh*, 39.
62. Warner, "'Where Angels Fear to Tread,'" 135–38.
63. Rubin, "Blood under the Bridge," 200–206; Robinson, "Passion, Politics, and Politically Incorrect Sex," 73–75; Warner, "'Where Angels Fear to Tread,'" 130–31; Vance, *Pleasure and Danger*, 431–32.
64. Reproduced in Robinson, "Passion, Politics, and Politically Incorrect Sex," 76–77.
65. Robinson, "Passion, Politics, and Politically Incorrect Sex," 80; Vance, *Pleasure and Danger*, 433–34.
66. Robinson, "Passion, Politics, and Politically Incorrect Sex," 93.
67. Robinson, "Passion, Politics, and Politically Incorrect Sex," 100.
68. Warner, "'Where Angels Fear to Tread,'" 143.
69. Fran Moira, "Lesbian Sex Mafia (L S/M) Speak Out," *Off Our Backs* 12, no. 6 (June 30, 1982): 23, accessed December 18, 2013, http://web.archive.org/web/20080306135008/http://www.geocities.com/wikispace/oob.1982b.html.
70. Warner, "'Where Angels Fear to Tread,'" 145–55.
71. Robinson, "Passion, Politics, and Politically Incorrect Sex," 102–3.
72. Linden, *Against Sadomasochism*.
73. Robinson, "Passion, Politics, and Politically Incorrect Sex," 105.
74. Rubin, "Blood under the Bridge," 211.
75. See also Warner, "'Where Angels Fear to Tread,'" 29–31.
76. Linden, *Against Sadomasochism*, 147, 164.
77. Linden, *Against Sadomasochism*, 7–8, 23, 29, 32–37, 87, 132.
78. Linden, *Against Sadomasochism*, 49, 51, 79, 83.

79. Linden, *Against Sadomasochism*, 22 (emphasis in original). See also 93.
80. Linden, *Against Sadomasochism*, 170–71.
81. Linden, *Against Sadomasochism*, 108.
82. R. Lewis and K. Adler, "Come to Me Baby, or What's Wrong with Lesbian SM," as cited in Robinson, "Passion, Politics, and Politically Incorrect Sex," 117.
83. Robinson, "Passion, Politics, and Politically Incorrect Sex," 117–18.
84. Robinson, "Passion, Politics, and Politically Incorrect Sex," 132.
85. Robinson, "Passion, Politics, and Politically Incorrect Sex," 134, 142.
86. Irene Reti and Pat Parker, *Unleashing Feminism: Critiquing Lesbian Sadomasochism in the Gay Nineties* (Santa Cruz, CA: HerBooks, 1993).
87. Kathy Miriam, "From Rage to All the Rage: Lesbian-Feminism, Sadomasochism, and the Politics of Memory," in Reti and Parker, *Unleashing Feminism*, 66–69.
88. Jamie Lee Evans, "Rodney King, Racism and the S/M Culture of America," in Reti and Parker, *Unleashing Feminism*, 74.
89. Evans, "Rodney King, Racism and the S/M Culture of America," 75.
90. Miriam, "From Rage to All the Rage," 39–40.
91. Robinson, "Passion, Politics, and Politically Incorrect Sex," 136–39; Warner, "'Where Angels Fear to Tread,'" 166–67.
92. Robinson, "Passion, Politics, and Politically Incorrect Sex," 140.
93. Also, both sides wrote dystopian science fiction stories prophesying the worst if the other side won, such as Patrick Califia's "The Hustler" in the short story collection *Macho Sluts* and Sharon Lim-Hing's story "The Rules of Love" in *Unleashing Feminism*.
94. Warner, "'Where Angels Fear to Tread,'" 169, 181–86.
95. Warner, "'Where Angels Fear to Tread,'" 174.
96. Robinson, "Passion, Politics, and Politically Incorrect Sex," 144–45.
97. Stein, "S/M's Copernican Revolution," 149.
98. Stein, "S/M's Copernican Revolution," 146.
99. Gil Kessler, Philip Douglas, and Barry Douglas, "GMSMA's Three Pillars: Education, Social, Activism," GMSMA (Newsletter written for GMSMA Board retreat, courtesy of Gil Kessler).
100. David Stein, "'Safe Sane Consensual': The Making of a Shibboleth," Boybear, 2002, accessed January 2, 2014, www.boybear.us/ssc.pdf.
101. Stein, "S/M's Copernican Revolution," 155–56.

CHAPTER ELEVEN

1. Thomas S. Weinberg and Martha S. Magill, "Sadomasochistic Themes in Mainstream Culture," in *S&M: Studies in Dominance and Submission*, ed. Thomas S. Weinberg (Amherst, NY: Prometheus Books, 1995), 226.

2. Nathan Rambukkana, "Taking the Leather Out of Leathersex: The Internet, Identity, and the Sadomasochistic Public Sphere," in *Queer Online: Media Technology and Sexuality*, ed. Kate O'Riordan and David J. Phillips (New York: Peter Lang, 2007), 72.

3. Rambukkana, "Taking the Leather Out of Leathersex," 74.

4. Tom Boellstorff, *Coming of Age in Second Life: An Anthropologist Explores the Virtually Human* (Princeton, NJ: Princeton University Press, 2008), 156–57; David Steinberg, "Comes Naturally #34: Sex on the Net: Thoughts on a Culture Being Born," *Spectator Magazine*, June 2, 1995, accessed September 23, 2014, http://sexuality.org/authors/steinberg/cn34.html; Mark Bennet, "Digital Kinks," in *The Best of Skin Two*, ed. Tim Woodward (New York: Masquerade Books, 1993), 99.

5. Marian Palandri and Lelia Green, "Image Management in a Bondage, Discipline, Sadomasochist Subculture: A Cyber-Ethnographic Study," *Cyberpsychology & Behavior* 3, no. 4 (2000): 633.

6. Gloria G. Brame, "How a Nice Jewish Girl Like Me Became an Unrepentant Pervert," *Fetish Alliance*, accessed September 25, 2014, http://www.fetishalliance.net/Stories/Other_Stories/nicejewishgirlbecameunrepentantpervert.htm.

7. Brame, "How a Nice Jewish Girl Like Me."

8. Richard Kadrey, "alt.sex.bondage," *Wired*, June 1994, accessed September 26, 2014, http://archive.wired.com/wired/archive/2.06/alt.sex.bondage_pr.html.

9. Kadrey, "alt.sex.bondage."

10. Paulina Borsook, *Cyberselfish: A Critical Romp through the Terribly Libertarian Culture of High Tech* (New York: PublicAffairs, 2001), 104.

11. Rambukkana, "Taking the Leather Out of Leathersex," 73.

12. Rambukkana, "Taking the Leather Out of Leathersex," 76.

13. Gloria G. Brame, William D. Brame, and Jon Jacobs, *Different Loving: An Exploration of the World of Sexual Dominance and Submission* (New York: Villard Books, 1993), 34.

14. Stein, "S/M's Copernican Revolution," in *Leatherfolk: Radical Sex, People, Politics, and Practice*, ed. Mark Thompson (Boston: Alyson Publications, 1991), 144.

15. Keith F. Durkin, "The Internet as a Milieu for the Management of a Stigmatized Sexual Identity," in *Net.seXXX: Readings on Sex, Pornography, and the Internet*, ed. Dennis D. Waskul (New York: Peter Lang, 2004), 131.

16. Durkin, "The Internet as a Milieu," 134–43.
17. Polly Peachum, "Defining The BDSM Life Style: The Essential Prerequisite," accessed September 23, 2014, http://gos.sbc.edu/p/peachum.html.
18. Boellstorff, *Coming of Age in Second Life*, 160–65.
19. Cleo Odzer, *Virtual Spaces: Sex and the Cyber Citizen* (New York: Berkley Books, 1997), 200–203.
20. Odzer, *Virtual Spaces*, 64–68, 222–24.
21. Odzer, *Virtual Spaces*, 185–92.
22. S. Bardzell and J. Bardzell, "Docile Avatars: Aesthetics, Experience, and Sexual Interaction in Second Life," *People and Computers* 1, no. 21 (2007): 6, 8.
23. Shannon McRae, "Flesh Made Word: Sex, Text, and the Virtual Body," in *Internet Culture*, ed. David Porter (New York: Routledge, 1997), 77–78.
24. Julian Dibbell, "A Rape in Cyberspace; or, How an Evil Clown, A Haitian Trickster Spirit, Two Wizards, and a Cast of Dozens Turned a Database into a Society," *Flame Wars: The Discourse of Cyberculture*, ed. Mark Dery (Durham, NC: Duke University Press, 1994), 237–61; see also Odzer, *Virtual Spaces*, 198–200.
25. Boellstorff, *Coming of Age in Second Life*, 162–64.
26. Artemis Fate, "The Problems of Gor—Part 1," *Alphaville Herald*, November 27, 2006, accessed November 14, 2014, http://alphavilleherald.com/2006/11/the_problems_of.html.
27. Tjarda Sixma, "The Gorean Community in Second Life: Rules of Sexual Inspired Role-Play," *Journal of Virtual Worlds Research* 1, no. 3 (2008): 10–11.
28. Jeremy Wilson, "Behind Gor, a 'Slave Master' Subculture of Sexual Deviance," *Daily Dot*, March 31, 2014, accessed November 27, 2014, http://www.dailydot.com/lifestyle/gor-gorean-slaves-history/.
29. Borsook, *Cyberselfish*, 100–101.
30. Katherine Mieszkowski, "Geek Love," *San Francisco Bay Guardian*, August 20, 1997.
31. Shadow, "History of Munches," *House of de Sade*, October 22, 2012, accessed January 15, 2015, https://web.archive.org/web/20101203010254;http://www.houseofdesade.com/munchhistory/history.
32. Margot Danielle Weiss, *Techniques of Pleasure: BDSM and the Circuits of Sexuality* (Durham, NC: Duke University Press, 2011), 34–35, 51.
33. Andrea Zanin, "Facebook for the Kinky: Montreal-Based FetLife.com Networks Fetishists of the World," *Montreal Mirror*, September 4–10, 2008, accessed November 14, 2014, http://web.archive.org/web/20120630172329;http://www.montrealmirror.com/2008/090408/news1.html.
34. John Baku, "FetLife.com Launches—The First Social Network for Kinksters," Sexual Deviants Living in a Web 2.0 World, January 10, 2008, accessed

November 14, 2014, http://web.archive.org/web/20120228192556;http://sexualdeviants20.com/2008/01/10/fetlifecom-launches-the-first-social-network-for-kinksters/.

CHAPTER TWELVE

1. Gayle Rubin, "Thinking Sex: Notes for a Radical Theory of the Politics of Sexuality," in *Culture, Society and Sexuality: A Reader*, ed. Richard G. Parker and Peter Aggleton (London: UCL Press, 1999), 163.

2. See Lynda Hart, *Between the Body and the Flesh: Performing Sadomasochism* (New York: Columbia University Press, 1998), 38.

3. Michel Foucault, *The History of Sexuality, Volume 1: An Introduction*, trans. Robert Hurley (New York: Pantheon Books, 1978), 103.

4. Richard B. Krueger, "The DSM Diagnostic Criteria for Sexual Masochism," *Archives of Sexual Behavior* 39 (2010): 354.

5. Richard B. Krueger, "The DSM Diagnostic Criteria for Sexual Sadism," *Archives of Sexual Behavior* 39 (2009): 341.

6. Krueger, "Sexual Sadism," 341–42; Krueger, "Sexual Masochism," 354.

7. Krueger, "Sexual Sadism," 342.

8. Krueger, "Sexual Masochism," 354.

9. Krueger, "Sexual Sadism," 342.

10. Krueger, "Sexual Masochism," 354.

11. Krueger, "Masochism," 18.

12. Race Bannon, "Kink Aware Professionals," accessed December 17, 2014, http://bannon.com/kap. KAP was handed over to the National Coalition for Sexual Freedom in 2006.

13. Krueger, "Masochism," 18; Krueger, "Sadomasochism," 8–9.

14. American Psychiatric Association, *Diagnostic and Statistical Manual of Mental Disorders: DSM-5* (Washington, DC: American Psychiatric Association, 2014), 686.

15. American Psychiatric Association, *Diagnostic and Statistical Manual of Mental Disorders*, 694.

16. American Psychiatric Association, *Diagnostic and Statistical Manual of Mental Disorders*, 701.

17. American Psychiatric Association, *Diagnostic and Statistical Manual of Mental Disorders*, 703.

18. National Coalition for Sexual Freedom, "NCSF History," accessed December 18, 2014, https://ncsfreedom.org/who-we-are/about-ncsf.html.

19. Susan Wright, "Susan Wright," accessed December 17, 2014, http://www.susanwright.info/author.html.

20. Tiamatsvision, "Interview with Author Susan Wright," Technoccult, November 24, 2008, accessed December 17, 2014, http://technoccult.net/archives/2008/11/24/interview-with-author-susan-wright; Sensuous Sadie, "SCENEprofiles Interview with Susan Wright, Founder of the National Coalition for Sexual Freedom (NCSF)," SCENEprofiles, accessed December 17, 2014, http://67.159.222.79/interviews/susanwrightinterview.

21. Diane Mehta, "The Rumpus Interview with Susan Wright," *The Rumpus*, May 22, 2013, accessed December 18, 2014, http://therumpus.net/2013/05/the-rumpus-interview-with-susan-wright/.

22. Brian Flaherty, "DSM Revisions: The Impact on BDSM," *Fearless Press*, July 26, 2013, accessed December 18, 2014, http://www.fearlesspress.com/2013/07/26/dsm-revisions-the-impact-on-bdsm/.

23. Melissa Meinzer, "More on Sex Blogger Kendra Holliday's Custody Challenge," *Riverfront Times*, December 21, 2010, accessed December 18, 2014, http://blogs.riverfronttimes.com/dailyrft/2010/12/the_beautiful_kind_custody_challenge_sex_blogger.php; see also "Interview with Kendra Holliday from the Sex Positive Movement," *Lovesick Love*, accessed December 18, 2014, http://www.lovesicklove.com/2012/03/interview-with-kendra-holliday-from-the-sex-positive-movement.html.

24. Robert Ridinger, "Negotiating Limits: The Legal Status of SM in the United States," in *Sadomasochism: Powerful Pleasures*, ed. Peggy J. Kleinplatz and Charles Moser (Binghamton, NY: Harrington Park Press, 2006), 204–5.

25. Marty Klein and Charles Moser, "SM (Sadomasochistic) Interests as an Issue in a Child Custody Proceeding," in Kleinplatz and Moser, *Sadomasochism: Powerful Pleasures*, 233–42.

26. People v. Samuels, 250 Cal. App. 2D 501, 513, 58 Cal. Rptr. 439, 447 (1967), accessed December 8, 2014, http://scholar.google.ca/scholar_case?case=16311354488091574089&hl=en&as_sdt=2006&as_vis=1.

27. Kenneth Anger (dir.), *Fireworks*, 1947; Kenneth Anger (dir.), Ernest D. Glucksman (wri.), *Scorpio Rising* (Puck Film Productions, 1963). Anger was charged with obscenity for both films, and ultimately exonerated by the California Supreme Court.

28. State v. Battista, Case Nos. CA 4815 & CA 4816, Court of Appeals of Ohio, Fifth Appellate District, Stark County, Ohio, Slip Opinion (8 November 1978), accessed December 10, 2014, http://www.csun.edu/~hfspc002/PoliceFreeGaySlaves.html.

29. Emma Wilkins, "Jury Throws Out Student Rape Case," *Times* (London), December 1, 1994, 3, accessed December 10, 2014, http://www.holysmoke.org/sdhok/rape020.htm.

30. Ben Attias, "'Police Free Gay Slaves': Some Juridico-Legal Consequences of the Discursive Distinctions between the Sexualities" (master's thesis, California State University, Northridge), accessed December 21, 2014, http://www.csun.edu/~hfspc002/PoliceFreeGaySlaves.html.

31. Ridinger, "Negotiating Limits," 198–99.

32. Anil Aggrawal, *Forensic and Medico-Legal Aspects of Sexual Crimes and Unusual Sexual Practices* (Boca Raton, FL: CRC Press, 2009), 157–59.

33. Chris White, "The Spanner Trials and the Changing Law on Sadomasochism in the UK," in Kleinplatz and Moser, *Sadomasochism: Powerful Pleasures*, 171.

34. R v. Brown and Others (1992) 94 Cr. App. R 302 CA.

35. Philip Jenkins, *Intimate Enemies: Moral Panics in Contemporary Great Britain* (New York: Aldine de Gruyter, 1992), 85–86.

36. The Spanner Trust, "The History of the Spanner Case," accessed December 23, 2014, http://www.spannertrust.org/documents/spannerhistory.asp.

37. White, "The Spanner Trials," 176–77.

38. European Commission on Human Rights, 1997, paragraphs 45, 47, 50, and 51. Quoted in White, "The Spanner Trials," 179.

39. Times Law Report, 1996, 2 Cr app R 241, quoted in White, "The Spanner Trials," 181.

40. Ellsworth A. Fersch, *Thinking about the Sexually Dangerous: Answers to Frequently Asked Questions, with Case Examples* (New York: iUniverse, 2006), 73–78.

41. Michelle Chihara, "Paddleboro," *Nerve*, September 27, 2000, accessed December 28, 2014, http://www.nerve.com/dispatches/chihara/paddleboro.

42. Michelle Chihara, "Spank You Very Much," *Boston Phoenix*, September 28–October 5, 2000, accessed December 28, 2014, http://www.bostonphoenix.com/archive/features/00/09/28/S_M.html.

43. Ridinger, "Negotiating Limits," 200–201. See also Cheryl Hanna, "Sex Is Not a Sport: Consent and Violence in Criminal Law," *Boston College Law Review* 42, no. 2 (2001): 268, 272, accessed August 20, 2015, http://lawdigitalcommons.bc.edu/bclr/vol42/iss2/1/.

44. Law Reform Commission, 1995, section 10.39, quoted in White, "The Spanner Trials," 185.

45. Margaret Quigley, "The Mapplethorpe Censorship Controversy," Political Research Associates, accessed December 29, 2014, http://www.politicalresearch.org/1991/05/01/the-mapplethorpe-censorship-controversy/.

46. Wayne Overbeck and Genelle Irene Belmas, *Major Principles of Media Law* (Boston: Wadsworth Cengage Learning, 2012), 429.

47. Quoted in Judd Handler, "Can David Beat Goliath in the Battle of Obscenity? Part 2" *Ynot News*, January 2, 2002, accessed December 29, 2014, https://ncsfreedom.org/resources/communications-decency-act/item/419-ynot-news-january-2-2002.html.

48. Julia Scheeres, "New Suit Targets Obscenity Law," *Wired*, December 2001, accessed December 29, 2014, http://archive.wired.com/culture/lifestyle/news/2001/12/49044.

49. Darren Roberts, *The Unsexpected Story: The Real Story about the Billion-Dollar Adult Entertainment Industry* (West Hills, CA: Clearly Confused, 2012), 164.

50. Glenn A. Fine, *Investigation into the Removal of Nine U.S. Attorneys in 2006*. (Washington DC: US Department of Justice, 2009), 204–8, 237, 241.

51. "United States v. Fletcher," Digital Media Law Project, 2008, accessed December 11, 2014, http://www.dmlp.org/threats/united-states-v-fletcher.

52. Clay Calvert and Robert D. Richards, "A War over Words: An Inside Analysis and Examination of the Prosecution of the Red Rose Stories and Obscenity Law," *Journal of Law and Policy* 16, no. 1 (2008): 198–99.

53. National Coalition for Sexual Freedom, "2002 Incident Response Report," accessed December 22, 2014, https://ncsfreedom.org/component/k2/item/369-2002-incident-response-report.html.

54. National Coalition for Sexual Freedom, "2003 Incident Response Report," accessed December 22, 2014, https://ncsfreedom.org/component/k2/item/480-2003-incident-response-report.html.

55. "Cancel Sexual Torture Convention, CWA Urges Adam's Mark Chicago-Northbrook Hotel," Concerned Women for America of Illinois, February 6, 2003, accessed December 22, 2014, http://www.cwfa.org/images/content/Cancel%20Sexual%20Torture%20Convention.pdf.

56. Evelyn Schlatter, "18 Anti-Gay Groups and their Propaganda," Southern Poverty Law Center, accessed December 12, 2014, http://www.splcenter.org/get-informed/intelligence-report/browse-all-issues/2010/winter/the-hard-liners.

57. Peter LaBarbera, "VIDEO: LaBarbera Notes Fake Masculinity of Homosexuality—PFAW's Right Wing Watch Reacts," Americans for Truth about Homosexuality, June 25, 2014, accessed December 12, 2014, http://americansfortruth.com/2014/06/25/labarbera-notes-fake-masculinity-of-homosexuality-pfaw-right-wing-watch-reacts/.

58. Peter LaBarbera, "From 'Gay Pride' to 'Poly Pride'—Tristan Taormino," Americans for Truth about Homosexuality, February 6, 2009, accessed December 12, 2014, http://americansfortruth.com/2009/02/06/from-gay-pride-to-poly-pride-tristan-taormino/.

59. Peter LaBarbera, "Thank You for Helping to Restrict the Perversions and Health Hazards at 'Winter Wickedness,'" Americans for Truth about Homosexuality, February 10, 2009, accessed December 12, 2014, http://americansfortruth.com/2009/02/10/thank-you-for-helping-to-restrict-the-perversions-at-winter-wickedness/.

60. LaBarbera, "From 'Gay Pride' to 'Poly Pride.'"

61. Peter LaBarbera, "Democrat Party Helps Gay Task Force Honor Sadomasochistic Slavery Advocate Guy Baldwin," Americans for Truth about Homosexuality, February 8, 2008, accessed December 12, 2014, http://americansfortruth.com/2008/02/08/democrat-party-sponsors-event-honoring-sadomasochistic-slavery-advocate/.

62. Peter LaBarbera, "BREAKING: Obama Champions Gay Task Force's 'Creating Change' Conference—Which Promotes 'Kinky Sex' (Sadomasochism) and Multi-Partner Unions; Event Funded by Southwest Airlines, Office Depot, AARP and Wells Fargo," Americans for Truth about Homosexuality, January 25, 2013, accessed December 12, 2014, http://americansfortruth.com/2013/01/25/breaking-obama-champions-gay-task-force-creating-change-conference-which-promotes-sadomasochism-multi-partner-unions/.

63. Peter LaBarbera, "New York City Plays Host to Folsom-East Deviant Sex-Fest—Violating Lewdness Laws," Americans for Truth about Homosexuality, June 24, 2009, accessed December 12, 2014, http://americansfortruth.com/2009/06/24/breakingnew-york-city-plays-host-to-folsom-east-deviant-sex-fest-violating-city-lewdness-laws/.

64. Peter LaBarbera, "WATCH: Planned Parenthood Video Promotes Sexual Sadism & Masochism—BDSM—to Youth," Americans for Truth about Homosexuality, July 31, 2009, accessed December 12, 2014, http://americansfortruth.com/2014/07/31/planned-parenthood-video-promotes-sexual-sadism-bdsm-to-youth/.

65. Peter LaBarbera, "Breaking News: Doubletree Hotel in D.C. Plays Host to Homosexual 'Pig Sex' Orgy during Inaugural Weekend," Americans for Truth about Homosexuality, January 14, 2009, accessed December 12, 2014, http://americansfortruth.com/2009/01/14/breaking-newsdoubletree-hotel-in-dc-plays-host-to-homosexual-pig-sex-orgy/.

66. Peter LaBarbera, "Folsom Street Fair 2012 Poster Epitomizes San Francisco Homosexual Deviance and Folly of Liberal 'Tolerance,'" Americans for Truth about Homosexuality, August 13, 2012, accessed December 12, 2014, http://americansfortruth.com/2012/08/13/folsom-street-fair-2012-poster-epitomizes-san-francisco-homosexual-deviance/.

67. Alex Henderson, "Fighting the Culture War with Hate, Violence and Even Bullets: Meet the Most Extreme of the Radical Christians," Alternet.org, June 27,

2011, accessed September 15, 2014, http://www.alternet.org/story/151436/fighting_the_culture_wars_with_hate,_violence_and_even_bullets:_meet_the_most_extreme_of_the_radical_christians.

68. Forrest Wilder, "He Who Casts the First Stone," *Texas Observer*, February 24, 2010, accessed September 15, 2014, http://www.texasobserver.org/he-who-casts-the-first-stone/.

69. "Facts," PlannedParenthoodExposed.com, accessed December 14, 2014, http://plannedparenthoodexposed.com/facts/.

70. "Planned Parenthood Exposed Peddling BDSM to Teens in Oregon," July 22, 2014, PlannedParenthoodExposed.com, accessed December 14, 2014, http://plannedparenthoodexposed.com/2014/07/22/planned-parenthood-exposed-peddling-bdsm-to-teens-in-oregon/.

71. Unless otherwise stated, quotes from McGeorge come from telephone interviews conducted on June 8–10, 2008.

72. Kerry Lauerman, "A Taste of the Whip for Saddam," *Salon*, December 3, 2002, accessed January 3, 2015, http://www.salon.com/2002/12/04/un_sm/.

73. David Rennie, "UN Weapons Inspector Is Leader of S&M Sex Ring," *Telegraph*, November 30, 2002.

74. McGeorge died during cardiac surgery on August 18, 2009.

CONCLUSION

1. The binding of Isaac, Genesis 22, KJV.

2. David Macey, *The Lives of Michel Foucault* (London: Hutchinson, 1993), 368–69.

3. David Stein, "How to Do the Right Kinky Thing—Ethical Principles for BDSM," *Leatherati*, September 2013 (bold and italics in original), accessed February 20, 2015, http://www.leatherati.com/2013/09/how-to-do-the-right-kinky-thing/.

4. Michael Hiley and Arthur Joseph Munby, *Victorian Working Women: Portraits from Life* (Boston: D. R. Godine, 1980), 32 (italics in original).

5. Donna Minkowitz, *Ferocious Romance: What My Encounters with the Right Taught Me about Sex, God, and Fury* (New York: Free Press, 1998), 3.

6. Minkowitz, *Ferocious Romance*, 129–30.

7. Minkowitz, *Ferocious Romance*, 127–28.

8. The *Fifty Shades* trilogy was a rewrite of "Master of the Universe," a fan-fiction series based on Stephanie Meyers's *Twilight* series of vampire romance novels, published 2005–2008.

9. Margot D. Weiss, "Mainstreaming Kink: The Politics of BDSM Representation in U.S. Popular Media," *Journal of Homosexuality* 50, nos. 2–3 (2006): 103 (emphasis in original).

10. Weiss, "Mainstreaming Kink," 105.

11. Weiss, "Mainstreaming Kink," 111 (emphasis in original).

12. Weiss, "Mainstreaming Kink," 114.

13. Weiss, "Mainstreaming Kink," 116.

14. Lindsay Anne Hallam, *Screening the Marquis de Sade: Pleasure, Pain and the Transgressive Body in Film* (Jefferson, NC: McFarland, 2012), 170.

15. Weiss, "Mainstreaming Kink," 119.

16. Weiss, "Mainstreaming Kink," 126.

Bibliography

Aggrawal, Anil. 2009. *Forensic and Medico-Legal Aspects of Sexual Crimes and Unusual Sexual Practices.* Boca Raton, FL: CRC Press.

Allison, Dorothy. 2013. *Skin: Talking about Sex, Class and Literature.* New York: Open Road Integrated Media. http://public.eblib.com/choice/publicfullrecord.aspx?p=1807449.

Ålvik, Jon Mikkel Broch. 2008. "Modalities of Desire : Representations of Sadomasochism in Popular Music." Master's thesis, University of Oslo http://urn.nb.no/URN:NBN:no-20057.

American Psychiatric Association 2013. *Diagnostic and Statistical Manual of Mental Disorders: DSM-5.* Washington, DC: American Psychiatric Association Publishing.

Anger, Kenneth (dir.). 1947. *Fireworks.*

Anger, Kenneth (dir.), Ernest D. Glucksman (wri.). 1963. *Scorpio Rising.* Puck Film Productions.

Apter, Emily S. 1991. *Feminizing the Fetish: Psychoanalysis and Narrative Obsession in Turn-of-the-Century France.* Ithaca, NY: Cornell University Press.

Aravamudan, Srinivas. 1999. *Tropicopolitans: Colonialism and Agency, 1688–1804.* Durham, NC: Duke University Press.

Atkinson, Diane. 2003. *Love and Dirt: The Marriage of Arthur Munby and Hannah Cullwick.* London: Macmillan.

Bardzell, S., and J. Bardzell. 2007. "Docile Avatars: Aesthetics, Experience, and Sexual Interaction in Second Life." *People and Computers* 1 (21): 3–12.

Barker-Benfield, G. J. 1996. *The Culture of Sensibility: Sex and Society in Eighteenth-Century Britain.* Chicago: University of Chicago Press.

Barkun, Michael. 2013. *Culture of Conspiracy: Apocalyptic Visions in Contemporary America.* Berkeley: University of California Press.

Barraclough, Geoffrey. 1981. *The Christian World: A Social and Cultural History.* New York: Harry N. Abrams.

Basu, Biman. 2012. *The Commerce of Peoples: Sadomasochism and African American Literature*. Lanham, MD: Lexington Books.

Beetham, Margaret, and Kay Boardman. 2001. *Victorian Woman's Magazines: An Anthology*. Manchester: Manchester University Press.

Bernheimer, Charles. 1989. *Figures of Ill Repute: Representing Prostitution in Nineteenth-Century France*. Cambridge, MA: Harvard University Press.

Bersani, Leo. 1996. *Homos*. Cambridge, MA: Harvard University Press.

Bienvenu, Robert V. 1998. "The Development of Sadomasochism as a Cultural Style in the Twentieth-Century United States." PhD diss. Indiana University.

Boellstorff, Tom. 2008. *Coming of Age in Second Life: An Anthropologist Explores the Virtually Human*. Princeton, NJ: Princeton University Press.

Borsook, Paulina. 2001. *Cyberselfish: A Critical Romp through the Terribly Libertarian Culture of High Tech*. New York: PublicAffairs.

Brame, Gloria G., William D. Brame, and Jon Jacobs. 1993. *Different Loving: An Exploration of the World of Sexual Dominance and Submission*. New York: Villard Books.

Brass, Tinto (dir.), Antonio Colantuoni et al. (wri.). 1976. *Salon Kitty*. Coralta Cinematografica, Cinema Seven Film, Les Productions Fox Europa.

Breitwieser, Mitchell Robert. 1990. *American Puritanism and the Defense of Mourning: Religion, Grief, and Ethnology in Mary White Rowlandson's Captivity Narrative*. Madison: University of Wisconsin Press.

Brill, Dunja. 2008. *Goth Culture: Gender, Sexuality and Style*. Oxford: Berg.

Brissenden, R. F. 1974. *Virtue in Distress: Studies in the Novel of Sentiment from Richardson to Sade*. New York: Barnes and Noble.

Brown, Carolyn E. 1986. "Erotic Religious Flagellation and Shakespeare's Measure for Measure." *English Literary Renaissance* 16 (1): 139–65.

Brownmiller, Susan. 1975. *Against Our Will: Men, Women and Rape*. New York: Simon & Schuster.

Bullough, Vern, Dwight Dixon, and Joan Dixon. 1994. "Sadism, Masochism, and History, or When Is Behaviour Sado-Masochistic?" In *Sexual Knowledge, Sexual Science: The History of Attitudes to Sexuality*, edited by Roy Porter and Mikuláš Teich. Cambridge: Cambridge University Press.

Buttsworth, Sara, and Maartje Abbenhuis. 2010. *Monsters in the Mirror: Representations of Nazism in Post-War Popular Culture*. Santa Barbara, CA: Praeger Publishers.

Byrne, Romana. 2013. *Aesthetic Sexuality: A Literary History of Sadomasochism*. New York: Bloomsbury.

Califia, Pat. 1994. *Public Sex: The Culture of Radical Sex*. Pittsburgh, PA: Cleiss Press.

Callois, Roger. 1961. *Man, Play and Games*, translated by Meyer Barash. Chicago: University of Chicago Press.

Cavani, Liliana (dir.), Liliana Cavani et al. (wri.). 1974. *The Night Porter.* Lotar Film Productions.

Clarke, John R., and Michael Larvey. 2003. *Roman Sex: 100 B.C. to 250 A.D.* New York: Harry N. Abrams.

Cleugh, James. 1967. *The First Masochist; A Biography of Leopold von Sacher-Masoch.* New York: Stein and Day.

Clissold, Stephen. 1977. *The Barbary Slaves.* Totowa, NJ: Rowman & Littlefield.

Cohn, Norman Rufus Colin. 1993. *The Pursuit of the Millennium: Revolutionary Millenarians and Mystical Anarchists of the Middle Ages.* London: Pimlico.

Cole, Shaun. 2000. *Don We Now Our Gay Apparel: Gay Men's Dress in the Twentieth Century.* Oxford: Berg.

Corbin, Alain. 1990. *Women for Hire: Prostitution and Sexuality in France after 1850.* Cambridge, MA: Harvard University Press.

Cromwell, John (dir.), Erich Maria Remarque, and Talbot Jennings (wri.). 1941. *So Ends Our Night.* David L. Loew-Albert Lewin.

Cruickshank, Dan. 2010. *London's Sinful Secret: The Bawdy History and Very Public Passions of London's Georgian Age.* New York: St. Martin's Press.

Cullwick, Hannah, and Liz Stanley. 1984. *The Diaries of Hannah Cullwick, Victorian Maidservant.* New Brunswick, NJ: Rutgers University Press.

Daley, Brittany A., and Stephen J. Gertz. 2005. *Sin-a-Rama: Sleaze Sex Paperbacks of the Sixties.* Los Angeles: Feral House.

Damian, Peter. 2005. *Peter Damian: Letters 151–180.* Washington, DC: Catholic University of America Press.

Darnton, Robert. 1995. *The Forbidden Best-Sellers of Pre-Revolutionary France.* New York: W.W. Norton.

Davenport-Hines, R. P. T. 1999. *Gothic: Four Hundred Years of Excess, Horror, Evil, and Ruin.* New York: North Point Press.

Davis, Robert C. 2004. *Christian Slaves, Muslim Masters: White Slavery in the Mediterranean, the Barbary Coast, and Italy, 1500–1800.* London: Palgrave Macmillan.

Deforges, Régine, and Pauline Réage. 1979. *Confessions of O: Conversations with Pauline Réage.* New York: Viking Press.

Deleuze, Gilles, and Leopold Sacher-Masoch. 1991. *Masochism: Coldness and Cruelty.* New York: Zone Books.

DelPlato, Joan. 2002. *Multiple Wives, Multiple Pleasures: Representing the Harem, 1800–1875.* Madison, NJ: Fairleigh Dickinson University Press.

Dennis, Donna. 2009. *Licentious Gotham: Erotic Publishing and Its Prosecution in Nineteenth-Century New York.* Cambridge, MA: Harvard University Press.

Dery, Mark. 1994. *Flame Wars: The Discourse of Cyberculture.* Durham, NC: Duke University Press.

Dmytryk, Edward (dir.), Emmet Lavery, and Gregor Ziemer (wri.). 1943. *Hitler's Children*. RKO Radio Pictures.

Doherty, Thomas Patrick. 1999. *Pre-code Hollywood: Sex, Immorality, and Insurrection in American Cinema, 1930–1934*. New York: Columbia University Press.

Dolan, Frances E. 2007. "Why Are Nuns Funny?" *Huntington Library Quarterly* 70 (4): 509–35.

Easton, Martha. 2002. "Pain, Torture and Death in the Huntington Library *Legenda aurea*." In *Gender and Holiness: Men, Women and Saints in Late Medieval Europe*, edited by Samantha J. E. Riches and Sarah Salih, 49–64. London: Routledge.

Edmonds, Don (dir.), Jonah Royston, and Glen Rowland. 1975. *Ilsa: She Wolf of the SS*. Aeteas Filmproduktions.

Edmonds, Don (dir.), Langston Stafford (wri.). 1976. *Ilsa, Harem Keeper of the Oil Sheiks*. Mount Everest Enterprises Ltd.

Ehrenreich, Barbara, Elizabeth Hess, and Gloria Jacobs. 1986. *Re-making Love: The Feminization of Sex*. Garden City, NY: Anchor Press/Doubleday.

Ekins, Richard, and Dave King. 2002. *Blending Genders: Social Aspects of Cross-Dressing and Sex-Changing*. London: Routledge.

Evans, Stewart P., and Keith Skinner. 2001. *Jack the Ripper: Letters from Hell*. Stroud, UK: Sutton.

Farren, Mick. 1985. *The Black Leather Jacket*. New York: Abbeville Press.

Fersch, Ellsworth A. 2006. *Thinking about the Sexually Dangerous: Answers to Frequently Asked Questions, with Case Examples*. New York: iUniverse, Inc.

Fessenden, Tracy. 2000. "The Convent, the Brothel, and the Protestant Woman's Sphere." *Signs* 25 (2): 451–78.

Finaldi, Gabriele, and Susanna Avery-Quash. 2000. *The Image of Christ*. London: National Gallery.

Fine, Glenn A. 2009. *Investigation into the Removal of Nine U.S. Attorneys in 2006*. Washington, DC: US Department of Justice.

Fisher, Trevor. 1997. *Prostitution and the Victorians*. New York: St. Martin's Press.

Foley, James (dir.), Niall Leonard, and E. L. James (wri.). 2017. *Fifty Shades Darker*. Universal Pictures, Perfect World Pictures (Beijing).

Foucault, Michel. 2001. *Madness and Civilization: A History of Insanity in the Age of Reason*. London: Routledge.

Foucault, Michel. 1978. *The History of Sexuality*. New York: Pantheon Books.

Franco, Jess (dir., wri.), Erwin C. Dietrich (wri). 1977. *Wanda, the Wicked Warden* (aka *Ilsa, the Wicked Warden*). Cinépix, Elite Film.

Freud, Sigmund, James Strachey, Anna Freud, Alix Strachey, and Alan Tyson. 2001. *The Standard Edition of the Complete Psychological Works of Sigmund Freud (1917–1919), Vol. 17*. London: Vintage.

Friedländer, Saul. 1993. *Reflections of Nazism: An Essay on Kitsch and Death*. Bloomington: Indiana University Press.

Frost, Laura Catherine. 2002. *Sex Drives: Fantasies of Fascism in Literary Modernism*. Ithaca, NY: Cornell University Press.

Fuller, Jean Overton. 1971. *Swinburne*. New York: Schocken Books.

Fulton, Rachel. 2002. *From Judgment to Passion: Devotion to Christ and the Virgin Mary, 800–1200*. New York: Columbia University Press.

Gay, Peter. 1984. *Education of the Senses: The Bourgeois Experience*. Vol. 1. New York: Oxford University Press.

Gibson, Ian. 1978. *The English Vice: Beating, Sex, and Shame in Victorian England and After*. London: Duckworth.

Gibson, Ian. 2002. *The Erotomaniac: The Secret Life of Henry Spencer Ashbee*. London: Faber.

Glucklich, Ariel. 2001. *Sacred Pain: Hurting the Body for the Sake of the Soul*. Oxford: Oxford University Press.

Gordon, Mel. 2006. *Voluptuous Panic: The Erotic World of Weimar Berlin*. Port Townsend, WA. Feral House.

Gossett, Thomas F. 1985. *Uncle Tom's Cabin and American Culture*. Dallas, TX: Southern Methodist University Press.

Goswin. 2006. *Send Me God: The Lives of Ida the Compassionate of Nivelles, Nun of La Ramée, Arnulf, Lay Brother of Villers, and Abundus, Monk of Villers*. University Park: Pennsylvania State University Press.

Gray, Francine du Plessix. 1998. *At Home with the Marquis de Sade: A Life*. New York: Simon & Schuster.

Hallam, Lindsay Anne. 2012. *Screening the Marquis de Sade: Pleasure, Pain and the Transgressive Body in Film*. Jefferson, NC: McFarland.

Hancock, Joseph, Toni Johnson-Woods, and Vicki Karaminas. 2013. *Fashion in Popular Culture: Literature, Media and Contemporary Studies*. Bristol, UK: Intellect.

Hanly, Margaret Ann Fitzpatrick, ed. 1995. *Essential Papers on Masochism*. New York: NYU Press.

Hanson, Dian. 2006. *The History of Girly Magazines: 1900–1969*. Hong Kong: Taschen.

Hart, Lynda. 1998. *Between the Body and the Flesh: Performing Sadomasochism*. New York: Columbia University Press.

Harvey, J. R. 1996. *Men in Black*. Chicago: University of Chicago Press.

Heller, Tamar. 1997. "Flagellating Feminine Desire: Lesbians, Old Maids, and New Women in 'Miss Coote's Confession,' a Victorian Pornographic Narrative." *Victorian Newsletter* 92: 9–15.

Hickman, Katie. 2003. *Courtesans: Money, Sex, and Fame in the Nineteenth Century*. New York: Morrow.

Hiley, Michael, and Arthur Joseph Munby. 1980. *Victorian Working Women: Portraits from Life*. Boston: D. R. Godine.

Hodes, Martha Elizabeth. 1997. *White Women, Black Men: Illicit Sex in the Nineteenth-Century South*. New Haven, CT: Yale University Press.

Hofstadter, Richard. 2008. *The Paranoid Style in American Politics* (1952; reprinted) New York: Vintage.

Horn, Pamela. 2004. *The Rise and Fall of the Victorian Servant*. Stroud, UK: Sutton.

Horton, James Oliver, and Lois E. Horton. 2005. *Slavery and the Making of America*. Oxford: Oxford University Press.

Hudson, Derek, and Arthur Joseph Munby. 1972. *Munby, Man of Two Worlds: The Life and Diaries of Arthur J. Munby, 1828–1910*. London: J. Murray.

Hughes, Kathryn. 1993. *The Victorian Governess*. London: Hambledon Press.

Hughes, Kathryn. 2005. *The Short Life and Long Times of Mrs. Beeton*. London: Fourth Estate.

Hughes, Robert. 1997. *American Visions: The Epic History of Art in America*. New York: Alfred A. Knopf.

Jacopetti, Gualtiero, and Franco Prosperi (dir., wri.). 1971. *Goodbye Uncle Tom*. Euro International Film (EIA).

Jeffreys, Sheila. 1994. *The Lesbian Heresy: A Feminist Perspective on the Lesbian Sexual Revolution*. London: Women's Press.

Jenkins, Philip. 1992. *Intimate Enemies: Moral Panics in Contemporary Great Britain*. New York: Aldine de Gruyter.

Johnson, Walter. 1999. *Soul by Soul: Life Inside the Antebellum Slave Market*. Cambridge, MA: Harvard University Press.

Jones, Robert Kenneth. 1975. *The Shudder Pulps: A History of the Weird Menace Magazines of the 1930's*. New York: New American Library.

Jullian, Philippe. 1977. *The Orientalists: European Painters of Eastern Scenes*. Oxford: Phaidon.

Kabbani, Rana. 2008. *Imperial Fictions: Europe's Myths of the Orient*. London: Saqi.

Kadrey, Richard. 1994. "alt.sex.bondage." *Wired*, June.

Kendrick, Walter M. 1987. *The Secret Museum: Pornography in Modern Culture*. New York: Viking.

Khan, Ummni. 2008. "Sadomasochism Once Removed: S/m in the Socio-Legal Imaginary." SJD diss., University of Toronto.
Kilpatrick, Nancy. 2004. *The Goth Bible: A Compendium for the Darkly Inclined.* New York: St. Martin's Griffin.
Kleinplatz, Peggy J., and Charles Moser. 2006. *Sadomasochism: Powerful Pleasures.* Binghamton, NY: Harrington Park Press.
Krafft-Ebing, R. von, and Domino Falls. 1997. *Psychopathia Sexualis.* London: Velvet Publications.
Krueger, Richard B. 2010. "The DSM Diagnostic Criteria for Sexual Masochism." *Archives of Sexual Behaviour* 39 (2): 346–56.
Krueger, Richard B. 2009. "The DSM Diagnostic Criteria for Sexual Sadism." *Archives of Sexual Behavior* 39 (2): 325–45.
Kunzle, David. 1973. *History of the Comic Strip / Narrative Strips and Picture Stories in the European Broadsheet from c. 1450 to 1825. Vol. 1.* Berkeley: University of California Press.
Kunzle, David. 2004. *Fashion and Fetishism: Corsets, Tight-Lacing and Other Forms of Body-Sculpture.* Stroud, UK: Sutton.
LaFleur, Jean (dir.), Marven McGara (wri.). 1977. *Ilsa, the Tigress of Siberia.* Mount Everest Enterprises Ltd.
Largier, Niklaus. 2007. *In Praise of the Whip: A Cultural History of Arousal.* New York: Zone Books.
Larkin, Oliver W. 1960. *Art and Life in America.* New York: Holt, Rinehart and Winston.
Leigh, Michael, and Louis Berg. 1963. *The Velvet Underground.* New York: Macfadden.
Leonard, Amy E., Karen L. Nelson, Sarah R. Cohen, Alexandra Shepard, and Margaret Ferguson. 2011. *Masculinities, Childhood, Violence: Attending to Early Modern Women—and Men.* Newark: University of Delaware Press.
Levine, Martin P., Peter M. Nardi, and John H. Gagnon. 1997. *In Changing Times: Gay Men and Lesbians Encounter HIV/AIDS.* Chicago: University of Chicago Press.
Linden, Robin Ruth, ed. 1982. *Against Sadomasochism: A Radical Feminist Analysis.* East Palo Alto, CA: Frog in the Well.
Linnane, Fergus. 2003. *London: The Wicked City; A Thousand Years of Vice in the Capital.* London: Robson.
Lunning, Frenchy. 2013. *Fetish Style.* New York: Bloomsbury.
Macey, David. 1993. *The Lives of Michel Foucault.* London: Hutchinson.
Magilow, Daniel H., Elizabeth Bridges, and Kristin T. Vander Lugt. 2012. *Nazisploitation! The Nazi Image in Low-Brow Cinema and Culture.* New York: Continuum.

Mails, Thomas E. 1998. *Sundancing: The Great Sioux Piercing Ritual*. Tulsa, OK: Council Oak Books.

Mains, Geoffrey. 1984. *Urban Aboriginals: A Celebration of Leather Sexuality*. San Francisco: Gay Sunshine Press.

Marcus, Sharon. 2009. *Between Women: Friendship, Desire, and Marriage in Victorian England*. Princeton, NJ: Princeton University Press.

Marcus, Steven. 1966. *The Other Victorians: A Study of Sexuality and Pornography in Mid-Nineteenth-Century England*. New York: Basic Books.

Martin, Charles D. 2002. *The White African American Body: A Cultural and Literary Exploration*. New Brunswick, NJ: Rutgers University Press.

Mason, Michael. 1994. *The Making of Victorian Sexuality*. Oxford: Oxford University Press.

McClintock, Anne. 1995. *Imperial Leather: Race, Gender, and Sexuality in the Colonial Contest*. New York: Routledge.

McInnis, Maurie Dee. 2011. *Slaves Waiting for Sale: Abolitionist Art and the American Slave Trade*. Chicago: University of Chicago Press.

McKenzie, P. R. 1997. *Hail Orisha! A Phenomenology of a West African Religion in the Mid-Nineteenth Century*. Leiden: Brill.

Melton, J. Gordon. 2007. *The Encyclopedia of Religious Phenomena*. Detroit: Visible Ink.

Miller, Nancy Ava. 2009. *Pervert: Notes from the Sexual Underground*. Peplove Press.

Mills, Robert. 2002. "Ecce Homo." In *Gender and Holiness: Men, Women and Saints in Late Medieval Europe*, edited by Samantha J. E. Riches and Sarah Salih, 152–73. London: Routledge.

Minkowitz, Donna. 1998. *Ferocious Romance: What My Encounters with the Right Taught Me about Sex, God, and Fury*. New York: Free Press.

Molineux, Catherine. 2005. "Hogarth's Fashionable Slaves: Moral Corruption in Eighteenth-Century London." *ELH* 72 (2): 495–520.

Morgan, David. 1998. *Visual Piety: A History and Theory of Popular Religious Images*. Berkeley: University of California Press.

Mormando, Franco. 2011. *Bernini: His Life and His Rome*. Chicago: University of Chicago Press.

Morrison, Toni. 1992. *Playing in the Dark: Whiteness and the Literary Imagination*. New York: Vintage Books.

Móynahan, Brian. 2002. *The Faith: A History of Christianity*. New York: Doubleday.

Murray, Thomas E., and Thomas R. Murrell. 1989. *The Language of Sadomasochism: A Glossary and Linguistic Analysis*. New York: Greenwood Press.

Nitke, Barbara, and A. D. Coleman. 2003. *Kiss of fire: A Romantic View of Sadomasochism*. Heidelberg: Kehrer.

Odzer, Cleo. 1997. *Virtual Spaces: Sex and the Cyber Citizen*. New York: Berkley Books.

O'Malley, Patrick R. 2006. *Catholicism, Sexual Deviance, and Victorian Gothic Culture*. Cambridge: Cambridge University Press.

Oosterhuis, Harry. 2000. *Stepchildren of Nature: Krafft-Ebing, Psychiatry, and the Making of Sexual Identity*. Chicago: University of Chicago Press.

O'Riordan, Kate, and David J. Phillips. 2007. *Queer Online: Media Technology and Sexuality*. New York: Peter Lang.

Overbeck, Wayne, and Genelle Irene Belmas. 2012. *Major Principles of Media Law*. Boston: Wadsworth Cengage Learning.

Palandri, Marian, and Lelia Green. 2000. "Image Management in a Bondage, Discipline, Sadomasochist Subculture: A Cyber-Ethnographic Study." *Cyberpsychology and Behavior* 3 (4).

Parfrey, Adam. 2003. *It's a Man's World: Men's Adventure Magazines, The Postwar Pulps*. Los Angeles: Feral House.

Parker, Richard G., and Peter Aggleton. 1999. *Culture, Society and Sexuality: A Reader*. London: UCL Press.

Pasolini, Pier Paolo (dir., wri.). 1975. *Salò, or the 120 Days of Sodom*. Produzioni Europee Associate (PEA), Les Productions Artistes Associés.

Peakman, Julie. 2003. *Mighty Lewd Books: The Development of Pornography in Eighteenth-Century England*. Houndmills, Basingstoke, UK: Palgrave Macmillan.

Peakman, Julie. 2009. *Sexual Perversions, 1670–1890*. Basingstoke, UK: Palgrave Macmillan.

Peschier, Diana. 2009. "Religious Sexual Perversion in Nineteenth-Century Anti-Catholic Literature." In *Sexual Perversions, 1670–1890*, edited by Julie Peakman, 202–20. Basingstoke, UK: Palgrave Macmillan.

Philip, Neil. 1991. *Working Girls: An Illustrated History of the Oldest Profession*. London: Bloomsbury.

Pilcher, Tim, and Gene Kannenberg. 2008. *Erotic Comics: A Graphic History from Tijuana Bibles to Underground Comix*. New York: Abrams.

Pinchevski, Amit, and Roy Brand. 2007. "Holocaust Perversions: The Stalags Pulp Fiction and the Eichmann Trial." *Critical Studies in Media Communication* 24 (5): 387–407.

Popoff, Martin. 2007. *Judas Priest: Heavy Metal Painkillers: An Illustrated History*. Toronto: ECW Press.

Porter, David. 1997. *Internet Culture*. New York: Routledge.

Porter, Roy, and Mikuláš Teich. 1994. *Sexual Knowledge, Sexual Science: The History of Attitudes to Sexuality.* Cambridge: Cambridge University Press.

Pratchett, Terry. 2002. *Eric*, New York: HarperCollins.

Praz, Mario. 1956. *The Romantic Agony.* New York: Meridian Books.

Quilleriet, Anne-Laure. 2003. *The Leather Book.* Paris: Editions Assouline.

Rachilde. 1994. *The Marquise de Sade.* Translated by Liz Heron. Sawtry, UK: Dedalus.

Ramsland, Katherine M. 1991. *Prism of the Night: A Biography of Anne Rice.* New York: Dutton.

Reay, Barry. 2002. *Watching Hannah: Sexuality, Horror and Bodily Deformation in Victorian England.* London: Reaktion.

Reed, Rebecca Theresa, Nancy Lusignan Schultz, and Maria Monk. 1999. *A Veil of Fear: Nineteenth-Century Convent Tales by Rebecca Reed and Maria Monk.* West Lafayette, IN: Notabell.

Reich, Wilhelm. 1946. *The Mass Psychology of Fascism.* Translated by Theodore P. Wolfe. New York: Orgone Institute Press.

Reti, Irene, Pat Parker, Kathy Miriam, Anna Livia, Jamie Lee Evans, Sharon Lim-Hing, and D. A. Clark. 1993. *Unleashing Feminism: Critiquing Lesbian Sadomasochism in the Gay Nineties.* Santa Cruz, CA: HerBooks.

Reynolds, David S. 2012. *Mightier Than the Sword: Uncle Tom's Cabin and the Battle for America.* New York: W.W. Norton.

Riches, Samantha, and Sarah Salih. 2002. *Gender and Holiness: Men, Women and Saints in Late Medieval Europe.* London: Routledge.

Ridgely, J. V. 1974. "George Lippard's *The Quaker City*: The World of the American Porno-Gothic." *Studies in the Literary Imagination* 7 (1).

Roberts, Darren. 2012. *The Unsexpected Story: The Real Story about the Billion-Dollar Adult Entertainment Industry.* West Hills, CA: Clearly Confused.

Roberts, Diane. 1994. *The Myth of Aunt Jemima: Representations of Race and Region.* London: Routledge.

Robinson, Anna. 2015. "Passion, Politics, and Politically Incorrect Sex: Towards a History of Lesbian Sadomasochism in the USA 1975–1993." Master's thesis, Central European University, Budapest.

Rubin, Gayle. 2011. *Deviations: A Gayle Rubin Reader.* Durham, NC: Duke University Press.

Rubin, Gayle. 1996. "The Outcasts: A Social History," in *The Second Coming*, ed. Pat Califia and Robin Sweeney. Boston: Alyson.

Rubin, Gayle. 1994. *The Valley of the Kings: Leathermen in San Francisco, 1960–1990.* Two vols. Ann Arbor: University of Michigan Press.

Sacher-Masoch, Wanda von. 1990. *The Confessions of Wanda von Sacher-Masoch*, translated by Marian Phillips, Caroline Hébert, and V. Vale. San Francisco: Re/Search Publications.

Samois (Organization), editors. 1987. *Coming to Power: Writings and Graphics on Lesbian S/M.* Boston: Alyson Publications.

Schick, İrvin Cemil. 1999. *The Erotic Margin: Sexuality and Spatiality in Alteritist Discourse.* London: Verso.

Seves, Richard Pérez. 2017. *Charles Guyette: Godfather of American Fetish Art.* N.p.: Richard Pérez Seves.

Shainberg, Steven (dir.), Erin Cressida Wilson (wri.). 2003. *Secretary.* DVD. Santa Monica, CA: Studio Home Entertainment.

Sidén, Hans, and Donald H. Gilmore. 1972. *Sadomasochism in Comics: A History of Sex and Violence in Comic Books.* San Diego, CA: Greenleaf Classics.

Sigel, Lisa Z. 2005. *International Exposure: Perspectives on Modern European Pornography, 1800–2000.* New Brunswick, NJ: Rutgers University Press.

Silverman, Lisa. 2001. *Tortured Subjects: Pain, Truth, and the Body in Early Modern France.* Chicago: University of Chicago Press.

Sixma, Tjarda. 2009. "The Gorean Community in Second Life: Rules of Sexual Inspired Role-Play." *Journal of Virtual Worlds Research.* http://journals.tdl.org/jvwr/article/view/330.

Sontag, Susan. 1980. *Under the Sign of Saturn.* New York: Farrar, Straus & Giroux.

Spring, Justin. 2010. *Secret Historian: The Life and Times of Samuel Steward, Professor, Tattoo Artist, and Sexual Renegade.* New York: Farrar, Straus and Giroux.

Stanton, Eric. 1998. *The Dominant Wives and Other Stories.* Köln: Taschen.

Steele, Valerie, and Jennifer Park. 2008. *Gothic: Dark Glamour.* New Haven, CT: Yale University Press.

Steele, Valerie. 2001. *The Corset: A Cultural History.* New Haven, CT: Yale University Press.

Stone, Lawrence. 1992. "Libertine Sexuality in Post-Restoration England: Group Sex and Flagellation among the Middling Sort in Norwich in 1706–07." *Journal of the History of Sexuality* 2 (4): 511–26.

Taylor-Johnson, Sam (dir.), Kelly Marcel, E. L. James (wri.). 2015. *Fifty Shades of Grey.* Focus Features, Michael De Luca Productions, Trigger Street Productions.

Terpstra, Nicholas. 1995. *Lay Confraternities and Civic Religion in Renaissance Bologna.* Cambridge: Cambridge University Press.

Thomas, Donald. 1979. *Swinburne, the Poet in His World.* New York: Oxford University Press.

Thompson, Hunter S. 1966. *Hell's Angels: A Strange and Terrible Saga.* New York: Ballantine Books.

Thompson, Mark. 1991. *Leatherfolk: Radical Sex, People, Politics, and Practice.* Boston: Alyson Publications.

Trunk, Jonny. 2010. *Dressing for Pleasure in Rubber, Vinyl and Leather: The Best of Atomage, 1972–1980.* London: FUEL Design & Publishing.

Tupper, Peter, ed. 2016. *Our Lives, Our History: Consensual Master/slave Relationships from Ancient Times to the 21st Century.* New York: Perfectbound Press.

Turan, Kenneth, and Stephen F. Zito. 1974. *Sinema: American Pornographic Films and the People Who Make Them.* New York: Praeger.

Turner, Victor W. 1995. *The Ritual Process: Structure and Anti-Structure.* New York: Aldine de Gruyter.

Vance, Carole S. 1984. *Pleasure and Danger: Exploring Female Sexuality.* Boston: Routledge & Kegan Paul.

Waddell, Helen. 1998. *The Desert Fathers: Translations from the Latin.* New York: Vintage Books.

Warner, Alex Ellis. 2011. "'Where Angels Fear to Tread': Feminism, Sex and the Problem of SM, 1969–1993." PhD diss., Rutgers University.

Waskul, Dennis D. 2004. *Net.seXXX: Readings on Sex, Pornography, and the Internet.* New York: Peter Lang.

Webster, J. Carson. 1983. *Erastus D. Palmer: Sculpture—Ideas.* Newark: University of Delaware Press.

Weinberg, Thomas S. 1995. *S & M: Studies in Dominance and Submission.* Amherst, NY: Prometheus Books.

Weinberg, Thomas S., and G. W. Levi Kamel. 1983. *S and M: Studies in Sadomasochism.* Buffalo, NY: Prometheus Books.

Weiss, Margot. 2005. "Mainstreaming Kink: The Politics of BDSM Representation in U.S. Popular Media." *Journal of Homosexuality* 50 (2–3): 103–32.

Weiss, Margot Danielle. 2011. *Techniques of Pleasure: BDSM and the Circuits of Sexuality.* Durham, NC: Duke University Press.

Wood, Marcus. 2000. *Blind Memory: Visual Representations of Slavery in England and America, 1780–1865.* Manchester: Manchester University Press.

Wood, Marcus. 2002. *Slavery, Empathy, and Pornography.* Oxford: Oxford University Press.

Woodward, Tim. 1993. *The Best of Skin Two.* New York: Masquerade Books.

Index

abjection, 102
The Abolition of the Slave Trade (Cruikshank, I.), 93
abortion, 245
Abu Ghraib, 170
abuse, 3
Addio Zio Tom (Goodbye Uncle Tom) (1971), 160
AFTAH. *See* Americans for Truth about Homosexuality
Against Our Will (Brownmiller), 153, 207
Against Sadomasochism: A Radical Feminist Analysis (Linden), 166, 210, 212
ageplay, 117
aggregation (ritual phase), 17, 20
agon, 8
agricultural society, 116
AIDS, 200, 201
alea, 8
Alexander (Prince of Orange), 141
algolagnia, 131
Allison, Dorothy, 206, 210
alternative sexuality, 9
alt.sex.bondage (asb), 219–21, 226; validation provided by, 222
American Decency Association, 243
American Family Association, 243
American Psychiatric Association (APA), 231; Sexual and Gender Identities Workgroup, 234
Americans for Truth about Homosexuality (AFTAH), 243
The Anatomy of the English Nunnery at Lisbon in Portugall (Rowlandson, T.), 43
anesthesia, 143
"The Angel in the House" (Patmore), 137
Anger, Kenneth, 235
Anglican Church, 42
Ann Veronica (Wells, H. G.), 115
anti-Catholicism, 39–41, 62; Gothic novels and, 64; Orientalism and, 87
Antoniou, Laura, 10
APA. *See* American Psychiatric Association
Arabian Nights, 135
Ariadne, 16
aristocratic authority, 125
Arnett, Chuck, 182
Arnulf (Cistercian lay brother), 23
asb. *See* alt.sex.bondage
ascetics, 23–24
Ashbee, Henry Spencer, 9, 10, 134

Ashcroft, John, 240
atheism, 67
Atkinson, Ti-Grace, 207, 208
Atmeare, John, 49
austerities, 14
authoritarianism, 150, 211
autonomy, 109, 112, 119
The Avengers (television show), 190, 191
Awful Disclosures of Maria Monk (Monk), 45–46

Baku, John, 226
Baldwin, Guy, 199, 200, 232, 244
Bannon, Race, 232, 244
Barbary Coast, 73, 78
Barnard Conference, 209, 210
Barnum, P. T., 83
Baron, Hal, 174
Barrin, Jean, 42
BBSes. *See* bulletin board systems
BDSM community lore, 226
BDSM organizations, 196, 213; established, 233; first generation of, 215; private newsletters published by, 218
Bean, Joseph W., 181
"Beating Fantasies and Daydreams" (Freud, A.), 4–5
Beeton, Isabella, 128
Beeton, Sam, 96, 128
Berkley, Theresa, 117
Bernardino of Siena, 34
Bernini, Gian Lorenzo, 34
Bersani, Leo, 151
biblical law of Solomon, 123
biker culture, 2, 89; mainstream fashion and, 191; post–World War II, 10
Bilbrew, Gene, 187, 188

bildungsroman, 41
Binet, Alfred, 143
birching, 122–23
bisexuality, 198
The Bitter Draught of Slavery (Normand), *81*
Bizarre (magazine), 185
black clothing, 177–78
black persons: caricatures of, 94; sexual use of, 91
Blake, William, 93, 97, 251, 262
body modification, 7, 185
Bogden, Daniel, 241–42
Boileau, Abbe Jacques, 38
Bond, Pat, 196–97
bondage, 8, 20, 84, 120, 143, 190; fetish fashion instead of, 188; look of, 183; magazines for, 185; Page and, 187; self-bondage, 246; whimsy combined with, 186
Boulton, Ernest "Fanny," 177
bourgeois classes: bourgeois family, 43; flagellation and, 49; massive power differential in bourgeois homes, 106
Brame, Gloria, 219
Brando, Marlon, 179, 180
Brass, Tinto, 161–62
British rockers, 179
British Union of Fascists, 178
brothels, 50, 120
Brown, William Wells, 98
Brownmiller, Susan, 153, 207–8
Buchanan, Mary Beth, 242
Buchenwald, 160
Buddhists, 256–57
bulletin board systems (BBSes), 218–19
BurgerMunch, 226
Burke, Edmund, 58

burlesque, 11
Burnaby, Fred, 80
Burtman, Leonard "Lennie," 188–89
Burton, Richard Francis, 9, 10, 74, 79–80, 134–35
Bush, George W., 240–41
Butler, Samuel, 52
Byron (Lord), 108

Cabanel, Alexandre, 80
Cabaret (1972), 163
Cadiere, Mary Catherine, 40
Califia, Patrick, 198, 204–5
Callois, Roger, 8
camp, 164
capitalism, 121, 130
Carmilla (Fanu), 126
Carrington, Charles, 101
Carter-Johnson Memorial Library, 9
Cartoonists and Illustrators School, 187
Casimir III, 138
The Castle of Otranto (Walpole), 62
A Catalogue of Jilts, Cracks & Prostitutes, Nightwalkers, Whores, She-friends, Kind Women and other of the Linnen-lifting Tribe (anonymous pamphlet), 54
Catholicism, 137; Catholic hierarchy, 24; Protestants contention with Catholics over flagellation, 39; tales of women menaced by, 45. *See also* anti-Catholicism
censorship: "Miller test" for, 239; relaxed, 190
Charlton, Paul, 241–42
chastity, 60
chat rooms, 218
"A Child Is Being Beaten" (Freud, S.), 4

The Children of the Chapel (Leith), 133
chimney sweeping, 106–7, 110
Christ after the Flagellation Contemplated by the Christian Soul (Velazquez), 27
Christianity, 23, 38; Christian devotion, 47; Christian Europe, 73; Christian mystics, 22; Christian slaves, 76; consensual sadomasochism and, 21; flagellation and, 24; seduction and, 41; self-flagellation and, 11; women and, 26
Christian martyrs, 138
Churchill, Winston, 124
"Circassian beauties," 82–83
citizenship, 83
City of Night (Rechy), 180–81
Clarissa (Richardson), 60–61, 68
Clarke, D. A., 169
class transgression, 140
Cleland, John, 52–54
Clement VI (Pope), 25
Cleopatra Trying Out Poisons on Her Lovers (Cabanel), 80
Clotel; or, the President's Daughter (Brown), 98—99
Coalition for a Feminist Sexuality Against Sadomasochism, 209
Cockburn (Lord Chief Justice), 44
Colin, Rodney, 154
coming out, 195–96
Communications Decency Act of 1996, 240
Communism, 155
communitas, 253
Comstock, Anthony, 9
Concerned Women for America, 240, 242

The Confessional Unmasked; Shewing the Depravity of the Romanish Priesthood, the Iniquity of the Confessional and the Questions put to Females in Confession (Protestant Electoral Union), 44
Confessions (Rousseau), 55–56, 144, 146
The Confessions of Wanda von Sacher-Masoch (Rümelin), 140
confessors, 44
Congress to Unite Women, 203
Connor, Sarah, 90
consensual sadomasochism, 3, 11, 21
consent, 8, 53, 208, 211, 222, 224, 231, 232, 233, 235, 236, 252, 256
contact sports, 257
Coote, Edward, 125
corporal punishment, 3, 52, 56, 65, 90; in English education, 122–23; erotic books on, 124; Victorians and, 117
corsairs, 73
corsets, 121–22
Council of Trent, twenty-fifth session of, 33
courtesans, 119
Coutts, John A. S., 185, 186, 187
The Cremorne (adult magazine), 100
criminal-class, 175
cross-dressing, 127
Crown of Thorns, 23
The Crucifixion (Grünewald), 27
Cruikshank, George, 96
Cruikshank, Isaac, 93
cuckold fantasy, 49
Cullwick, Hannah, 9, 102–3, 104–13, *105*, *111*, 124, 141, 254
Cumberland, Richard, 93

Damian, Peter (Saint), 22–23, 24
d'Antigny, Blanche, 119–20
d'Aranda, Emanuel, 73
d'Argens, Marquis, 41–42
Day of Ashura, 14
decadent writers, 143
democracy, 160
depersonalization, 165
derogatory terms, 20
Desclos, Anne, 2, 152
Despréaux, Nicolas Boileau, 38
Diagnostic and Statistical Manual of Mental Disorders (DSM) (APA), 231–35
Dickens, Charles, 178
Diderot, Denis, 40–41
Dietrich, Marlene, 156
Different Loving (Brame), 219
disciplina, 23
divorce law, 141
Dominic (hermit), 23
Dr. Magnus Hirschfeld's Institute of Sexology, 9
Dr. Pusey's Insane Project Considered, 43
Drummer (magazine), 163–64
DSM. *See Diagnostic and Statistical Manual of Mental Disorders*

Easton, Dossie, 199
East Village Other (magazine), 196
Ecstasy of Saint Teresa (Bernini), 34
Eichmann, Adolf, 164
electrotherapy, 145
Emile, ou l'éducation (Rousseau), 56
emotion, 58–59
emotional manipulation, 137
England: attitudes toward American slavery in, 102, 107; corporal

punishment in English education, 122–23
England, Lynndie, 170
"the English vice," 117
Enlightenment, 39, 57
epistolary novels, 124
equestrianism, 118
eroticism, 151; eroticization of slavery, 92–93; of nuns, 44; pain and, 33
The Erotomaniac (Gibson), 9
An Essay Concerning Human Understanding (Locke), 50, 57
The Ethical Slut (Easton), 199
ethics, 220, 235, 252, 253; hedonism, ethical, 50
Eton College, 122–23
"Etonensis," 126, 128
European civilization, 72, 73, 78, 80
European Commission on Human Rights, 237
Evans, Jamie Lee, 168, 212
Evo (magazine), 197
"Execution of Breaking on the Rack" (Blake), 93
exhibitionism, 74
Exotique (magazine), 188
Experimental Lecture by Colonel Spanker, 126–27

fagging system, 123
Faithfull, Marianne, 191
families, 95
Family Herald (magazine), 127
Fanny Hill (Cleland), 52–54
fantasizer, 5
fantasy, 3, 61; cuckold fantasy, 49; cultural anxieties and fantasy pleasures, 6; embarrassing, 116; rape fantasy, 5

Fanu, Sheridan Le, 126
"Fascinating Fascism" (Sontag), 165
fascism, 3, 161; British Union of Fascists, 178; Foucault on sexual deviance and, 151; political dynamic of, 150; primitivism and, 153; professed ideals of, 162; sadomasochism and, 166–70; sexual deviance and, 162, 166
fashion designers, 122
fasting, 14
The Female Eunuch (Greer), 154
The Feminine Mystique (Friedan), 154
feminism, 210; Brownmiller feminist analysis of rape, 153, 207; orthodoxy of radical lesbian-feminists, 212; second-wave, 155, 203, 208
Feminist Perspectives on Pornography conference, 209
femme fatales, 120, 191
Ferocious Romance (Minkowitz), 255
FetLife, 226–27
Fifty Shades of Grey (James), 258, 259, 261
First Amendment, U. S. Constitution, 241
fisting, 1, 200, 203, 230
flagellation, 22–23, 26, 37–38, 39, 55; bourgeois classes and, 49; erotic, 117; flagellant novels, 124, 126, 133; flagellant processions, 24–25; Gothic novels and, 70; instability of meaning attached to, 52; institutional, 126; marriage and, 17; mutual, 14; paradox of, 125; in Pompeii, 15; prostitutes and, 54; recontextualization of, 48; Rousseau and, 55–56; self-flagellation, 11; *"le vice Anglaise"*,

116–17; voluntary, 35, 56. *See also* flogging
"Flagellation of a Female Samboe Girl" (Blake), 93
De flagorum usu in re veneria et lumborum renumque officio (Meibom), 37
Fleming, Ian, 124
Fletcher, Karen, 242
flogging, 123, 132, 198
The Flogging Block (Swinburne), 132
Forcible Appeal for the Abolition of the Slave Trade (Newton), 93
Foucault, Michel, 2, 3, 48, 231; on fascism and sexual deviance, 151
François, Donatien Alphonse, 65
Freeman, Theophilus, 90
French Revolution, 59; Sade and, 69
Freud, Anna, 4–5, 169
Freud, Sigmund, 4, 56, 144
Friedan, Betty, 154, 203
Friedman, David F., 159
Fritscher, Jack, 164, 198, 240
"From Rage to All the Rage: Lesbian-Feminism, Sadomasochism, and the Politics of Memory" (Miriam), 212
Frost, Laura, 171
furries, 224

Gay Community Services Center, 236
Gay Freedom Day Parade, 1979, 206
Gay Male S/M Activists (GMSMA), 206, 213–15
Gay Officers Action League, 214
Genet, Jean, 171
Gerson, Jean, 34
Gervex, Henri, 121
Gibson, Ian, 9
Ginsberg, Allen, 239

Girard, John Baptist, 40
Gladstone (Prime Minister), 117
Glucklich, Ariel, 19
GMSMA. *See* Gay Male S/M Activists
Golden Legend (Huntington Library), 27
Goldstein, Richard, 164
Gone with the Wind (Mitchell), 98
gonorrhea, 49
Gonzales, Alberto, 241
Goodbye Uncle Tom (Addio Zio Tom) (1971), 160
Gor novels (Norman), 88, 224
Gothic novels, 62; anti-Catholicism and, 64; elements of, 67; flagellation and, 70; Orientalism and, 84; in post-Revolutionary U. S., 63; slavery abolitionist movement and, 95
government surveillance, 66
Goz, Jutka, 189
The Great Dictator (1940), 164
Greece, 83
The Greek Slave (Powers), *85*, *86*, 87
Greenwood, John, 83
Greer, Germaine, 154
Grimaldi, John, 245–46, 247
Grounds, Ellen, *103*
Grünewald, Mathias, 27
Guyette, Charles, 184–85

Halfway to Hell (1953), 159
handkerchief, 180
Hankey, Frederick, 10
harems, 74, 78, 80–82, 88
Harley-Davidson, 191
A Harlot's Progress (Hogarth), 54, *55*
harm, 252–53
Harris, Jack, 54

Harvey, John, 177
Hawthorne, Nathaniel, 63
hedonism, ethical, 50
hell, 78
Hell's Angels, 163, 179
Helms, Jesse, 240
Hemmings, Sally, 98
Henry (Cumberland), 93
heterosexuality: coitus, 7; European civilization and, 80; kink culture and, 199, 216, 249; rejection of, 125; sadomasochism and, 183, 193, 202
"Hicklin test," 44
Hildreth, Richard, 97
Hill, Aaron, 76
Historia flagellantium (Boileau), 38
Hitler, Adolf, 150
Hitler's Children (1943), 154
Hitler Youth, 161
Hoagland, Sarah Lucia, 166
Hocutt, Richard, 214
Hofstadter, Richard, 39
Hogarth, William, 54, *55*
Holliday, Kendra, 234
Holocaust, 156, 164, 168–70, 211
homophobia, 236–37
Homos (Bersani), 151
homosexuality, 7, 75, 143, 145, 182–83; reclaiming slurs for, 222. *See also* leatherman culture
Howard, Noni, 199
Howl (Ginsberg), 239
Hudibras (Butler), 52
Human Sexuality Forum's Variations II group, 219
Huntington Library, 27
hydrotherapy, 145
hyperesthesia, 143
hypnosis, 145

ilinx, 8
Ilsa: Harem Keeper of the Oil Sheiks (1976), 160
Ilsa: She Wolf of the SS (1974), 157, *158*, 159–60
Ilsa: The Tigress of Siberia (1977), 161
Ilsa: The Wicked Warden (1977), 160—161
impact play, 20
Incidents in the Life of a Slave Girl (Jacobs), 99—100
industrial society, 116
infanticide, 46
International Ms. Leather contest, 213
internet, 217–24
interwar period, 153
intimacy, 241
Introduction to the Devout Life (Sales), 25
Iraq, 170, 245, 246, 247, 248
Islam, 73, 74
Ismael, Muley, 76

Jack the Ripper, 129
Jacobs, Harriet, 99–100
James, E. L., 258, 259, 261
Jay, Karla, 203, 207
Jefferson, Thomas, 98
Jeffreys, Sheila, 167, 213
Jellinghaus, Rob, 221
Jesus Christ, 22; depictions of, 26–27
"Jesus Courting the Christian Soul" (*Die Minnende Seele*), *28, 29*–30
Jonel, Marissa, 211
Joynes, James Leigh, 132
Juliette (Sade), 67, 69
Justine (Sade), 67, 68, 70; *Le nouvelle Justine*, 69

Kama Sutra of Vatsyayana, 135
Kane, Reverend Jim, 199
Kantrowitz, Arnie, 163
Kavadi Attam dance, 14
Keller, Rose, 66
King, Rodney, 168, 212
kink, 6–7, 215; anti-kink police operation, 236; heterosexuality and, 199, 216, 249; increasing visibility of, 195, 218, 261; intimacy and, 241; kink-based social networks, 226; main media for, 184; medical discourse and, 248; online kink communities, 219; political struggles and, 231
Kink Aware Professionals, 232
"kinkies," 190
Kinsey, Alfred, 7, 175
Kinsey Institute, 9
Kiss Me Kate (1953), 190
Kiss of Fire: A Romantic View of Sadomasochism (Nitke), 241
Klaw, Irving and Paula, 186–87
Koch, Ilse, 160
Koch, Karl-Otto, 160
Kolb, Terry, 197
Kottowitz, Anna von, 139
Krafft-Ebing, Richard von, 56, 65, 142–47
Krueger, Richard, 234

Laaksonen, Touko, 180
LaBarbera, Peter, 243–44
Lady Chatterley's Lover (Lawrence), 239
LaLaurie, Delphine, 160
LambdaMOO, 224
Largier, Nicholas, 22
The Last of the Nuba (Riefenstahl), 165

Latent Image (magazine), 189
Latin, 142
Lautrec, Toulouse, 47
Lawrence, D. H., 171, 239
lay worshipers, 23
Lazenby, George, 100–101, 102
Leather Archives and Museum, 9
leather culture: early, 10; in mid-1970s, 164
leather jackets, 178–79; in mainstream fashion, 191
leatherman culture, 174, 175; New Guard of, 181–82; Old Guard of, 181–82; Tool Box leather bar, 182; women and, 199
Leatherman's Handbook (Townsend), 181
Leather Pride, 206
Leaves of Grass (Whitman), 94
leg shacklers, 154–55
Leigh, Michael, 192, 193
Leith, Mary, 133
Lesbia Brandon (Swinburne), 133
Lesbian Herstory Archives, 210
lesbianism, 42, 125, 126, 202–13
Lesbian Sex Mafia (LSM), 206, 210, 214
Lesbian Sex Wars, 209
les femmes tondues, 161
"Letter from a Former Masochist" (Jonel), 211
Lewis, Matthew G., 63
libertinism, 60; debauchery of, 69; government surveillance of libertines, 66
liminality (ritual phase), 17–19, 253; achieving, 22; transformation from, 65
Linden, Robin Ruth, 166
lingerie, 121

Lippard, George, 64, 95
Lipschutz, Barbara, 204
List of Covent Garden Ladies (Harris), 54
literacy, 116, 124
Live Action, 245
Locke, John, 50, 57
London Life (magazine), 184, 185
Love Camp Seven (1969), 156, 159
lower classes, unruly desires of, 124
LSM. *See* Lesbian Sex Mafia
ludus, 8
Ludwig II of Bavaria (King), 141
Lupercalia, 14–15
The Lustful Turk (anonymous English erotic novel), 9, 84
Lynch, Jessica, 170

Macho Sluts (Califia), 199
Magister, Thom, 176
mainstream culture, 235
mainstream fashion, 191
mainstream fiction, 127
maisons de tolérance, 120
Majdanek, 160
male concubines, 75
Man, Play, and Games (Callois), 8
Manet, Édouard, 121
Mapplethorpe, Robert, 240, 241
Marais (Inspector), 65–66
Marcus, Stephen, 9, 135
La Marquise de Sade (Rachilde), 120, 136
marriage, 17, 58, 110; marriage equality, 244; rejection of, 125
The Marriage of Heaven and Hell (Blake), 251
Married Women's Property Acts, 147

masculinity, 152; icons of, 180; masculine rapaciousness, 76; new model of, 58; normative, 177
masochism, 142, 143, 146, 207, 231–32; "childhood experience" explanation of, 36
Masochism in Modern Man (Reik), 197
mass media, 183
Master-slave relationships, 3, 116; consensual, 6, 102
materialism, 67; pleasure-seeking, 50; rationalism and, 58; secular, 47
Maturin, Charles, 63
McCord, Lydia, 98
McGeorge, Harvey John "Jack," 245–48
McLintock! (1963), 190
Measure for Measure (Shakespeare), 36–37, 150
Meibom, Johann Heinrich, 37, 38, 50
Melmoth the Wanderer (Maturin), 63
Melville, Herman, 63
Memoirs of a Woman of Pleasure (Cleland), 52–54
The Memoirs of Dolly Morton (Carrington), 9, 101
Men in Black (Harvey), 177
mercantile society, 50
metatropism, 131
Middle Passage, horrors of, 90
Mighty Lewd Books (Peakman), 39
Miksche, Mike, 175
military fashion, 89, 163
Miller, Nancy Ava, 201, 247
Millingen, Frederick, 80
Milne, Bob, 175
Milnes, Richard Monckton, 134
mimesis, 8
Minkowitz, Donna, 255–56

Die Minnende Seele ("Jesus Courting the Christian Soul"), *28*, 29–30
Mirandola, Pico della, 35, 37
Miriam, Kathy, 212, 213
Mishkin, Eddie, 187
Miss Coote's Confession (anonymous), 124–26
Mitchell, Margaret, 98
Monk, Maria, 45–46
The Monk (Lewis), 63
Mood Pictures, 169
MOOs (text-based virtual environment), 223
Morris, Jane, 49
Morris, Robert, 49
Morrison, Toni, 102
mortification, 23, 33; mild forms of, 26; self-mortification, 22, 24
Mosley, Oswald, 178
The Mother of God (Sacher-Masoch), 138
Moulin Rouge cabaret, 145
Mr. Benson (Preston), 181
MUDs (text-based virtual environment), 223
Munby, Arthur, 9, 103–13, *111*, 141, 254
Murugan, 14
Musafar, Fakir, 185, 199–200
MUSHes (text-based virtual environment), 223
MUVEs (text-based virtual environment), 223
Myles, Meg, 189
My Secret Life, 9
Mysteries of Verbena House ("Etonensis"), 126
The Mysteries of Verbena House; or, Miss Bellasis Birched for Thieving, 10

Nana (Manet), 121
Nana (Zola), 119–20, 136
National Coalition for Sexual Freedom (NCSF), 233, 234, 240, 241, 249
National Endowment for the Arts, 240
National Gay and Lesbian Task Force, 244
National Gay Task Force, 214
National Geographic, 80
National Organization for Women, 209, 234
Native Americans, 64; virtue in distress and, 87
Nazis, 9, 160; chic, 165; ideology, 162; imagery, 163; Nazisploitation, 154–57, 170, 190; SS dress uniform, 149
NCSF. *See* National Coalition for Sexual Freedom
necrophilia, 143, 231
neurasthenia, 143
The New Temptation of Saint Anthony (postcard), 121
Newton, Richard, 93
The Night Porter (1974), 156–57, 164
Nitke, Barbara, 240–41
Nitke v. Ashcroft, 241
"noble savage," 59
"normal" sex, 7
Norman, John, 88, 224
Normand, Ernest, *81*
Norris, Maryel, 211
"nudies," 190
The Nun (*La religieuse*) (Diderot), 41
nuns, 43, 45–46, 128; eroticism of, 44

Obama, Barack, 242, 244
Obscene Publications Act, 1857, 43–44, 124, 127

obscenity, 239–40; Cockburn on, 44; Gonzales on, 241; "Hicklin test" for, 44
Obscenity Prosecution Task Force, 241
O'Dell, Brian, 214
"Of the Innermost Soul, How God Chastises Her and Makes Her Suited to Him" (*Von der Ynnigen selen wy sy gott casteyet unnd im beheglich mach*), *31*
O'Hara, Scarlett, 98
Old Guard, 10
120 Days of Sodom (Sade), 67, 68, 71
On Horseback through Asia Minor (Burnaby), 80
On Our Backs (journal), 212, 213
Operation Spanner, 237, 238
"An Opinionated Piece on Sadomasochism" (Norris), 211
Opus Dei, 26
orgasm, 37
Orientalism, 76–78, 79, 113; anti-Catholicism and, 87; in erotica, 71; Gothic novels and, 84; locations and boundaries of "The Orient," 72; of *Uncle Tom's Cabin* (Stowe), 95; visual arts and, 80; women and, 75
Orwell, George, 124
The Other Victorians (Marcus), 135
Ottoman Empire, 83
Otway, Thomas, 51

Paddleboro, 238
paganism, 22, 137
Page, Bettie, 187
paidia, 8
pain, 13; eroticism and, 33; liminality and, 19; as physical indulgence, 35

Palmer, Erastus Dow, 87
papal bulls, 25
paradoxia, 143
The Paranoid Style in American Politics (Hofstadter), 39
paraphilia, 231, 233, 234
parenting, 123
paresthesia, 143
Pasolini, Pier Paolo, 161
Passion of Christ, 22, 26
passives, 131
passivism, 131
pastoralism, 113
patriarchy, 81, 160, 207, 208, 209, 210, 212–13
Payne, Frederick "Stella," 177
Peachum, Polly, 222–23
Peakman, Julie, 39
Pearse, Sophia Mable, 118
Peasant Justice (Sacher-Masoch), 138
Pellow, Thomas, 75
People Exchanging Power (PEP), 201–2
The Perfect Moment (Mapplethorpe), 240
The Perfumed Garden (Burton), 9, 135
perversion, 39, 145
Philosophy in the Bedroom (Sade), 67, 68
Photo Bits (magazine), 185
physical ordeals, 2, 8; commonality of, 13; voluntary, 17
The Picture of Dorian Gray (Wilde), 47
Pistor, Fanny, 137
Pitts, Joseph, 75, 76
Planet of the Apes (1968), 190
Planned Parenthood, 245
Plath, Sylvia, 171

play, modes of, 8
Plutarch, 14
Poe, Edgar Allan, 63
police, 237–39
polygyny, 46, 76, 80, 95
Pompeii, 9, 15, *15*, *16*
pornography, 6, 9; academic study of, 10; anti-pornography activists, 209; hardcore, 40; literary stars dabbling in, 130; mob-connected publishers of, 183–84; "whore dialogue" format of, 68, 125
Portrait of Hortense Mancini, Duchess of Mazarin (Gennari), 92
posture molls, 54
Potter, Sarah, 117
Powers, Hiram, *85*, 86, *86*, *87*
pre-Revolutionary France, 2
Preston, John, 181
primitivism, 59; fascism and, 153
"Princkazons," 188
privacy, 229–30, 237, 249
The Producers (1967), 164
propaganda, 152
property rights, 112
prostitutes, 54, 117; casual, 104; costumes and, 120; Sacher-Masoch never seeking, 139; upper crust of, 118
Protestant Electoral Union, 44
Protestantism, 42; Antebellum American Protestants, 44, 46; Catholics contention with Protestants over flagellation, 39; Protestant piety, 47; women and, 43
psychiatry, 142
Psychopathia Sexualis (Krafft-Ebing), 56, 142–43, 146, 148
Punch (magazine), 87

punishment, 1, 21; birching, 122–23; cross-dressing as form of, 127. *See also* corporal punishment
purgatory, 78

Quaker City; or, the Monks of Monk-Hall (Lippard), 64, 95
Quarterly Christian Spectator, 46
Quesnet, Constance, 69

Rachilde, 120
racial difference, 83, 98
racial mixing, 98
rakes, 50, 58, 60–61, 65
rape, 3, 135; Brownmiller feminist analysis of, 153, 207; imagery, 152; rape fantasy, 5
rationalism, materialism and, 58
ravishment, 5
Reage, Pauline, 102, 152
realist writers, 142–43
reason, 58–59
Rechy, John, 180–81
Redemptionists, 78
Reformation, 43
Regina v. Hicklin, 44
Reich, Wilhelm, 154
Reik, Theodore, 197
Relatos de Presidio ("Stockade Tales"), 170
La religieuse (The Nun) (Diderot), 41
religious authority, 57
religious experience, 14, 253–54; religious ecstasy, 33; religious ordeal, 29; sexual ecstasy and, 41–42
Repent Amarillo, 244
Resurrection of Christ, 26
Reti, Irene, 168–69
Ribalta, Francisco, 27

Rice, Anne, 230
Richardson, Samuel, 60–61, 68
Riefenstahl, Leni, 165
Rigg, Diana, 190
Rita of Cascia (Saint), 23
ritual, 18, 20–21, 253; pagan rituals, 22; three-step process of, 17, 26
The Ritual Process (Turner), 17
Roberts, Diane, 95–96
Roehm, Ernst, 153
Rolla (Gervex), 121
Roman Empire, 2
Romantic ideals, 62
Rose, Lila, 245
Rossetti, Dante Gabriel, 132
Rotten Row, 118–19
"roughies," 190
Rousseau, Jean-Jacques, 55–56, 116, 144, 146
Rowlandson, Mary, 87
Rowlandson, Thomas, 43
Rubin, Gayle, 205, 258
Rümelin, Aurora, 140–41

Sacher-Masoch, Leopold von, 2, 102, 136–42, 254
Sacred Pain (Glucklich), 19
Sade, Marquis de, 2, 65–70, 130; grotesque crimes of, 3
sadiques actives, 131
sadism, 143, 231–32
"Sadism, Masochism and Lesbian-Feminism" (Hoagland), 166
sadomasochism, 210; accessibility to, 221–22; asb on ethics and philosophy of, 220; authoritarianism and, 150; clinical and legal origins of, 131; definition of sex and, 252; difficulty in defining, 6; external attacks on, 230; fascism and, 166–70; heterosexuality and, 183, 193, 202; as historically contingent, 251; legal cases regarding, 236–37; mainstream culture and, 235; physical and mental safety and, 257; religion and, 254–55; Sontag on, 165–66; women in early sadomasochistic culture, 134. *See also* consensual sadomasochism
"Sadomasochism: The Erotic Cult of Fascism" (Jeffreys), 167
sadomasochistic imagination, 4; relationship between reality and, 6
"Safe, Sane and Consensual" (SSC), 8, 215, 252
safety, physical and mental, 257
Saint Francis Embracing the Crucified Christ (Ribalta), 27
Sala, George Augustus, 118
Sales, Francis de, 25
Salò (1975), 161
Salon Kitty (1976), 161–62
salvation, 102
Samois Collective, 205–6
Samuels, Marvin, 235–36
San Francisco Bay Guardian, Culture Shocked column in, 225
Sapphistry (Califia), 199
Sardanapalus (Byron), 108
Satan in High Heels (1962), 189
"scenes," 17, 20
Screw (magazine), 196, 197
Second Life, 223, 224
Secretary (2002), 258, 259–60, 261
The Secret Life of Linda Brent, a Curious History of Slave Life (Lazenby), 100–101, 102
"A Secret Side of Lesbian Sexuality" (Califia), 204

seduction, 5, 41
Self, Samuel, 49, 50
Self, Sarah, 49
sensation play, 20
sensibility, novel of, 65
sensibility theory, 57, 59, 92–93
sensory deprivation, 20
sentimentality, 59
separation (ritual phase), 17
servants: domestic, 147; exploitation of, 106; hierarchy of, 109
sex education, 245
sex scandals, 40
sexual abuse, 40
sexual anarchy, 78, 97, 99, 100
sexual arousal, 7, 18
sexual deviance, 97; categories of, 143; fascism and, 162, 166; Foucault on fascism and, 151; physicality of, 65; Sade compiling encyclopedia of, 68
sexual ecstasy, 41–42
sexual freedom, class and gender privilege and, 135
sexual mores, 252
sexual revolution, 193
sexual writings, 124
Shadwell, Thomas, 50–51
Shakespeare, William, 36–37, 150
shame, 9
Shaw, George Bernard, 123
Shiite Muslims, 14
The Sims Online, 223
Sioux, 13
Slater, Cynthia, 197, 198, 200, 205
The Slave, or Memoirs of Archy Moore (Hildreth), 97
slaveholders, governing fiction among, 90

slavery, 74, 102, 113; Christian slaves, 76; eroticization of, 92–93; illustrations of, 98; mulatto slave women and virtue in distress, 99; pro-slavery art, 94; racial difference and, 83; redeemed captives, 77; slave auctions, 71; "slave girl" gradually becoming white, 82; slave markets, 76; violence of, 92; "white slavery" moral panics, 79
slavery, American, 144; British attitudes toward, 102, 107; consensual Master-slave relationships and, 6; long term effects of, 89; open secret of, 98; *Punch* (magazine) on, 87; sexual access to slaves in, 90, 92; tyranny of, 3
slavery abolitionist movement, 61, 92–93, 144; Gothic novels and, 95; literature of, 96
"S&M: The Dark Side of Gay Liberation" (Goldstein), 164
sober contemplation, 43
social-constructivism, 211
social networks, kink-based, 226
social structure, 18
Society of Janus (SOJ), 197–200, 214
soc.subculture.bondage-bdsm, 221
sodomy, 40
So Ends Our Night (1941), 154
SOJ. *See* Society of Janus
Sontag, Susan, 165–66
Southern Poverty Law Center, 243
South of Market, 200, 201
South Plains Leatherfest, 10
spanking, 190, 223, 238
"spare the rod and spoil the child," 52

"The Spirit Is Feminist but the Flesh Is?" (Jay), 203
spiritual renewal, 13, 23–24; vicarious experience of, 26
SSC. *See* "Safe, Sane and Consensual"
stag film network, 184
Stalag novels, 155–56
Stanford Prison experiment, 166
Star, Susan Leigh, 166–67
Stein, David, 183, 215, 252
Steward, Samuel M., 174
Stewart, Potter, 6
St. Laurent, Yves, 191
Stonewall riots, 195
Story of O (Reage), 2, 102, 152
Stothard, Thomas, 90, *91*
Stowe, Harriet Beecher, 65, 94–97, 99, 107, 144
stress position, 170
Sturman, Reuben, 189
the sublime, 58–59
submission: "comedies" of, 145; to women, 136
Sun Dance, 13–14
suspension piercing, 7
Sutcliffe, John, 191
"Swastikas: The Street and the University" (Star), 166–67
Sweet Gwendoline (comic strip), 186
Swinburne, Algernon Charles, 117, 130, 132–34
swinging/swapping, 192, 196
switchables, 197
sympathy, 59
syphilis, 139

taboos, 149–50
Tarzan and the Slave Girl (1950), 190
Tassy, Laugier de, 76
Tatbir, 14
tawse, 115
Teresa of Ávila (Saint), 33–34, 41, 47
TES. *See* Till Eulenspiegel Society
Testard, Jeanne, 66
text-based virtual environments, 223
Thaipusam, 14
theater, 65, 66
Thérèse Philosophe (d'Argens), 41–42, 47
"Thinking Sex" (Rubin), 258
Thorne, Dyanne, 157, 160–61
Three Essays on Sexuality (Freud, S.), 56
Till Eulenspiegel Society (TES), 196–98, 207, 214
Tom of Finland, 162, 180, 193
Tool Box leather bar, 182
torture, 1, 74; in Iraq war, 170
Townsend, Larry, 181
transformation, 3; from liminality, 65; psychological, 19
transgression, 20, 193
transvestism, 112, 128
A Treatise on the Use of Flogging in Medicine and Venery (Meibom), 50
Triumph of the Will (1935), 164, 165
Turkish bogeyman, 79
Turner, Victor, 17, 18, 253
Twisted Monk, 11
tyrannism, 131

Uncle Tom's Cabin (Stowe), 65, 94–96, 99, 107, 144; fetishistic reading of, 97
uniform fetishes, 54, 115

United States (U. S.): Antebellum American Protestants, 44, 46; Gothic novels in post-Revolutionary America, 63; nativist sentiment of, 46; neo-colonialist narrative of U. S. as civilizing force in Iraq, 170. *See also* slavery, American
United States v. Fletcher, 242
Unleashing Feminism (1993), 168, 212, 213
UN mission to Iraq to search for weapons of mass destruction (UNMOVIC), 245, 246, 247
upper-classes, 37
U. S. *See* United States
US-Iraq war, 170, 248

vanilla sex, 6, 203, 204, 211, 212, 222, 226, 241, 258
vegetarianism, 256–57
Velazquez, Diego, 27
Velvet Underground (band), 193
The Velvet Underground (Leigh), 192
Velvet Underground and Nico (1967), 193
Venice Preserv'd (Otway), 51
Venus dans la cloitre (Barrin), 42
Venus in Furs (Sacher-Masoch), 102, 136–37, 140, 254
victimization, 8
victim-rake dyad, 60
Victoria (Queen), 115
Victorians, 116; corporal punishment and, 117; corsets and, 121–22; gentleman, 132; moralistic repression, 130; social hierarchy of, 106; women, 118
Vietnam War, 155
Village Voice (magazine), 197

Villa of the Mysteries, 15–17, *16*
Vincent, Gene, 179
violence, 178, 236; bodily, 64; images of, 27; in place of sexuality, 190; of slavery, 92; U. S. nativist sentiment leading to, 46
Virginian Luxuries (anonymous), 91–92
Virgin Mary, 24–25
virtue in distress, 58, 59–60, 86, 186; mulatto slave women and, 99; Native Americans and, 87; Sade and, 67
The Virtuoso (Shadwell), 50–51
visual arts, Orientalism and, 80
Von der Ynnigen selen wy sy gott casteyet unnd im beheglich mach ("Of the Innermost Soul, How God Chastises Her and Makes Her Suited to Him"), *31*
vore, 224
The Voyage of the Sable Venus, from Angola to the West Indies (Stothard), 90, *91*
voyeurism, 126

Walpole, Horace, 62
Walters, Catherine "Skittles," 118
war, 152
Ward, Brent, 241
waterboarding, 170
WAVPM. *See* Women Against Violence in Pornography and the Media
Weiss, Margot, 259
Wells, H. G., 115
Wells, Sarah, 49
The Whippingham Papers (Swinburne), 132
The White Captive (Palmer), 87

whiteness, 83
Whitman, Walt, 94
Wilde, Oscar, 47; trial of, 147, 177
Wild Life among the Koords (Millingen), 80
The Wild One (1953), 179, 180
Willie, John, 187
Wink (magazine), 186
Wiseman, Jay, 198, 199
Wodehouse, P. G., 127
Wollstonecraft, Mary, 61
women, 61, 116; bisexual, 198; Christianity and, 26; corsets and, 121–22; as domestic servants, 147; in early sadomasochistic culture, 134; eroticizing oppression of, 167; feminine vulnerability and modesty, 76; Krafft-Ebing on, 146; lacking property rights, 112; leatherman culture and, 199; mulatto slave women and, 99; Orientalism and, 75; propaganda of white women menaced by dark men, 84; Protestantism and, 43; rakes and, 60; Sacher-Masoch and, 139; sensibility theory and, 57; sexual access to women slaves, 90; sexual independence of, 126; submission to, 136; tales of women menaced by Catholicism, 45; unruly desires of, 124; Victorian, 118; working-class, 103–4
Women Against Violence in Pornography and the Media (WAVPM), 208–9, 210
women-in-peril scenarios, 190
working-classes, 103–4
World War I, 152
World War II: leather jackets and, 179; motorcycle gang culture after, 10
Wright, Susan, 234

Xanadu Pleasure Gardens, 199
xenophobia, 42

Yeager, Bunny, 187

Zola, Emile, 119–20

About the Author

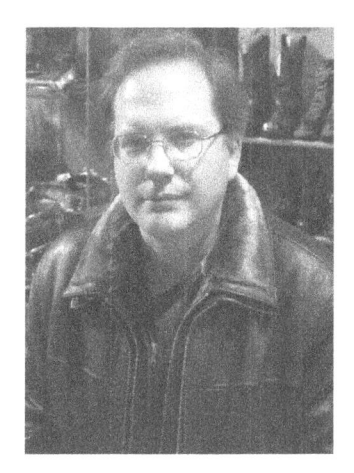

Peter Tupper was born and raised in Vancouver, British Columbia. He studied history at the University of British Columbia and journalism at Langara College. One of his first professional fiction sales was to Circlet Press's *S/M Futures* anthology. His nonfiction writing has appeared in *Wired* magazine, the *Canadian Medical Association Journal*, the *Globe and Mail*, the *Utne Reader*, and www.TheTyee.ca. He is a cofounder of Metro Vancouver Kink, a nonprofit BDSM community organization in Vancouver, and remains active in the BDSM scene. He has researched and blogged about the history of consensual sadomasochism since 2005, and has presented at The Art of Loving in Vancouver, the Centre for Sex Positive Culture in Seattle, Washington, and the 2012, 2013, and 2016 Master-slave Conferences. He has also been a guest on Graydancer's Ropecast, the Masocast, Jack Rinella's Leathercast, Erotic Awakening, and the People of Kink podcasts. He edited and contributed to *Our Lives, Our History: Consensual Master/slave relationships from Ancient Times to the 21st Century*, a nonfiction anthology sponsored by Master Taino's Training Academy. This won the 2017 Geoff Mains Nonfiction Book Award from the National Leather Association: International.